DESIGNING
AND CONDUCTING
gender,
sex,
health
research

Contents

Preface   vii

About the Editors and Contributors   ix

Acknowledgments   xvii

PART I: CONTEXT AND CONCEPTS   1

  1. **Why Put Gender and Sex Into Health Research?**   3
     Lorraine Greaves

PART II: DESIGN   15

  2. **Sex and Gender: Beyond the Binaries**   17
     Joy L. Johnson and Robin Repta

  3. **Implications of Sex and Gender for Health Research:**
     From Concepts to Study Design   39
     Joy L. Johnson, Robin Repta, and Shirin Kalyan

  4. **Approaches to the Measurement of Gender**   65
     Pamela A. Ratner and Richard G. Sawatzky

  5. **Measuring Biological Sex**   85
     Gillian Einstein

PART III: SEX AND GENDER RESEARCH   103

  6. **Fieldwork: Observations and Interviews**   105
     Cathy Chabot and Jean Shoveller

  7. **Visual Methods in Gender and Health Research**   127
     Rebecca J. Haines-Saah and John L. Oliffe

  8. **Secondary Analysis—Gender, Age, and Place: Gender, Place,**
     and the Mortality Gap Between Urban and Rural Canadians   145
     Aleck Ostry and Amanda Slaunwhite

  9. **Content and Discourse Analysis**   161
     Brendan Gough and Steve Robertson

10. **Approaches to Examining Gender Relations in Health Research**   175
    Joan L. Bottorff, John L. Oliffe,
    Mary T. Kelly, and Natalie A. Chambers

11. **Developing a Gender Role Socialization Scale**   189
    Brenda Toner, Taryn Tang, Alisha Ali, Donna Akman, Noreen Stuckless,
    Mary Jane Esplen, Cheryl Rolin-Gilman, and Lori Ross

PART IV: POLICY, PROCESS, AND PRODUCTS   201

12. **Gender, Health, Research, and Public Policy**   203
    Toni Schofield

13. **Boundary Spanning: Knowledge Translation as Feminist**
    Action Research in Virtual Communities of Practice   215
    Nancy Poole

14. **Design, Methods, and Knowledge Exchange:**
    Connections and Pathways   227
    John L. Oliffe

Afterword   243

Author Index   245

Subject Index   253

Preface

Ever present are questions about *how* to do gender, sex, and health research. Yet, generic study designs and methods do not always meet the specific needs or interests of students and health researchers who want to explicitly engage gender and/or sex in their work. Of course, there are a number of ways to thoughtfully guide the efforts of gender, sex, and health researchers. One strategy is to draw together established researchers and students to share their approaches and experiences as a means of building capacity while advancing the empirical, methodological, and theoretical aspects of the enterprise. Worthy of mention here is such a collective, the Canada-based research group NEXUS, from which this volume has emerged. During its tenure from 2003 to 2009, the NEXUS group brought together an interdisciplinary team of researchers and students to engage the concepts of gender, diversity, and place in a variety of health and illness issues. As the NEXUS infrastructure funds ended, so too did some of the formal collaborations the group had facilitated. Yet, from NEXUS came many great moments and achievements, and some synergistic collectives continue today, albeit less formally. As NEXUS ended, there was interest and energy to further share our insights about designing gender, sex, and health research. With the support of NEXUS, and the expertise and hard work of research manager Stephanie Coen, we developed a book proposal that eloquently made the case for this volume, *Designing and Conducting Gender, Sex, and Health Research.* When SAGE enthusiastically responded to the ideas put forward in that proposal, the chance to chronicle and extend the work of NEXUS was realized.

The philosophy of NEXUS had always been to develop capacity through sharing experiences and expertise with others, and those goals drive this volume. We were also interested in soliciting contributions from gender, sex, and health researchers who had not formally linked to NEXUS but with whom we had always wanted to work. Fortunately, we were able to recruit an array of expert contributors to ensure a high-quality volume for addressing design and methods issues. With the wonderful assistance of research assistant Christina Han, we were able to piece together and format all the authors' contributions and send a full first draft, and the revised finished product, to SAGE. What follows is a four-part, 14-chapter volume, a collection dedicated to advancing gender, sex, and health research.

Part I provides a historical overview detailing the trends and turns that led to the current state of research in gender, sex, and health. Part II includes four chapters that unpack design considerations to promote understandings about different conceptual and operational definitions, and the implications of these in building research design. Part III unveils six chapters that foreground various methods using empirical examples to contextualize those diverse strategies. Part IV engages issues around public policy and knowledge exchange processes and products to close out the volume.

In sum, what follows is a much needed collection that distills design, methods, and dissemination considerations for gender, sex, and health research. While each chapter and section has the strength and substance to stand alone, as a collection, the volume also has great potential to conceptually advance the field of gender, sex, and health research.

John L. Oliffe and Lorraine Greaves

About the Editors and Contributors

JOHN L. OLIFFE

John L. Oliffe is an associate professor at the University of British Columbia, Canada. His men's health research program includes studies addressing prostate cancer, depression, South Asian Canadian immigrant men, smoking patterns of fathers, and youth sexual health. He has published methodological, theory-based, and empirical articles and chapters describing linkages between masculinities and men's health promotion in the context of varying health practices and diverse illness experiences.

LORRAINE GREAVES

Lorraine Greaves is a senior investigator with the British Columbia Centre of Excellence for Women's Health, and a clinical professor in the School of Population and Public Health, Faculty of Medicine, University of British Columbia. She has a doctorate in medical sociology from Monash University and has published widely on a range of women's health issues and the integration of gender and women's health into program, policy, and practice. Her special areas of research interests focus on women, substance use, trauma, and violence. Her extensive research on women, gender, and tobacco use and policy has influenced national and international bodies. She has received numerous awards including an honorary doctorate from the University of Ottawa for her contributions to women's health in Canada.

About the Contributors

DONNA AKMAN

Donna Akman is a psychologist with the Women's Mental Health Program at the Centre for Addiction and Mental Health, and an assistant professor in the Department of Psychiatry at the University of Toronto, Canada. Her clinical and research interests focus on feminist issues in psychology and psychotherapy.

ALISHA ALI

Alisha Ali is an associate professor in the Department of Applied Psychology at New York University. Her research investigates social and cultural influences on women's depression, including the effects of emotional abuse, harassment, and discrimination. She is coeditor, along with Dana Crowley Jack, of the book *Silencing the Self Across Cultures: Depression and Gender in the Social World*, published in 2010 by Oxford University Press. She is currently principal investigator on a series of studies examining economic empowerment programs for survivors of domestic violence.

JOAN L. BOTTORFF

Joan L. Bottorff is a professor at the University of British Columbia and director of the Institute for Healthy Living and Chronic Disease Prevention. Her program of research in cancer prevention and health promotion includes studies addressing tobacco reduction in a variety of populations, cancer screening, and health promotion among cancer patients and their families. In her research she has explored the social context of health behavior and has published both methodological and empirical articles focusing on gender influences.

CATHY CHABOT

Cathy Chabot is an anthropologist and is employed as the research manager with the Youth Sexual Health Team based at the University of British Columbia. She has extensive fieldwork experience in the area of social inequities and health, particularly in British Columbian settings. She received her master's in anthropology from Simon Fraser University in 2002.

NATALIE A. CHAMBERS

Natalie A. Chambers is an interdisciplinary doctoral student at the University of British Columbia Okanagan. She has participated in health research studies and coauthored publications on women and men's tobacco cessation during pregnancy, tobacco use of youth, First Nations women and tobacco, South Asian Canadian women's experiences of breast cancer, the health behaviors of immigrants and refugees in Canada, and models of First Nations chronic disease self-management and health governance.

GILLIAN EINSTEIN

Gillian Einstein is an associate professor in the Department of Psychology and the Dalla Lana School of Public Health, as well as founder and director of the Collaborative Graduate Program in Women's Health, at the University of Toronto. Her cognitive neuroscience and women's health research program includes studies addressing the neurobiological effects of cultural practices such as female genital circumcision/mutilation/cutting (FGC), the effects on memory of prophylactic oophorectomy in women carrying the BRCA1/2 gene mutations, and sex differences in sensitivity to touch. She has published on vision, Alzheimer's disease, sex differences, FGC, and women's health. She has edited and annotated a book of classical papers in hormones and behavior called *Sex and the Brain* (2007, MIT Press).

MARY JANE ESPLEN

Mary Jane Esplen is a clinician-scientist and professor in the Department of Psychiatry, Faculty of Medicine, University of Toronto, and director of the de Souza Institute. She is a therapist and researcher working in psychosocial oncology. She has a strong interest in developing measurement tools and support groups or therapy interventions for cancer genetics populations and individuals with cancer. She also has an interest in women's health issues and works with individuals in the area of body image and sexual health. She is the recent past president of the Canadian Association of Psychosocial Oncology.

BRENDAN GOUGH

Brendan Gough was appointed as chair in social psychology at Nottingham Trent University in 2007. He is a qualitative researcher interested in gender issues, especially concerning men and masculinities. He has published various papers on gender identities and relations that draw on discursive and psychoanalytic concepts, including areas such as sexism, homophobia, and men's health. Gough is coeditor of *Qualitative Research in Psychology* (Taylor & Francis) and *Social & Personality Psychology Compass* (Critical Psychology Section) (Blackwell). He has coproduced three books with various colleagues: *Critical Social Psychology* (with M. McFadden), *Reflexivity in Qualitative Research* (with L. Finlay), and *Men, Masculinities, and Health* (with S. Robertson).

REBECCA J. HAINES-SAAH

While writing this chapter, Rebecca J. Haines-Saah was a postdoctoral fellow at the Centre for Nursing and Health Behaviour Research at the

University of British Columbia, with funding from the Social Sciences and Humanities Research Council of Canada and the Psychosocial Oncology Research Training Program (PORT). She holds a doctorate (2008) in behavioral health sciences from the Dalla Lana School of Public Health, University of Toronto. Her research interests include social theories of health and illness, gender and health, adolescent substance use, and analyses of tobacco and drug use in media and popular cultures.

JOY L. JOHNSON

Joy L. Johnson is the scientific director of the Canadian Institute of Health Research's Institute of Gender and Health and a professor in the School of Nursing at the University of British Columbia (UBC). Johnson's highly productive research program focuses on health promotion and health behavior change, and addresses social, structural, and individual factors that influence health behavior. A major thrust of her work focuses on sex and gender issues in substance use. Johnson has made extensive contributions in the field of tobacco research, and her work has been recognized with numerous awards including the UBC Killam Research Prize.

SHIRIN KALYAN

Shirin Kalyan received her doctorate in experimental medicine from the University of British Columbia in 2006, specializing in the stress-induced regulation of the immune system. Her research is concerned with sex and gender differences in the neuroendocrine control of the stress-response system that regulates chronic ailments such as osteoporosis, autoimmunity, and cardiovascular disease. As a translational scientist, Shirin facilitates knowledge sharing between disciplines and is able to design unique studies that bridge population, clinical, and basic sciences in the context of women's health research.

MARY T. KELLY

Mary T. Kelly is an independent research consultant and freelance writer. She holds a master of arts degree and provides qualitative-based services for health research investigators and their projects.

ALECK OSTRY

Aleck Ostry is a professor in the faculty of social sciences at the University of Victoria. He holds a Canada Research Chair in the Social

Determinants of Community Health and is also a Senior Scholar with the Michael Smith Foundation for Health Research in British Columbia. He has a master of science in health service planning, a master's in history (specializing in the history of public health), and a doctorate in epidemiology. He conducts an extensive program on the social determinants of health with a focus on rural health, food security, and nutrition policy.

NANCY POOLE

Nancy Poole is the director of research and knowledge translation for the British Columbia Centre of Excellence for Women's Health in Vancouver, British Columbia, Canada. Poole has extensive experience in research and knowledge exchange relating to policy and service provision for women with tobacco and other substance use problems. She is well known in Canada for leadership in piloting online, participatory methods for knowledge generation and exchange, including virtual networks, collaboratories, and communities of inquiry/practice.

PAMELA A. RATNER

Pamela A. Ratner is a professor of nursing at the University of British Columbia and holds a Senior Scholar Award from the Michael Smith Foundation for Health Research. She has led research initiatives to inform practice and policy through analyses of the social contexts that create barriers to health, affect health seeking, and influence health system responses. In particular, she has examined how gender and diversity influence health behavior. Her specific research program has focused on cardiovascular risk reduction and the psychosocial determinants of health risk behavior. Ratner has a particular interest in latent variable modeling and health measurement. She is a member of the Institute Advisory Board of the Canadian Institutes of Health Research, Institute of Circulatory and Respiratory Health, and was elected a Fellow of the Canadian Academy of Health Sciences in 2007.

ROBIN REPTA

Robin Repta is a social science researcher at the Centre for Nursing and Health Behaviour Research at the University of British Columbia (UBC). She received a master's degree in human kinetics from UBC in 2006 and has continued to conduct qualitative gender and health research. Her current work focuses on social inequalities among tobacco-smoking teens, the representation of marijuana in Canadian newspapers, and the integration of sex and gender as variables in health research.

STEVE ROBERTSON

Steve Robertson worked in the UK National Health Service (NHS) for more than 20 years before commencing a career in research. He secured an NHS Fellowship to complete his doctorate and an Economic and Social Research Council/Medical Research Council Interdisciplinary Fellowship to complete his period of postdoctoral study. His main interests and publications are around social theories of masculinity and their application to aspects of health and illness, but he has also worked on masculinity and disability; the sociology of (male) bodies; fathers and fatherhood; men, masculinity, and mental well-being; evaluating men's health programs; and men's engagement (or not) with health services. He has successfully completed two Florence Nightingale Foundation Travel Scholarships, and has worked with fellow academics, policymakers, and practitioners from Australia, the United States, and Canada. He has also acted as a consultant on gender and men's health to the UK Department of Health and the World Health Organization (Europe).

CHERYL ROLIN-GILMAN

Cheryl Rolin-Gilman is the advanced practice nurse for the Women's Mental Health Program and the Addictions Program at the Centre for Addiction and Mental Health (CAMH) and a lecturer for the Department of Psychiatry and Faculty of Nursing at the University of Toronto. She has been working at CAMH since April 1999, when she also completed her master's degree in nursing. In the course of her studies, she focused on women's issues, particularly integrating feminist principles into practice. Prior to her work at CAMH, she held various nursing leadership positions. She was the professional practice leader and educator of the Mental Health Patient Service Unit at Sunnybrook and Women's College Health Sciences Centre. In that area, she worked with war veterans and developed her interest in trauma.

LORI ROSS

Lori Ross is a research scientist in the Social, Equity and Health Research Section of the Centre for Addiction and Mental Health and an associate professor in the Department of Psychiatry, Dalla Lana School of Public Health, and Lawrence S. Bloomberg Faculty of Nursing of the University of Toronto. Her research focuses on mental health and health service experiences of marginalized communities, with a particular focus on lesbian, gay, bisexual, and transgender populations.

RICHARD G. SAWATZKY

Richard G. Sawatzky is an associate professor of nursing at Trinity Western University, Canada. His research focuses on methods of patient-reported outcomes and quality-of-life measurement, and the intersections of spirituality, religion, culture, and other sources of diversity in various health care contexts. He has a particular methodological interest in the use of latent variable mixture modeling for examining sample heterogeneity with respect to individuals' self-reports about their health status and quality of life. He is a member of the International Society for Quality of Life Research and the International Society for Quality of Life Studies.

TONI SCHOFIELD

Toni Schofield is an associate professor at the University of Sydney, Australia. She has published widely in the sociology of gender, focusing on public policy and health. Her current research projects are diverse, including large publicly funded studies of prosecution and deterrence in workplace health and alcohol use and harm minimization among young people. As in her previous work, the principal object of inquiry is the social dynamics involved in "the problem" and how they generate barriers to and opportunities for interventions to address and redress it.

JEAN SHOVELLER

Jean Shoveller is a professor at the University of British Columbia, Faculty of Medicine, School of Population and Public Health, where she coleads the Social and Life Course Determinants of Health theme. She holds a Canadian Institutes of Health Research/Public Health Agency of Canada Applied Public Health Chair and a Senior Scholar Award from the Michael Smith Foundation for Health Research. Her program of research and training focuses on the social contexts of youth health inequities, with a particular emphasis on intervention to improve youth sexual health.

AMANDA SLAUNWHITE

Amanda Slaunwhite is a doctoral student in the Department of Geography at the University of Victoria. Her research interests include gender-based analysis of mental health issues, health planning in northern communities, and occupational mental health. Slaunwhite is a recipient of the Canadian Institutes of Health Research Frederick Banting and

Charles Best Doctoral Award and is affiliated with the Western Regional Training Centre for Health Services Research. She is currently contributing to research related to the provision of mental health services in rural and remote communities, mental health care restructuring in British Columbia, and the utilization of health care services by persons with substance dependence issues.

NOREEN STUCKLESS

Noreen Stuckless is an assistant professor in the Department of Psychiatry at the University of Toronto. She teaches psychology of women and gender-related courses at York University and the University of Toronto. She has coauthored publications involving domestic violence and the scale development of measures including those on attitudes toward revenge, cognitive bowel disorders, and the psychosocial effects of diagnoses of genetic mutations. Her current research is on interpartner violence and, in particular, how the violence affects women and their children.

TARYN TANG

Taryn Tang is an assistant professor in the Women's Mental Health Program, Department of Psychiatry, University of Toronto. She is interested in the cumulative and intersecting social and psychological determinants of mental health. This approach recognizes that multiple factors, such as gender, income, and ethno-racial identity, come together in distinct ways to influence health outcomes for individuals and groups. Her areas of research have focused on gender differences in migrant socioeconomic integration and mental health and mental illness stigma among ethno-racial communities in Canada.

BRENDA TONER

Brenda Toner is the cohead of Social Equity and Health Research at the Centre for Addiction and Mental Health and a professor and head of the Women's Mental Health Program and the director of the Fellowship Program in the Department of Psychiatry at the University of Toronto. Toner has published and presented on a variety of health-related problems that are disproportionately diagnosed in women, including eating disorders, anxiety, depression, chronic pelvic pain, chronic fatigue, and irritable bowel syndrome. She is particularly interested in investigating factors in the lives of women that influence health and well-being, including gender role socialization, violence, discrimination, and body dissatisfaction.

Acknowledgments

The writing of **Chapter 1** and the editing of this volume, along with the development of many ideas underpinning this enterprise, were made possible by the support of colleagues and partners at the British Columbia Centre of Excellence for Women's Health whose activities are supported by Health Canada, via the Centres of Excellence for Women's Health Program. The impetus for this volume originated with NEXUS, a research team on the social context of health behavior that was supported by the Michael Smith Foundation for Health Research. The views expressed are my own.

Lorraine Greaves

The writing of **Chapter 4** was made possible by the career support provided to the first author by a Michael Smith Foundation for Health Research Senior Scholar Award.

Pamela A. Ratner

The author gratefully acknowledges the opportunity to think about and present many of her ideas first at the Institute of Gender and Health's Summer Institute in Vancouver, British Columbia, in June 2009. Thanks go also to the Committee on Degrees in Studies of Women, Gender, and Sexuality at Harvard University for the invitation of a visiting professorship and providing a fecund environment in which to revisit the ideas and write **Chapter 5** during Spring 2010.

Gillian Einstein

The writing of **Chapter 6** was made possible by the career support provided to the second author by a Canadian Institutes of Health Research (CIHR) and Public Health Agency of Canada (Applied Public Health Chair in Improving Youth Sexual Health) and Michael Smith Foundation for Health Research Senior Scholar Award. The empirical examples shared are drawn from the CIHR-funded projects—*Sex, Gender and Place: An Analysis of Youth's Experiences With Sexually Transmitted Infection Testing*—as well as research funded by the British

Columbia Medical Research Foundation—*Investigating the Experience of Teenage Pregnancy in Prince George, British Columbia.*

Cathy Chabot and Jean Shoveller

Rebecca J. Haines-Saah was a recipient of postdoctoral fellowships from the Social Sciences and Humanities Research Council of Canada and the Psychosocial Oncology Research Training program of the Canadian Institutes of Health Research while writing **Chapter 7**. The *Smoke in My Eyes* study was funded by a student research grant from the Canadian Tobacco Control Research Initiative.

Rebecca J. Haines-Saah

The development of the scale and the writing of **Chapter 11** were made possible by the support of a grant from the Social Sciences and Humanities Research Council. In addition, support to the Centre for Addiction and Mental Health for salary of scientists and infrastructure has been provided by the Ontario Ministry of Health and Long-Term Care. The views expressed in this chapter do not necessarily reflect those of the Ministry of Health and Long-Term Care.

Brenda Toner

Much of the conceptual material in **Chapter 12** was developed over more than a decade of research funded by the Australian Department of Health and Ageing, the Australian Research Council (ARC), and the Australian Health Policy Institute. Empirical examples are drawn from this work and further research supported by the Academy of the Social Sciences in Australia. The prodigious research and support of my colleague and friend Raewyn Connell have been central to the approach and methods outlined in the chapter. So, too, have the numerous discussions on this subject with Anthony Nolan. I am also indebted to my current colleagues working with me on a large ARC-funded study of alcohol use and harm minimization.

Toni Schofield

The writing of **Chapter 13** was made possible through a range of projects employing the use of virtual communities, which have been sponsored by the British Columbia Centre of Excellence for Women's Health (BCCEWH) in Vancouver, funded in part by Health Canada. The author thanks the Promoting Health in Women research team at BCCEWH for thoughtful discussions of the role of virtual communities as mechanisms for knowledge translation and feminist action research, and Mary Lasovitch for development editing support.

Nancy Poole

The editing of this volume, contributions to Chapters 7 and 10, and the writing of **Chapter 14** were made possible by the career support provided by a Canadian Institutes of Health Research (Institute of Gender and Health) New Investigator Award and a Michael Smith Foundation for Health Research Scholar Award. The empirical examples shared are drawn from a program funded by the Canadian Institutes of Health Research (Institute of Gender and Health)—*Families Controlling and Eliminating Tobacco (FACET)*. Special thanks to Mary Kelly, Christina Han, Anna Chan, and Tina Thornton for their assistance, edits, and thoughtful reviews of the earlier drafts of Chapter 14.

John L. Oliffe

Many thanks to the reviewers of our book proposal and volume for their thoughtful feedback, guidance, and enthusiasm for this work.

John L. Oliffe and Lorraine Greaves

Kate Hunt, University of Glasgow

Aaron D. Coe, University of Phoenix

Patricia P. Rieker, Boston University and Harvard Medical School

Sharon G. Portwood, University of North Carolina at Charlotte

Part I

Context and Concepts

Why Put Gender and Sex Into Health Research?

Lorraine Greaves

Putting gender and sex into health research design is a practice that is only recently being encouraged or adopted by researchers, their funders, and audiences. This chapter provides background and context on the rationale for and recent history of this late, but welcome, shift. It presages examples of health research that have incorporated gender and sex into design, and offers a commentary on the history and future of gender and sex in health research.

Why put sex and gender into health research? At heart, it is a matter of ethics to do so. As "every cell has a sex," according to the Institute of Medicine (Wizemann & Pardue, 2001, p. 4), and every person is gendered (in some way), both sex (biological characteristics) and gender (socially constructed factors) must be woven into any health research that deems itself to be complete and/or relevant. Integrating these concepts reveals and reinforces their incredible significance in producing more accurate, effective, and relevant research findings. Hence, in order to improve health in humans (or animals), it is critically important to attend to both the biological and the social aspects of growth, development, illness, and recovery.

It is unfortunate that most studies on aspects of human health do not yet explicitly consider sex and gender in their design, data collection, or analysis. While progress is being made, examples of research articles, books, presentations, and products that do not distinguish along these lines are rampant, thereby making their results less useful, and sometimes useless.

Currently, the concepts of both sex and gender (and their relationships, contexts, and meanings) are routinely overlooked, misused, misunderstood, confused, or conflated in health research (see Fishman, Wick, & Koenig, 1999, for a discussion of the use of these terms), creating a kind of underlying chaos in the existing health literature.

Most disconcerting, perhaps, are researchers and research users who do not notice this gap, and consequently acritically apply gender- and sex-blind results to all people, wherever they are on the sex and gender continuum. These practices involve health promotion, diagnosis and treatment of diseases, clinical practices, therapeutic choices, program design, health system organization, and health and social policies. These practices also influence the designing of subsequent research studies.

At best, these conflations and oversights lead to practices that are just approximate and neutral. At worst, however, they can cause or perpetuate harm, pain, or inequity.

Ultimately, a generic approach to health research when these essential distinctions fail to be made in the design, analysis, or transfer of publicly funded research is simply unethical. In an age when knowledge transfer and translation is *the* critical path for funders, members of the public, and practitioners, how can any confidence be ascribed to health research results that do not comprehensively consider, measure, analyze, and account for both sex and gender, such fundamental aspects of human life? This rhetorical question underpins the enterprise of doing current, effective, and ethical research.

But putting sex and gender into health research is a complex task as our understanding of these concepts and the context of the health research enterprise has evolved considerably over the past few decades, and promises to continue to evolve. In addition, both sex and gender are concepts that are tightly interrelated, exist on continua, and, simultaneously, *interact iteratively* with each other. Not to mention, these concepts exist in an important web of influences on health and well-being, such as ethnicity, culture and race-related factors, age, ability, income, education, housing, and literacy, affecting the lives and bodies of people and being affected by them on micro to macro levels.

"Fault Line" of Gender

Apart from these obvious health impacts of doing health research differently, there is a critical social context in which these practices exist. Most societies are built and maintained along a "fault line" of gender (Papanek, 1984), and most societies have historically developed on a scaffold of patriarchal assumptions and practices. With the reemergence of feminism in the 1960s in many developed countries, a robust women's health movement emerged, addressing these assumptions and practices. Women's health advocacy engaged with multiple issues including roles, labor force participation, sexism, and violence against women. However, a robust section of the second-wave women's movement centered on health issues.

The women's health movement focused its energies on the body and women's control over it. On the care and clinical side, women complained about sexism, paternalism, and overmedicalization with particular emphasis on the appropriation by male doctors of sexual and reproductive issues, including childbirth. Women's health advocates also called for an end to oversights and omissions in both clinical practice and research, making particular note of the omission of women in clinical trials, all the while decrying gender neutrality and blindness that resulted from having too few women in science and medicine. It is in this context that the recent developments in the field of sex and gender in health research have emerged (Greaves, 2009).

The arguments began to build for changing health research. By the 1990s various countries were grappling with arguments for changing the approach to reflect sex and gender. The arguments included the issue of biological "differences," making the point that women's and men's bodies are different. Social differences were increasingly evident as well, with more and more social scientists illustrating that being male and being female are gendered experiences and, relatedly, that femininities and masculinities have varied but palpable meanings.

There was an important political dimension as well. At bottom, there was an argument for redress, noting that research on women, with women, and by women had been overlooked and needed rebalancing by attention to sex and gender and indeed, specifically, women's health. The reasons range from social justice and equity arguments to error rectification. It became clear that mistakes had occurred, and could continue to occur, when research on men was applied to women.

The response to the AIDS epidemic in some countries in the 1980s marked a key turning point for gay men's health. More latterly, broader issues around men's health have surfaced, and a nascent men's health movement has emerged. In part driven by the example of documenting and theorizing women's health, some men's health researchers have focused on the impact of masculinities on men's health behavior and their interactions with health systems. Others have unearthed new knowledge and funding for sex-specific health issues such as prostate cancer, bringing attention to such male-specific disease in line with the huge public attention to issues such as breast cancer for women.

Separately, a broader men's movement has often reacted to funding and attention that have emphasized both women's issues and women's health. These initiatives have often made the political point about including men as well as women in sex- and gender-specific initiatives, funding, and programming. The men's movement has focused on issues such as custody and access for divorced fathers, along with high-level attention to men's health.

In the context of these cultural shifts that are de-emphasizing patriarchy in favor of more liberal, equitable organizational power systems (clearly occurring at faster rates in some societies than in others), the range of issues to consider in analyzing and measuring sex and gender is dizzying. If sex and gender interact to create health, and are affected by cultural and temporal factors, how do we proceed in putting sex and gender into health research? How do we measure these synergistic effects? Further, how do we capture these concepts, processes, and relationships to pin them down?

Recent History of the Concepts of Sex and Gender

At the outset of the "second wave" of feminism in the 1960s, just discussing the influence of sex on health was novel. Sex, then, became the label and concept taken into the field, and represented both biological and social controversies and agreements. Given this stance, most of the early discourse was focused on "sex differences" (between males and females, men and women) and underpinned a range of requests for sex-disaggregation of data, differential treatment of women in clinical practices, and consideration of social issues such as "sex roles" and "sex-role socialization." As can be seen from the list of concepts and labels below, the concept of gender followed, introduced by social scientists. Building on emerging notions of gender, the stage was set for an emerging differentiation of sex and gender as concepts and the recognition that both matter to women's health and, ultimately, men's health.

This differentiation was not evenly adopted across disciplines, fields, languages, and countries, however. This problem has been well described (Fishman et al., 1999) but, unfortunately, persists to this day. Nonetheless, both terms have been adopted in the literature and common discourse, even if used inconsistently between disciplines, or with different intentions. As the concepts of sex and gender became further developed, it emerged that a *differences model* was not accurately reflecting a continuum, or, at the very least, overlapping sets of characteristics that comprise sex and gender in human populations. Hence, the notion of *influences* of sex and gender captured this shift, along with the notion that certain *factors* such as bodily characteristics or social circumstances could affect human health.

Hence, the following linguistic layers are evident, at least in the North American context. While these layers represent shifts in thinking, and increasing sophistication, there are still uses for some of these early terms in certain circumstances as they offer precision to the field.

- Sex
- Sex differences

- Gender
- Sex and gender
- Sex and gender differences
- Sex differences and gender influences
- Sex- and gender-related factors

These evolving shifts in conceptualizing matched, reflected, or inspired a set of different analytic frameworks. As mentioned above, the notion of "sex differences" called for sex stratification, differentiation, and disaggregation, all techniques that indicated support for *comparing* men and women, or males and females. This assumed that the human population could be neatly divided into two, a binary or dimorphism that is no longer supportable. It also assumed that unless there was a "difference," there was unlikely to be a problem. This thinking was based on simple notions of equality, not the importance of equity or equal opportunity for health, and did not reflect evolving thinking about the continua of sex and gender.

Once the term *gender* was introduced, it became clear that a more complex process would be required to incorporate its full meaning, and gender analysis was born. Gender analysis frameworks stress *processes* of critical thinking to interrogate gender, and do not typically suggest concrete measures (see Clow, Pederson, Haworth-Brockman, & Bernier, 2009). Highlighting critical appraisals of gender encouraged identification of situational and temporal characteristics across cultures and time, entrenching gender as a social process. Ultimately, gender analysis surfaces the relational issues between males and females, men and women, or girls and boys in the context of social institutions.

Gender was, and is, a complex concept and social process. Many disciplines engaged in health research do not address such social scientific processes in training or practice. Perhaps because of this, gender did become conflated with sex in some discourses and disciplines. More troubling and distracting, gender became conflated with "women" in some political and policy contexts, perhaps to mask a focus on women when that proved unpopular politically. Hence, gender and health or gender concerns were widely interpreted as pertaining to women or women only. Once gender became more accurately and widely understood, it also had the effect of conflating men's concerns with women's concerns, a disservice to both women's health and men's health as explicit attention is needed to both.

In addition to these difficulties, gender, as a concept in health research, has had a varied ride in the past 20 years, as it is both more complex and resistant to measurement than is sex and more broadly and inaccurately used. Attempts to quantify gender are few as most scientists perceive gender as a multipronged concept and a social process that is tightly tethered to its context, thereby resisting universal measure. It has even been suggested that sex and gender need to be merged conceptually and measured accordingly, given their strong interactional component (see, for example, Phillips, 2005).

Nevertheless, several analytic frameworks contributed to our growing understanding of gender in health, notably the *determinants of health* and *social determinants of health* frameworks. These frames identified gender as a determinant of health, giving the field a strong boost. As thinking evolved, it became evident that the determinants of health operate together to create health, leading to new thinking about the necessity to indicate a clear and unambiguous incorporation of diversity into gender-based analysis. More recently, the concepts of health equity and inequity, identifying *opportunities for health* as the key measure, have helped to create actionable goals addressing diversities and disparities in health status. Finally, during all of this, more theoretical work on intersectional-type analyses has also emerged, identifying the myriad of features, factors, and processes that contribute to health, and contextualizing gender within those frameworks. These frameworks, more or less in order of emergence, are as follows:

- Sex stratification, differentiation, and disaggregation
- Gender (based) analysis and sex and gender (based) analysis
- (Social) Determinants of health
- Sex, gender, and diversity (based) analysis
- Disparities, (in)equities of health
- Intersectional-type analyses

The concept of diversity has had its own language evolution that has, in addition and by necessity, been different in different countries and regions. Over the past few decades, language, terminology, thinking, and a range of social and political events and movements have affected how diversity is interpreted, named, and understood. Terminology has also been determined by jurisdictional decisions about collection of census or other population-based data, resulting in different terms and classifications being used across jurisdictions, making comparisons difficult. In addition, there is growing imprecision as self-descriptions and multiple identities are measured. The concept of classification is a social construct, and many critics therefore debunk all efforts to collect such data. Nonetheless, relevant to health and other social opportunities and analyses, the following terms have been used and evolved over time:

- Race
- Nationality
- Minority group (visible or not)

- Ethnicity

- Ethnocultural identity

- Foreign born

- Indigenous

- Immigrant, migrant

- Racially classified social groups

Many of these terms have been variously either self-descriptions or externally imposed. Race, ethnic, and cultural labels are often contentious and contested. Nevertheless, in health, there is also often an interest and a need to identify health concerns, diseases, treatments, or policies that have a particular effect on groups according to their biological and social characteristics. Sometimes these requests are made by the group itself, seeking information; at other times they are descriptions of findings published as relevant to a particular group. There has been legitimate worry about such categorization being used for negative, prejudicial, and discriminatory purposes. However, these fears are being balanced by need and right to know as new techniques, knowledge, and technologies are resulting in new knowledge about genetics and other biological processes that shed light on difference. What is important, and again increasing the complexity of measurement in health research, is that many of the factors affecting diversity and health are in fact processes, such as the following:

- Biological processes

- Discrimination

- Experiences of sexism, racism, and heterosexism

- Identity formation

- Self-descriptions

- Labeling

This brief description of some of the key elements in evolving thinking about sex, gender, and diversity over the past several decades underscores the constantly evolving nature of this field. It also explains, to some extent, the emergence of the various fields of study listed below:

- Women's health

- Gender and women's health

- Gender and health

- Now (at least) three main fields:
  - Gender and health
  - Women's health
  - Men's health

Not surprisingly, the fields have multiplied and get more, not less, specific.

These stages of categorizing thinking in health reflect both political and sociological trends as well as their influence on global health organizations. As well, they represent the growing specificities and sophistication with which theoreticians and methodologists have approached these topics. This is not to ignore the nascent and emergent areas of study of intersex and transgendered and transsexual health (which, not incidentally, serves to starkly illuminate the complex and fluid conceptual issues surrounding sex and gender), but rather is to identify the areas affecting the majority of the human population.

Changing Practices to Support Sex and Gender in Health Research

Ultimately, the most compelling arguments for including sex and gender in health research became the ones made about ethics and the quality of science. Slowly but surely better science has been seen to include sex and gender, in the interests of increased validity, reliability, generalizability, and completeness. Without even seemingly getting "political," acknowledging past patriarchal influences, uneven funding practices, or even lack of interest, agreement about improving the quality of science is something that all responsible leaders and researchers could support (Greaves et al., 1999).

These slow and emergent shifts in thinking have manifested in the development or modification of research funding practices and organizations, or in the development of strategic links between policymaking and research. In Canada, for example, sex and gender analysis is a required element in research proposals to the Canadian Institutes of Health Research (Spitzer, 2006), and in the United States, evidence of attention to women, children, and minorities is required in research proposals to the National Institutes of Health (1993). In Canada, this effort is complemented and supported by a federal policy requiring gender-based analysis in policymaking across government, which was enacted in 2000 by Health Canada. This latter policy has put pressure on research users, in this case federal policymakers, to consider a wider range of issues and variables connected to sex and gender before making social, health, or economic policy. Internationally, these trends fit with a commitment to gender analysis at major international agencies, notably the World Health Organization (2002).

However, all of these initiatives and directives need to be understood in context and with caution. Two illustrations from North America highlight different approaches to institutionalizing gender analysis. The federal gender-based analysis policy in Canada was audited by the Auditor General in a report issued in 2009. This report indicated that compliance with this policy was minimal across seven chosen departments including Health Canada. Even more troubling is that even when it was performed and gender impacts were analyzed, there was no indication that *the analysis was considered* in the development of policy decisions or assessed and reported to the Cabinet in policy documents (Auditor General of Canada, 2009).

A very different approach was taken in the United States, where the General Accounting Office analyzed compliance to the 1993 *mandatory* policy requiring research proposals to include women, minorities, and children in research funded by the National Institutes of Health (NIH), or else justify why not. Its 1999 assessment indicated that while there was 97% compliance with the directive for inclusion in the year 1997, there remained a strong need for production of data that were going to lead to valid analysis by sex and gender, resulting in specific additional recommendations regarding the necessity for analysis (General Accounting Office, 2000).

In countries such as Australia and Canada, strategies to guide policy-making in gender and health have been developed. Most recently, in Australia a men's health strategy has been developed to parallel ongoing strategic activity in women's health. Over the years, many of these strategic developments in policymaking have relied on simplistic sex differentiation between categories of men and women, with less attention to gender and its effects, or the differences among women or men. Clearly, as all of these organizational initiatives and directives show, there is a long and rocky road between directives to improve either research or policymaking and effective results in the field of gender and health.

To support these institutional and organizational changes, capacity building for both researchers and research users has been required in the provision of tools, primers, and books. Research users can be frustrated in incorporating gender into policy and program development if inadequate or incomplete research exists and issues of gender and sex are unacknowledged or unexplored. To remedy this, the Canadian primer *Better Science With Sex and Gender: A Primer for Health Research* (Johnson, Greaves, & Repta, 2007) was recently released. This primer sets out in simple terms the challenges of incorporating sex and gender into health research, suggests some methods and options for starting out, and illustrates the importance of doing so. In that spirit there have been numerous attempts to outline gender analysis both at national and at international levels. There is a hunger among researchers, trainees, and well-established researchers alike, as well as research users, for more examples and information, and more support for experimentation and conceptual development.

GOING FORWARD WITH SEX AND GENDER AND HEALTH RESEARCH

Given the complexity of the tasks in putting sex and gender into health research, what are some reasonable goals going forward? Shall we continue to address the different language usage by discipline, culture, and place, and over time? Can we get agreement on definitions? Do we need to? Can we ever accurately measure sex and gender and their interactivity? What would a synthesized measure of both look like? Is the synergistic effect greater than either? Is this quantifiable? Is it better captured with qualitative or mixed-method research? Do these questions only apply to humans? And further, how do we measure diversity and its interaction with sex and gender? What influence do intersectional-type analyses have on the way sex and gender are integrated into health research? How will scientific and technological advances herald the potential for "postgenderism" (Dvorsky & Hughes, 2008) where the material bodies of individuals are so diverse or modified by technology or interventions that gender becomes a malleable and possibly elusive and yet liberating concept? These and related questions are increasingly top of mind for health researchers interested in gender, sex, and health.

As important, though, are the practical and advocacy goals inherent in this area. How do we generate more interest in sex, gender, and health research? Which arguments will resonate with the widest group of researchers, students, and funders? What will training look like? And finally, how can we institutionalize sex and gender in health research in more universities, hospitals, health authorities, governments, and countries? Can we encourage a surge of scientific advocacy to require sex and gender analyses at proposal development, at peer review, and in analysis and reporting in scholarly and nonacademic writing? Can we create such a demand in users of research for these very basic issues to be adequately addressed that ultimately all health research will acknowledge and measure the effect of sex and gender in human health? All of these questions and challenges underpin this field.

The design of research studies cannot practically be separated from knowledge translation activity. There are many points on the continuum of developing research when key decisions get made, and where investigators can either fail or succeed in producing sex- and gender-relevant research. These include decisions about how to generate and frame research questions, objectives, goals, or designs. Do these processes have consideration of sex and gender built in, and do they, ideally, engage with research users from the beginning? Does the research design assume that simple sex-based disaggregation of data based on the binary categories of males and females, men and women, and boys and girls is enough? Does the research design limit itself to categorical sex-based classifications with no overlay of gender analysis or explanation or data collection about gender? Or worse (though, as we have seen, common), does the research take sex and/or gender into account, collect the data, and fail to analyze and report such findings?

So why put sex and gender into health research? The utility of sex- and gender-based health research is in its contribution to improving understanding of all aspects of health, disease, treatment, and health system design and policy. Ultimately we aim to acquire more knowledge and information on the influences of sex and gender on health. In the process, however, it is important to generate more precision in sex, gender, and health research by evolving more accurate and complex measures of sex and gender. This requires that we engage with a range of disciplines and highly conceptual and theoretical work in order to fully understand all the components of gender and their implications in human life.

While perhaps any step on the road toward full sex and gender integration into health research is to be encouraged, the challenges are to embrace all aspects of this journey and to become exemplars and mentors to both colleagues and students. The notion of automatically asking whether or not a piece of new knowledge (or old, for that matter) applies equally and equitably across the spectrum of sexes and genders, in a range of diversities of bodies, practices, identities, ages, locations, and geographies, is new. It is essential to support a burgeoning field, attempting to make this kind of question automatic, and, ultimately, answerable.

References

Auditor General of Canada. (2009). *The spring 2009 report of the auditor general of Canada, Chapter 1*. Gatineau, QC, Canada: Minister of Public Works and Government Services of Canada.

Clow, B., Pederson, A., Haworth-Brockman, M., & Bernier, J. (2009). *Rising to the challenge: Sex- and gender-based analysis for health planning, policy and research in Canada*. Halifax, NS, Canada: Atlantic Centre of Excellence for Women's Health.

Dvorsky, G., & Hughes, J. (2008). *Postgenderism: Beyond the gender binary*. IEET White Paper 3. Hartford, CT: Institute for Ethics and Emerging Technologies. Retrieved December 11, 2010, from http://ieet.org/archive/IEET-03-Post Gender.pdf

Fishman, J. R., Wick, J. G., & Koenig, B. A. (1999). The use of sex and gender to define and characterize meaningful differences between men and women: A report of the task force on the NIH women's health research agenda for the

21st century [Executive summary]. *National Institutes of Health, Office of Research on Women's Health, 1,* 15–19.

General Accounting Office. (2000). *Women's health: NIH has increased its efforts to include women in research.* Retrieved December 11, 2010, from http://www .gao.gov/new.items/he00096.pdf

Greaves, L. (2009). Women, gender and health research. In P. Armstrong & J. Deadman (Eds.), *Women's health: Intersections of policy, research and practice* (pp. 3–20). Toronto, ON, Canada: Women's Press.

Greaves, L., Hankivsky, O., Amaratunga, C., Ballem, P., Chow, D., De Koninck, M., et al. (1999). CIHR 2000: *Sex, gender and women's health.* Vancouver, BC, Canada: British Columbia Centre of Excellence for Women's Health, Canadian Institutes for Health Research.

Health Canada. (2000). *Gender based analysis policy.* Ottawa, ON, Canada: Author.

Johnson, J. L., Greaves, L., & Repta, R. (2007). *Better science with sex and gender: A primer for health research.* Vancouver, BC, Canada: Women's Health Research Network.

National Institutes of Health. (1993). *NIH Revitalization Act of 1993: Public Law 103-43.* Retrieved December 11, 2010, from http://grants.nih.gov/grants/ olaw/pl103-43.pdf

Papanek, H. (1984). *Women in development and women's studies: Agenda for the future.* East Lansing: Office of Women in International Development, Michigan State University.

Phillips, S. P. (2005). Defining and measuring gender: A social determinant of health whose time has come. *International Journal for Equity in Health, 4*(11), 4–15.

Spitzer, D. (2006). *Gender and sex-based analysis in health research: A guide for CIHR researchers and reviewers.* Ottawa, ON, Canada: Canadian Institutes of Health Research.

Wizemann, T. M., & Pardue, M. (Eds.). (2001). *Exploring the biological contributions to human health: Does sex matter?* [Executive summary]. Washington, DC: National Academies Press, Institute of Medicine.

World Health Organization. (2002). *Integrating gender perspectives in the work of WHO: WHO gender policy.* Retrieved December 11, 2010, from http://www .who.int/gender/documents/engpolicy.pdf

Part II

Design

This section of the book addresses the key concepts from Chapter 1 and delves into these concepts in the context of design and measurement issues. This section is challenging, but essential reading; it addresses the theoretical and sometimes contradictory and confusing issues connected to putting sex and gender into health research.

Johnson and Repta, in Chapter 2, address the age-old binary question in sex, gender, and health research and put to rest the utility of binary or dimorphic thinking in the contemplation of the field. Fundamentally, they argue that such binary thinking, in addition to being theoretically unsound, excludes the lived realities of some human beings. They address and demolish the binary on two counts: first, that standard distinctions between male and female are moribund and stuck, and second, that the distinctions between sex and gender are similarly too rigid and limited. The key elements of dimorphic

thinking assume and concretize sex- and gender-related classifications, rather than opening them up for fluidity and development. Similarly, Johnson and Repta argue, the distinctions between sex and gender ignore the social construction of sex, as it develops over time and differs from place to place. This chapter challenges all of us to examine our emerging notions of sex and gender in research and search for a higher level of theorizing to underpin our designs going forward.

In Chapter 3, Johnson, Repta, and Kalyan address a wider set of concepts and examine their implications for study design. In this chapter, they build on the notion that including sex and gender in health research is a matter of ethics, and that it is essential. However, this chapter recognizes that sex and gender do not exist in a vacuum, but rather interact sometimes in complex ways with other factors and determinants of health. Hence, this chapter elucidates some of the analytic frameworks and terms mentioned in Chapter 1 and takes apart not only the social determinants of health but also the essential components of biology, such as hormones, metabolism, genes, and so on. Finally, Johnson et al. address the implications of all of this complexity for research design, examining approaches such as intersectionality, multilevel and system modeling, and epigenetics as diverse examples of incorporating sex, gender, and diversity into health research design.

Ratner and Sawatzky, in Chapter 4, address the critical issues of the measurement of gender. This chapter is an important attempt to clarify what is meant by gender by examining how gender has been measured and operationalized in health research. It also seeks to bring order to this underdeveloped and undertheorized element of sex, gender, and health research. Again, Ratner and Sawatzky address some of the language and concepts mentioned in Chapter 1 but dig deeply into how gender can be operationalized based on examinations of cases in which this has been accomplished. These reflect some very different design approaches. Ratner and Sawatzky offer some stark reminders

that measurement involves a set of theoretical assumptions inseparable from theory building. Finally, by highlighting a study examining the modern relevance of the Bem Sex Role Inventory developed in 1981, they address the conceptual challenge of measuring gender without examining its operations. This chapter takes us on an intriguing journey through thinking about the links between theory and method, and at the same time challenges us to root our efforts in concrete questions about health.

Einstein, in Chapter 5, contributes a detailed and comprehensive assessment of measuring biological sex. She traces the issues in measurement from reproductive to nervous system and illustrates the paradigms. Sex differences research has offered a structure for building the field and acquiring important new knowledge for health research. Einstein argues that such comparative research has an important role to play in highlighting the roles of various bodily systems in determining health and illness. She also articulates the issues that arise when gender affects sex, addressing the critical questions connected to the links between society and biology and arguing that influences both inside and outside the body work together to create the category "sex."

Sex and Gender 2

Beyond the Binaries

Joy L. Johnson

Robin Repta

> Research variables—"sex" polarized as "females" and "males," "sexuality" polarized as "homosexuals" and "heterosexuals," and "gender" polarized as "women" and "men"—reflect unnuanced series that conventionalize bodies, sexuality, and social location. Such research designs cannot include the experiences of hermaphrodites, pseudo-hermaphrodites, transsexuals, transvestites, bisexuals, third genders, and gender rebels as lovers, friends, parents, workers, and sports participants. Even if the research sample is restricted to putative "normals," the use of unexamined categories of sex, sexuality, and gender will miss complex combinations of status and identity, as well as differently gendered sexual continuities and discontinuities. (Lorber, 1996, p. 144)

For more than a decade researchers such as Lorber (1996, 2005) have challenged us to carefully reconsider the ways that we use the terms *gender* and *sex* in research. Despite these challenges, health researchers, on those occasions when they have considered sex and gender in their research, have tended to rely on conceptually stagnant notions of gender and sex that contrast masculine males with feminine females. "Moving beyond the binary" involves two important elements: first, reconsidering how we have conceptualized distinctions between masculine/feminine and male/female, and second, rethinking conceptualizations of gender as strictly social and of sex as strictly biological. A serious problem faced by

17

researchers is that our methods have not kept pace with our theoretical work in the area of sex and gender. A research design provides a blueprint for a research project. The way sex and gender are conceptualized has implications for all aspects of the design including the methodological approach, the data collection procedures, and analytic techniques. Incorporating gender and sex into a research design therefore requires consideration of all these elements. For example, while gender is typically theorized as a multidimensional, context-specific factor that changes according to time and place, it is routinely assumed to be a homogeneous category in research, measured by a single check box (Knaak, 2004). Furthermore, even in social science research where theories of gender originated, dangerous and static associations between women and femininity and men and masculinity are often assumed, eroding much of the diversity that exists within and among these categories (Dworkin, 2005). If the science of gender and health research is to advance, we must also consider ways not only to continually refine our base concepts, but also to promote interplay and praxis between theory and method.

With respect to sex, in health research, when it is conceptualized as a binary biological category (male and female), studies are often designed to compare two groups on particular parameters. While this approach is appropriate in some studies, it obfuscates the variation that occurs within and across sex with respect to genetics, anatomy, and physiology and also detracts from the fluid continuum of sex-related characteristics (Johnson, Greaves, & Repta, 2007). The same holds true for gender: If a study is guided by a conceptualization of gender that focuses on the roles that women and men hold in society, this will have implications for the research design. As Addis and Cohane (2005) attest, "Understanding the social context of masculinity (and gender more broadly) is similar to understanding the social context of race and ethnicity. Approaching important questions from only one perspective of difference is a bit like assuming we can only understand one racial, cultural, or ethnic group by comparing it with another. . . . Gender is about much more than sex differences between men and women on interesting dependent variables" (p. 635). To date, in health research there has been a lack of precision related to conceptual definitions of sex and gender and subsequent design. Researchers have tended to indicate that they are using a gender analysis or focusing on sex differences without appropriately delineating which aspects of gender or sex are of interest. Researchers need to move toward increased conceptual clarity and methodological precision. In this chapter we discuss various ways that sex and gender can be conceptualized and the implications of these conceptualizations for research design.

Before proceeding, it is important to reflect on research as a gendered practice. Science is a social enterprise, not created in a vacuum but influenced by societal opinions and politics. Scholars have investigated the ways that science has changed over the years, drawing attention to women's involvement in the scientific enterprise and detailing how societal shifts in gender roles have contributed to different research foci, methods, and epistemologies (Schiebinger, 1999). The fact that these changes have occurred emphasizes the socially constructed nature of research. Research design is similarly gendered as the questions we ask and the methodologies and methods we use are influenced by our gender as researchers and by gendered ideas about "hard" and "soft" research approaches. These types of distinctions underlie power dynamics in science, claims about the legitimacy of various scientific approaches, and distinctions made between biomedical/clinical research and social science research. For example, while clinical trials are now the universally accepted standard for clinical and health policy and practice, this is only one "way" of knowing, which has been shown to serve the financial interests of the physicians and research institutions that conduct this type of research (Mykhalovskiy & Weir, 2004). In light of the gendered nature of the scientific process, it behooves us to consider not only the ways that conceptualizations of gender influence design but also the ways that our research processes and research institutions are imbued with gender bias.

Sex

Sex is a biological construct that encapsulates the anatomical, physiological, genetic, and hormonal variation that exists in species. Our knowledge and understanding of sex has changed as we have come to appreciate the great diversity that exists within populations. For example, previous conceptions of sex assumed chromosomal arrangements XX and XY as the typical makeup for women and men, respectively, while we now understand that chromosomal configurations XXX, XXY, XYY, and XO exist, as well as XX males and XY females (de la Chapelle, 1981; McPhaul, 2002). The existence of these chromosomal arrangements has led to greater understanding of the genetic contributions of X and Y chromosomes to human phenotypic development and health (de la Chapelle, 1981) and indicates the need for research to expand narrow conceptualizations of sex to include this type of diversity. Within and across sex categories, variation also exists with respect to metabolic rate, bone size, brain function, stress response, and lung capacity. This variation cannot be captured by simple "male" and "female" designations, which is why it is important to think about sex in more than binary terms.

Conceptualizing sex accurately is important because of the great influence it has on health. There are many sex differences in the development of diseases such as coronary heart disease, Alzheimer's disease, and lung cancer, but the causal mechanisms that account for these differences are not always clear. To begin to identify these mechanisms we must conceptualize sex more precisely. Sex affects health, beginning with the different chromosomal compositions assigned to the sexes, which leads to variation in body shape and size, metabolism, hormonal and biochemical profiles, fat and muscle distribution, organ function, and brain structure, among other differences (Clow, Pederson, Haworth-Brockman, & Bernier, 2009; Johnson et al., 2007). These differences have profound influences on disease etiology, susceptibility, and development. There are numerous examples of this influence. Sex-based differences exist with respect to prescription and illicit drug uptake and response due to differences in metabolism, blood chemistry, and hormonal composition. For similar reasons, the effect of anesthetics varies according to sex. An individual's risk for myocardial infarction is greatly influenced by his or her levels of estrogen, which is a function of sex. In this way, research has confirmed both subtle and vast biological differences between and among the sexes, which has led to the realization that "every cell is sexed" (Institute of Medicine, 2001), affirming the importance of including sex variables in all types of health research.

While we often like to think of sex as biological and gender as social, both concepts are socially constructed and therefore subject to change over time. The ways we parse the categories *male, female, intersex,* and *other* are not biologically inherent but relative to place and time. Different cultures conceptualize sex variation in different ways, and our understandings of sex have changed over time (and continue to change) as biological variation is discovered and measurement techniques are refined. For example, procedures for assessing babies' sex at birth have evolved in recent years, particularly in the wake of the intersex movement that actively advocates for those whose reproductive or sexual anatomy is not clearly male or female, and can now include genetic and chromosomal reviews in addition to visual assessment of the genitals (Fausto-Sterling, 2000). Furthermore, in the space of a few decades, the treatment of intersex bodies has changed; assignment surgery at birth (where genitals and secondary sex characteristics are made to look male or female) is no longer widespread due to controversy over the physical, emotional, and sexual harm it can cause (Fausto-Sterling, 2000). Conceptualizing sex as a changing and fluid multidimensional construct ensures that these types of important biological variations are captured in research, ensuring that the needs of all individuals are considered. Comprehensive conceptualizations of sex are also essential for ensuring that more accurate and rigorous science gets carried out in order to identify the causes and importance of sex-related differences across the continuum (Clow et al., 2009).

Gender

Like sex, gender is a multidimensional construct that refers to the different roles, responsibilities, limitations, and experiences provided to individuals based on their presenting sex/gender. Gender builds on biological sex to give meaning to sex differences, categorizing individuals with labels such as *woman, man, transsexual,* and *hijra,*[1] among others. These categories are socially constructed, as humans both create and assign individuals to them. Thus, like sex, ideas about gender are also culturally and temporally specific and subject to change. Gender is often an amorphous concept. When we use the term in everyday conversation, it is not always clear what is being referred to. In what follows we describe approaches to conceptualizing gender: institutionalized gender, gender as constrained choice, gender roles, gender identity (including masculinities and femininities), gender relations, and gender as performance (embodied gender). We also discuss postgenderism as a means of thinking beyond the dyadic gender order. We recognize that there are other conceptualizations but offer these particular angles of vision to illustrate the ways that gender spans the micro to the macro and how conceptualizations vary in specificity and theoretical application.

INSTITUTIONALIZED GENDER

Gender is both produced and shaped by institutions such as the media, religion, and educational, medical, and other political and social systems, creating a societal gender structure that is deeply entrenched and rarely questioned, but hugely influential. Institutionalized gender refers to the ways that gender is rooted in and expressed through these large social systems, through the different responses, values, expectations, roles, and responsibilities given to individuals and groups according to gender (Johnson et al., 2007). For example, women are often paid less than men for similar work, and workplaces are often gendered, with certain departments and even entire occupations dominated by a particular gender. While gender is context-specific and subject to change, in almost every society in the world, men are more highly regarded than women and given greater power, access, money, opportunities, and presence in public life. The fact that these differences exist on such a large scale points to the embeddedness of institutionalized gender. Institutionalized gender also interacts with systems related to race, class, sexual identity, and other social constructs to further organize individuals and groups into hierarchies of privilege. Institutionalized gender is an important concept to consider in health research as it structures people's lives in ways that both permit and limit health by influencing, for example, experiences within and access to health care systems, resulting in different exposure risks and care received. Furthermore, vast differences

---

[1] *Hijra* is a South Asian term that refers to a third gender that is considered neither male nor female, although *hijra* are typically phenotypic men who wear female clothing (Reddy, 2005).

exist among the genders with respect to power and privilege within society, which affects health on a number of levels (e.g., financial stability is related to food security, safe neighborhoods, and good health care). For example, a Canadian study by Borkhoff et al. (2008) found that two times more men than women received total knee arthroplasty (TKA) despite similar levels of disability and symptoms. The authors' assertion that physicians consciously or unconsciously judge who is more likely to need and benefit from TKA based on presenting gender can be seen as an example of institutionalized gender as the findings indicate a systemic advantage associated with male gender (Borkhoff et al., 2008). Furthermore, Borkhoff et al. hypothesize that gender roles influence physician-patient interactions and that women's narrative speaking style is not as effective as men's factual and direct style when seeking help for injured knees. In both cases, gender biases affect health at the institutional level.

GENDER AS CONSTRAINED CHOICE

Bird and Rieker (2008) conceptualize gender as a series of constrained choices that impact health in complex ways. They contend that individuals make decisions about health within broader contexts of power and privilege where gender, in addition to other social determinants, affords varying levels of influence, control, access, and opportunity. So while individuals are likely aware of how to improve their health, structural factors such as time, money, and power can encourage or discourage healthy behavior (Bird & Rieker, 2008). Bird and Rieker's model of gender and health is unique in that it acknowledges the impact of both biological and social health influences and addresses how both intersect to produce health. Bird and Rieker argue that research on gender differences in health that focuses on biological processes needs to account for sociostructural constraints, while social research needs to acknowledge the ways that people's "choices" are mediated by biology. For example, women's role as caregiver can influence the amount of time they have to spend on health-promoting behaviors and activities (Bird & Rieker, 2008). Stress resulting from time constraints can affect and are affected by present cardiovascular and immune health, illustrating some of the interplay between sex and gender (Bird & Rieker, 2008). When investigating the impact of gender as a constrained choice, Bird and Rieker encourage asking the following questions: "Whose responsibility is health? Are protective measures, preventative behaviours, and the costs and consequences of poor health practices the province of individuals, families, the workplace, communities, states or some combination of these?" (p. 214). Viewing gender as a constrained choice therefore involves addressing the health restrictions that occur at many levels (individual, family, community, society) and acknowledging that healthy "choices" are limited by these overarching and intersecting constraints.

Andersson (2006; Andersson, Cockcroft, & Shea, 2008) uses a similar concept to constrained choice in his work on HIV/AIDS prevention in southern African countries, arguing that current prevention initiatives incorrectly assume that individuals are free to make "healthy choices." Andersson (2006) argues that promoting abstinence, condom use, microbicides, male circumcision, and the reduction of concurrent partnerships (all of which have been recommended in the literature) does not address the needs of individuals who are "choice disabled," or unable to use prevention tools as a result of power inequities. For example, individuals who are victims of sexual violence are unable to remain abstinent or insist on condom use, and health messages about limiting the number of sexual partners are rendered useless in the face of violence (Andersson, 2006). The notion of "choice disability" (Andersson, 2006) has applicability beyond the HIV/AIDS realm as many health behaviors and perceived health "choices" are in fact structured by contextual dynamics such as power, gender, socioeconomics, and so forth.

GENDER ROLES

Gender roles can be described as social norms, or rules and standards that dictate different interests, responsibilities, opportunities, limitations, and behaviors for men and women (Johnson et al., 2007; Mahalik et al., 2003). Gender roles structure the various "parts" that individuals play throughout their lives, impacting aspects of daily life from choice of clothing to occupation. Informally, by virtue of living in a social world, individuals learn the appropriate or expected behavior for their gender. While individuals can accept or resist traditional gender roles in their own presentation of self, gender roles are a powerful means of social organization that impact many aspects of society. For this reason, individuals inevitably internalize conventional and stereotypic gender roles, irrespective of their particular chosen gender, and develop their sense of gender in the face of strong messaging about the correct gender role for their perceived body. Gender roles shape and constrain individuals' experiences; men, women, and other genders are treated differently and have diverse life trajectories as a result of their ascribed role and the degree to which they conform.

Conventional, dualistic understandings of gender roles are problematic, inasmuch as they are not representative of the diversity that exists within and across populations. The embeddedness of dyadic gender roles in society also contributes to the discrimination of individuals who do not conform to these prescribed roles. Furthermore, the notion of gender as a role obfuscates the performative and distinctive nature of gender, instead suggesting a situated and static function (West & Zimmerman, 1987). Despite these issues, many scales have been developed to measure aspects of gender roles, the degree to which individuals take up these roles, and the effects of these roles on human health, well-being, and relationships (Bem, 1981; Eisler, Skidmore, & Ward, 1988; Mahalik et al., 2003; O'Neil, Helms, Gable, David, & Wrightsman, 1986). For example, Leech (2010) used data from the National Longitudinal Survey of Youth in the United States, which included a scale of attitudes toward traditional gender roles, and found that moderate gender role attitudes were associated with safer sex practices among sexually active young women. Leech theorizes that by having more fluid and egalitarian gender roles, young women challenge traditional conceptions of femininity, which promote subservience in sexual relationships, and instead bring greater awareness to their negotiations about safer sex. It is important to note that the more nuanced measure of gender used in this study enabled Leech to identify moderate gender role attitudes as a protective factor; Leech emphasizes that "scholars who remain interested in gender role orientations as an explanation for various social differences . . . should take particular care to measure the concept of gender role attitudes on a spectrum" (p. 442).

When considering the measurement of gender roles, it is also important to recognize that many measures are criticized for being "crude" or imprecise (Choi & Fuqua, 2003), and for a lack of reliability and validity (yielding inconsistent results across scales that purport to measure similar constructs) (Beere, 1990). Many scales also confuse the terms *sex* and *gender*, using them synonymously and thus incorrectly (e.g., the Bem Sex Role Inventory actually measures gender). Finally, recent research suggests that societal perceptions of appropriate feminine and masculine traits have changed in North America somewhat (Seem & Clark, 2006), which calls the accuracy of decades-old scales into question and highlights the temporal nature of socially constructed categories. Despite these issues, the prevalence of psychological research using gender role scales makes this aspect of gender one of the most frequently cited within the literature, although again, due to insufficient conceptualizations, the scales may actually measure phenomena other than gender roles.

GENDER IDENTITY

A great deal of feminist theorizing on gender identity is based on philosophical understandings of identity as reflexive self-relation (Butler, 2004; de Beauvoir, 1953/1974). Gender identity is similar to other social identities in that it relates to physical embodiment, and is mediated by people's relative location within their social environment and how they are judged by others, but ultimately is concerned with how people view themselves with respect to gender. Individuals' inner feelings impact how they present themselves as a man, a woman, or another gender. Gender identities develop within gendered societies, where the pressure to adopt the "correct" and "corresponding" gender according to presenting sex is strong.

Consequences exist for individuals who defy the gender order: In many parts of the world having an unclear gender presentation can result in discrimination, violence, and even death (Whittle, 2006).

Furthermore, even within societies where different and fluid gender presentations are more accepted, authors have discussed the uncomfortable evaluation that occurs when a person's gender is unclear and the seemingly human need to "sort" individuals according to the two-gender system (Namaste, 2009). Individuals thus internalize aspects of institutionalized gender and gender roles and negotiate their own gender identity in relation to the dyadic gender model. In this way, the conventional gender order is reinforced. The combined influence of internal feelings and social pressures guides gender identity development, impacting how individuals feel as gendered persons and constraining their behavior based on what they think and experience as acceptable for their given gender.

For example, Oliffe (2006), in his study of older men's experiences of androgen deprivation therapy (ADT) for advanced prostate cancer, found that the men's experiences of illness impacted the way they felt about themselves and their feelings of masculinity. After receiving ADT and experiencing subsequent body and mind changes, the men renegotiated their gender identities. While still constructed against hegemonic ideals of masculinity, the men's masculine selves were altered by physical, social, and sexual changes, which prevented them from "doing" their masculinity in conventional ways (Oliffe, 2006). Oliffe's study examines the socially constructed interpretation of men's physical changes as a result of ADT and therefore offers a unique means of approaching health issues where both sex and gender are at play. This example also demonstrates the interaction between sex and gender. Physiological sex affects social gender and vice versa, blurring the distinct categories that feminists fought so hard to separate and distinguish. While we discuss this in more depth later in the chapter, it is important to recognize here that sex and gender are dependent on each other for both meaning and the production of health. Because sex and gender interact to affect health status and generate health outcomes, research designs that are able to capture physiological and social measures are very useful. Furthermore, research that is able to theorize about the mechanisms behind sex and gender health interactions is particularly relevant.

MASCULINITY

Masculinity is a socially constructed component of gender that is typically associated with men and male characteristics, though this strict association has been problematized. Instead of associating masculinity with particular bodies, it is instead popularly theorized to be a range of behaviors, practices, and characteristics that can be taken up by anyone.

For example, Halberstam (1998) has made the case for female masculinity. Masculinity is therefore not a singular concept; multiple and conflicting masculinities have been identified that have varying degrees of power and that are born from different social contexts (Connell, 2005). For example, Connell (2005) has described the subordination of gay men by heterosexual men as a function of differing levels of power among the masculinities, with subordinate masculinities often conflated with femininity. Hegemonic masculinity is a particularly dominant form of masculinity, and while not static in any way, in most cultures it emphasizes strength, aggression, courage, independence, and virility (Connell & Messerschmidt, 2005). Hegemonic masculinity is also associated with heterosexual, White, middle-class status in Western cultures (Noble, 2004; Schippers, 2007). Masculinity is not stagnant and must be constantly maintained and reproduced through various gendered practices and behaviors. In this way, masculinity is best understood as a "floating signifier," given meaning by human-constructed language and the bodies that reproduce it (Schippers, 2007).

Masculinity can affect health. "Risky" health behaviors have been linked to hegemonic masculinity, as masculine individuals are encouraged to be strong in the face of illness, deny ill health or "weakness," and decline health services or interventions as a means of "being tough" (Connell & Messerschmidt, 2005; Lyons, 2009; Moynihan, 1998). As previously discussed, understandings and experiences of masculinity vary according to other social locations. In this way, Mullen, Watson, Swift, and Black (2007) note the emergence of multiple masculinities in their study of young men, masculinities, and alcohol consumption in Glasgow, Scotland. The authors discuss the ways in which different drinking cultures (e.g., mixed-sex clubs as opposed to traditional male-dominated pubs) and varying socioeconomic and educational backgrounds result in more flexible masculine roles and drinking behaviors for young men today, particularly when compared with the experiences of previous generations. For example, the young men's attitudes toward drinking tended to change with age, as their definitions of an enjoyable evening became affected by work responsibilities, finances, family obligations, and sports (Mullen et al., 2007). The authors contend that "we are witnessing a move away from the conventional hegemonic masculine role to a more pluralistic interpretation" (Mullen et al., 2007, p. 162). Health behaviors can thus be implicated in the construction and maintenance of the gender order.

FEMININITY

Like the connections often made between masculinity and maleness, femininity is often associated with femaleness, when it in fact is not inherently attached to any particular bodies and instead is constructed and reproduced through individuals' practices and behaviors in their everyday lives. While "emphasized femininity," along with multiple other overlapping femininities, has been described, these concepts are less developed than masculinities and require additional theoretical and empirical work (Connell & Messerschmidt, 2005; Schippers, 2007). While it has been suggested that no femininity is hegemonic, Connell (1987) offers the concept of "emphasized femininity" as a prioritized form of femininity, characterized by its domination by masculinity, which is a crucial component in men's supremacy over women in the gender order. In this way, all femininities are constructed as subordinate to masculinities (in particular hegemonic masculinity), and it is through this subordination that gender hegemony is created and maintained (Connell, 1987). It is important to note that while masculinity is prioritized as the "gold standard," both masculinity and femininity are constructed through their differences to each other. This is an important aspect of gender hegemony.

While femininity can affect health by encouraging individuals to take an interest in their health, it can also encourage feminine individuals to prioritize the health of children or other family members above their own, as part of a nurturing and caring ideal. Research has also demonstrated that high levels of masculinity but not femininity are associated with good mental health among adolescents, which is posited to be the result of many accumulated privileges associated with masculinity throughout the teenage years (Barrett & White, 2002). In finding that characteristics typically associated with boys and men improve the mental health of both sexes, interesting questions are raised about the way we value femininity in our society. In this way, scholars have problematized the positioning of femininity as "other," distinctly different from masculinity as opposed to a function of the gender system in its own right, both within society and reproduced in gender theorizing and research (Schippers, 2007). Research on femininities needs to interrogate the way in which femininities are oppressed and subjugated by masculinity.

GENDER RELATIONS

Gender operates relationally by influencing our expectations and understandings of others, and the ways in which we relate to and interact with them (Johnson et al., 2007). For example, within romantic relationships, ideas about who should initiate contact, pay for dinner, and drive on dates are all gendered. Gender relations describe the ways that relationships are guided by gendered expectations and understandings that can limit or expand our opportunities in various situations. In research, acknowledging the relational impact of gender is important in order to assess how health behaviors and relationships change in the presence of shifting gender dynamics. As Clow et al. (2009) contend, "Because gender is relational, we need to consider both the variety and hierarchy of gender roles and identities when we explore the links between gender and health" (p. 13).

In their study of couple interactions on women's tobacco reduction postpartum, Bottorff, Kalaw, et al. (2006) found that the gendered relationships between men and women affect women's rates of quit relapse. For example, when both partners smoke, women's tobacco reduction or cessation is often mediated by their partner's support or hindrance and strongly influenced by the social shame associated with women's smoking during pregnancy (Bottorff, Kalaw, et al., 2006). Furthermore, women's tobacco reduction during pregnancy and postpartum often offers their male partners an opportunity to reduce or quit smoking, which positions expectant and new fathers as uniquely primed to receive tobacco reduction or cessation messages (Bottorff, Oliffe, Kalaw, Carey, & Mróz, 2006). In light of these gendered findings, intervention efforts can consider the gendered roles of new parents when designing tobacco reduction or cessation programs, while also focusing on the health of the expectant and new mothers and fathers and not just the well-being of the fetus or infant (Bottorff, Kalaw, et al., 2006; Bottoff, Oliffe, et al., 2006).

GENDER AS PERFORMANCE (EMBODIED GENDER)

Gender has been theorized as a performance, constructed through the everyday practices of individuals (Butler, 1988; Lyons, 2009). Gender is manifested in the ways that individuals style their bodies and carry themselves, and also in how they speak and move (Butler, 1988, 2004). In this way, gender is not only produced by and on particular bodies but is also located within particular activities, behaviors, and practices. It is through the "stylized repetition" of these gendered practices (e.g., body gestures, mannerisms) that gender is performed (Butler, 1988, 2004). Furthermore, as Lyons (2009) explains, "Through engagement in these behaviours or practices, gender becomes accountable and assessed by others, and aspects of gendered identity become legitimated" (p. 395). Therefore, gender becomes embodied.

West and Zimmerman (1987, 2009) use the idea of gender performance in their highly regarded paper, "Doing Gender." West and Zimmerman's linguistic emphasis on the way gender is "done" underscores the conscious and unconscious production of gender in all social interactions and relationships. They also emphasize the accountability of gender within the dichotomous sex/gender system where individuals must perform gender if they wish to make themselves, and their actions, accountable. West and Zimmerman (1987) articulate that "actions are often designed with an eye to their accountability, that is, how they might look and how they might be characterized. The notion of accountability also encompasses those actions undertaken so that they are specifically unremarkable and thus not worthy of more than a passing remark, because they are seen to be in accord with culturally approved standards" (p. 136). While this may appear to make gender a solely personal and conscious endeavor, West and Zimmerman point out that gender is also implicated in all social relationships and at the institutional level, which enforces the production of gender. Everyone is therefore complicit in the maintenance of the gender order. Finally, "doing gender" reinforces essentialist arguments about differences between men and women, concealing the socially constructed nature of such differences and perpetuating the status quo subordination of women and femininities (West & Zimmerman, 1987, 2009). Using the concept of "doing gender" in research can direct attention to the ways in which health practices can be seen as forms of gender performance and the visceral enactment of gender hierarchies.

POSTGENDERISM

> Postgenderism confronts the limits of a social constructionist account of gender and sexuality, and proposes that the transcending of gender by social and political means is now being complemented and completed by technological means. (Hughes & Dvorsky, 2008, p. 2)

Some theorists argue that to address concerns with the conventional dyadic gender system, we need to move beyond it. The concept of postgenderism arose within feminist discussions of gender. Postgender perspectives typically advocate the dissolution of narrow and restricting gender roles as a means of emancipating women from patriarchy (Haraway, 1991). Postgenderism also posits that technologies, especially bio- and reproductive technologies, can erode strict binary gender roles to help create a postgender society (Haraway, 1991; Hughes & Dvorsky, 2008). The idea that technology has the potential to alter social norms and relationships is not new. For example, it is well established that the birth control pill contributed, in part, to White, middle-class North American women's liberation from the home and their increased participation in the workforce in the 1960s. Hughes and Dvorsky (2008) argue that "our contemporary efforts at creating gender-neutral societies have reached the limits of biological gender" (p. 13), and thus they discuss a range of technologies and medical advancements that have the potential to radically blur the distinctions between categories of gender, sex, and sexuality. The possibility of artificial wombs, parthenogenesis (a type of asexual reproduction that occurs in female animal and plant species where fertilization occurs without males), cloning, and same-sex reproduction are offered as examples of technologies that can change the way we reproduce and therefore classify human beings (Hughes & Dvorsky, 2008). Furthermore, surgeries that can create and modify genitals, electronic sex toys that connect participants via computer (teledildonics), and the psychopharmacological possibility of "de-gendering" the human brain using hormones all provide ways of thinking about a postgender world and highlight the breadth and variety of human gender, sex, and sexuality (Hughes & Dvorsky, 2008).

Postgenderism is often believed to offer a more egalitarian and just system, where individuals are not sexed at birth and instead are classified according to other means, for example, age, talents, and interests (Lorber, 2005). Postgender theories raise provocative questions about the role of gender and ethical concerns about the impact of technologies. If we are indeed able to (even in part) dismantle or move beyond the conventional gender order, does this mean gender will no longer impact human health? In research terms this question can also be raised with respect to measurement: Is it possible to independently measure all the aspects that contribute to gender differences in health (e.g., power, income, household responsibilities)? If so, can this fully account for the effects of gender? Or is there something about gender and gendered bodies, in whatever form they exist, that influences health?

Sexual Identity

Gender and sexual identity are often confounded within the literature, and for good reason. Matters of gender identity and sexual identity are closely linked. However, it is problematic to use these terms synonymously as there are important conceptual differences. Gender and sexual identity are different because people who hold a particular sexual identity (e.g., lesbian) can take on a range of gender identities.

The effects of sexual identity are all too commonly ignored or narrowly constructed in health research. Categorical limitations that are in part created by limited language and exacerbated by negative societal stereotypes diminish the sexual variation that exists within populations, which is reproduced within research. *Compulsive heterosexuality* (Rich, 1994) is a term that refers to heterosexuality as the default sexual orientation and as an organizing principle within societies that privileges and normalizes heterosexual relationships while discriminating against and discouraging all other sexual orientations and relationships. In health research, heterosexuality is usually the assumed default, which ignores the influence of sexual identity and the ways that sexual identity interacts with gender to produce unique health outcomes. Furthermore, Butler (1999) contends that heterosexual desire plays an important role in constructing masculinity and femininity as opposing genders. She argues that within dominant heterosexuality, the object of masculine desire is inherently feminine, while the object of feminine desire is inherently masculine (Butler, 1999). Hence, sexuality is linked to the construction of gender identity.

Matters of sexual identity force us to think about gender in new ways and have pushed the frontiers of queer/gender theory.

Implications for Research Design

The feminist sex/gender distinction has had unintended consequences. Underlying this conceptual dichotomy is the idea that sex is a fixed natural binary; sex is not seen as a process but as a self-evident fact. . . . [U]ntil gender scholars theorize sex as a social construction, notions of naturally binary sex will continue to act as a lodestone in our thinking and essentialist arguments will retain persuasive power. (Friedman, 2006, p. 1)

As the above quote describes, feminist theorizing about sex and gender has resulted in conceptualizations of singular "natural" binary categories. Unfortunately, the complexity of sex and gender is rarely captured in health research, where sex is typically measured using two categorical options and gender is neglected, limiting the scope and relevance of research results (Bird & Rieker, 2008; Hughes & Dvorsky, 2008). Recognizing that sex and gender are complex concepts, many elements of which exist on continua, influences the ways in which research is framed and organized. Relying on the male-female/masculine-feminine binary invariably homogenizes research participants and results, masking the variation that is inherent in populations. With growing calls for inclusivity and rigor in research, it is important to capture the variation within and across groups in order to study and account for these differences.

It is also important to acknowledge the ways that sex and gender, while distinct concepts, are inextricably linked and related. The social aspects of gender can map onto biology to create, maintain, or exacerbate physiological differences that are already established (Bird & Rieker, 2008). Sex and gender also mutually influence each other as feedback loops. For example, the incidence of melanoma is influenced by gendered bathing suit styles that expose different areas of the body, leading men to develop more trunk and midback lesions than women (Bulliard, Cox, & Semenciw, 1999; Pérez-Gómez et al., 2008). Sun exposure is further gendered by the different occupations and outdoor activities taken up by individuals, as well as by different clothing styles, gendered ideas about sunscreen use, and socioeconomic status that enables travel to sunny locations (Bulliard et al., 1999; Pérez-Gómez et al., 2008). This shapes who develops melanoma and where. These gender-specific factors are further compounded by both biological and gendered factors, as once melanoma has developed, the presence of estrogen is believed to affect the progression of the disease, while gendered dynamics related to body awareness, surveillance, and prioritizing health prompt individuals to seek medical attention differentially, which affects prognosis (Brady et al., 2000; Institute of Medicine, 2001; Pérez-Gómez et al., 2008). In this way, most health-related differences between men and women have both social and biological antecedents, confounding the distinction between sex and gender. This makes it challenging to distinguish whether sex or gender is at play and also complicates the search for the mechanisms that cause health differences. In research, it is important to acknowledge the conceptual differences between sex and gender, but also to recognize the ways that these concepts work in tandem to produce health.

When incorporating sex or gender into a research study, it is important to identify which specific aspects of these concepts are of interest. What is it about sex that is relevant to your particular topic? What relationship or aspects of gender are you interested in studying? Identifying the relevant aspects of sex and gender for a study is important as this will shape the measures and means of data collection as well as the types of analytic approaches used. In getting started, one might begin by considering the question: What sex- or gender-based mechanism influences the outcome of interest? Considering this question helps us to theorize about the relevant aspects of sex and gender that may be at play. These theoretical tenets or hypotheses lay the conceptual foundation for a study focused on sex and/or gender and health. For example, in considering sex and gender and health outcomes related to depression, one might ask if the different symptoms reported by men and women are related to biological factors (e.g., hormones) or social factors (e.g., hegemonic masculinities that influence the reporting of symptoms) or biases inherent in our measures of depression (e.g., a form of institutionalized gender). These are but three of many possible mechanisms that might account for observed difference. Again, the more precise we can be about the mechanisms, the better we will be able to capture these elements in our research design.

Bridging the Solitudes of Theory and Design

As has been emphasized in this chapter, the way we conceptualize sex and gender has implications for all elements of design including measurement. While this is addressed in Chapters 4 and 5, suffice it to say that underlying every measure of gender, and there are many measures, are particular conceptualizations. For example, the Bem Sex Role Inventory, a commonly used crude measure of gender, measures gender role perception and cannot ascertain elements of institutionalized gender or gender relations (Bem, 1981). Where researchers often fail in developing coherent research designs is in ensuring that the measures specified are in line with the broader conceptualization of gender being used in a study. Thus, theory and design often exist as two solitudes in research that are not adequately integrated or resolved. Incorrect or incomplete conceptualizations of sex and gender lead to insensitive and inaccurate analysis. A lack of sophisticated and precise methods and measures also contributes to poor research designs.

Bringing Sex, Gender, and Sexuality Together: The Body as a Contested Frontier

The human body is an important site of academic theorizing and scholarship. Many theorists have argued that the body serves as a metaphor for culture and society and, as such, that the body can and should be read as a text onto which societal norms and systems such as gender are inscribed (Howson, 2004; Hargreaves & Vertinsky, 2006; Shilling, 2005). Scholarship on the body raises provocative questions about the intersections and conceptualizations of gender, sex, and sexuality and interrogates assumptions about the connectedness of these categories. Trans- and intersex bodies in particular have disrupted strict and static categories of gender and sex, as these "uncategorizable" bodies highlight the limitations of current conceptualizations (Fausto-Sterling, 2000). For example, both the interpretation of sex differences with respect to endocrine function and the conception process in mammals are gendered narratives that reflect and reinforce different gender roles according to phenotypic sex (Martin, 1991). Because ideas of sex, sexuality, and gender can collide when it comes to the body, research that attempts to bridge the solitudes of theory and design is challenging. Theories of gender, sex, and sexuality constantly shift, making it difficult to implement theories in concrete ways. In this way, the body serves as a final frontier in sex and gender scholarship as it pushes us to think about sexed and gendered bodies and their distinctions and relationships differently.

It is important to note that while transgendered bodies can call our categories of sex and gender into question, they can also confirm and reinforce the conventional gender system in the way that transgendered bodies are judged and evaluated for sex reassignment surgery. Often transgendered individuals desiring surgery conform to strict heteronormative roles in order to legitimize their transition (Hughes & Dvorsky, 2008). In this way, the medical system restricts individuals' ability to make gender transitions that do not produce normative sexed and gendered bodies (Spade, 2006). For this reason, while most theorists appreciate that the medical system's recognition of gender variance has its benefits (e.g., access to safe treatments and surgeries, insurance coverage), they also acknowledge the ways in which this system reifies a dyadic and rigid view of gender and denigrates bodies that cannot be neatly organized into one of the two conventional gender categories: masculine male and feminine female

(Fausto-Sterling, 2000; Spade, 2006). Restricting the creation of "postgender" bodies therefore reinforces the conventional gender order.

Conclusion

Sex and gender are both important and mutually reinforcing concepts. The importance of these two concepts to issues of health cannot be overstated, which is why both need to be considered in health research. Improved theories about the relationships between gender, sex, and health are required in order to develop better methodologies. At the same time, methodologies and methods must keep up with theoretical progress; new and updated and improved methods for gender and health research are required.

References

Addis, M. E., & Cohane, G. H. (2005). Social scientific paradigms of masculinity and their implications for research and practice in men's mental health. *Journal of Clinical Psychology, 61*(6), 633–647.

Andersson, N. (2006). Prevention for those who have freedom of choice—or among the choice-disabled: Confronting equity in the AIDS epidemic. *AIDS Research and Therapy, 3*(1), 23.

Andersson, N., Cockcroft, A., & Shea, B. (2008). Gender-based violence and HIV: Relevance for HIV prevention in hyperendemic countries of southern Africa. *AIDS, 4,* S73–S86.

Barrett, A. E., & White, H. R. (2002). Trajectories of gender role orientations in adolescence and early adulthood: A prospective study of the mental health effects of masculinity and femininity. *Journal of Health and Social Behaviour, 43*(4), 451–468.

Beere, C. A. (1990). *Sex and gender issues: A handbook of tests and measures.* New York: Greenwood Press.

Bem, S. L. (1981). *Bem sex role inventory: Professional manual.* Palo Alto, CA: Consulting Psychologists Press.

Bird, C. E., & Rieker, P. P. (2008). *Gender and health: The effects of constrained choices and social policies.* Cambridge, UK: Cambridge University Press.

Borkhoff, C. M., Hawker, G. A., Kreder, H. J., Glazier, R. H., Mahomed, N. N., & Wright, J. G. (2008). The effect of patients' sex on physicians' recommendations for total knee arthroplasty. *Canadian Medical Association Journal, 178*(6), 681–687.

Bottorff, J. L., Kalaw, C., Johnson, J. L., Stewart, M., Greaves, L., & Carey, J. (2006). Couple dynamics during women's tobacco reduction in pregnancy and postpartum. *Nicotine & Tobacco Research, 8*(4), 499–509.

Bottorff, J. L., Oliffe, J., Kalaw, C., Carey, J., & Mróz, L. (2006). Men's constructions of smoking in the context of women's tobacco reduction during pregnancy and postpartum. *Social Science & Medicine, 62*(12), 3096–3108.

Brady, M. S., Oliveria, S. A., Christos, P. J., Berwick, M., Coit, D. G., Katz, J., et al. (2000). Patterns of detection in patients with cutaneous melanoma. *Cancer, 89*(2), 342–347.

Bulliard, J., Cox, B., & Semenciw, R. (1999). Trends by anatomic site in the incidence of cutaneous malignant melanoma in Canada, 1969–93. *Cancer Causes and Control, 10*(5), 407–416.

Butler, J. (1988). Performative acts and gender constitution: An essay in phenomenology and feminist theory. *Theatre Journal, 40*(4), 519–531.

Butler, J. (1999). *Gender trouble: Feminism and the subversion of identity.* London: Routledge.

Butler, J. (2004). *Undoing gender.* New York: Routledge.

Choi, N., & Fuqua, D. R. (2003). The structure of the Bem sex role inventory: A summary report of 23 validation studies. *Educational and Psychological Measurement, 63*(5), 872–887.

Clow, B., Pederson, A., Haworth-Brockman, M., & Bernier, J. (2009). *Rising to the challenge: Sex- and gender-based analysis for health planning, policy and research in Canada.* Halifax, NS, Canada: Atlantic Centre of Excellence for Women's Health.

Connell, R. (1987). *Gender and power.* Cambridge, UK: Polity Press.

Connell, R. (2005). *Masculinities* (2nd ed.). Berkeley: University of California Press.

Connell, R. W., & Messerschmidt, J. W. (2005). Hegemonic masculinity: Rethinking the concept. *Gender & Society, 19*(6), 829–859.

de Beauvoir, S. (1974). *The second sex* [Deuxième sexe]. New York: Vintage Books. (Original work published in 1953)

de la Chapelle, A. (1981). The etiology of maleness in XX men. *Human Genetics, 58*(1), 105–116.

Dworkin, S. L. (2005). Who is epidemiologically fathomable in the HIV/AIDS epidemic? Gender, sexuality, and intersectionality in public health. *Culture, Health & Sexuality, 7*(6), 615–623.

Eisler, R. M., Skidmore, J. R., & Ward, C. H. (1988). Masculine gender-role stress: Predictor of anger, anxiety, and health-risk behaviours. *Journal of Personality Assessment, 52*(1), 133–141.

Fausto-Sterling, A. (2000). The five sexes, revisited. *Sciences, 40*(4), 18.

Friedman, A. (2006). Unintended consequences of the feminist sex/gender distinction. *Genders Online Journal, 43.* Retrieved December 11, 2010, from http://www.genders.org/g43/g43_friedman.html

Halberstam, J. (1998). *Female masculinity.* Durham, NC: Duke University Press.

Haraway, D. J. (1991). *Simians, cyborgs, and women: The reinvention of nature.* New York: Routledge.

Hargreaves, J., & Vertinsky, P. A. (2006). *Physical culture, power, and the body.* Abingdon, Oxon, UK: Routledge.

Howson, A. (2004). *The body in society: An introduction.* Cambridge, UK: Polity.

Hughes, J., & Dvorsky, G. (2008). *Postgenderism: Beyond the gender binary.* IEET White Paper 3. Hartford, CT: Institute for Ethics and Emerging

Technologies. Retrieved December 11, 2010, from http://ieet.org/archive/IEET-03-PostGender.pdf

Institute of Medicine. (2001). Committee on understanding the biology of sex and gender differences. In T. M. Wizemann & M. Pardue (Eds.), *Exploring the biological contributions to human health: Does sex matter?* Washington, DC: National Academy Press.

Johnson, J. L., Greaves, L., & Repta, R. (2007). *Better science with sex and gender: A primer for health research.* Vancouver, BC, Canada: Women's Health Research Network.

Knaak, K. (2004). On the reconceptualizing of gender: Implications for research design. *Sociological Inquiry, 74*(3), 302–317.

Leech, T. G. J. (2010). Everything's better in moderation: Young women's gender role attitudes and risky sexual behaviour. *The Journal of Adolescent Health, 46*(5), 437–443.

Lorber, J. (1996). Beyond the binaries: Depolarizing the categories of sex, sexuality, and gender. *Sociological Inquiry, 66*(2), 143–160.

Lorber, J. (2005). *Breaking the bowls: Degendering and feminist change.* New York: Norton.

Lyons, A. C. (2009). Masculinities, femininities, behaviour and health. *Social and Personality Psychology Compass, 3*(4), 394–412.

Mahalik, J. R., Locke, B. D., Ludlow, L. H., Diemer, M. A., Scott, R. P. J., Gottfried, M., et al. (2003). Development of the conformity to masculine norms inventory. *Psychology of Men & Masculinity, 4*(1), 3–25.

Martin, E. (1991). The egg and the sperm: How science has constructed a romance based on stereotypical male-female. *Signs: Journal of Women in Culture & Society, 16*(3), 485.

McPhaul, M. J. (2002). Androgen receptor mutations and androgen insensitivity. *Molecular and Cellular Endocrinology, 198*(1–2), 61–67.

Moynihan, C. (1998). Theories in health care and research: Theories of masculinity. *British Medical Journal, 317*(7165), 1072–1075.

Mullen, K., Watson, J., Swift, J., & Black, D. (2007). Young men, masculinity and alcohol. *Drugs: Education, Prevention and Policy, 14*(2), 151–165.

Mykhalovskiy, E., & Weir, L. (2004). The problem of evidence-based medicine: Directions for social science. *Social Science & Medicine, 59*(5), 1059–1069.

Namaste, V. (2009). Undoing theory: The "transgender question" and the epistemic violence of Anglo-American feminist theory. *Hypatia, 24*(3), 11–32.

Noble, J. B. (2004). *Masculinities without men? Female masculinity in twentieth-century fictions.* Vancouver, BC, Canada: UBC Press.

Oliffe, J. (2006). Embodied masculinity and androgen deprivation therapy. *Sociology of Health & Illness, 28*(4), 410–432.

O'Neil, J., Helms, B., Gable, R., David, L., & Wrightsman, L. (1986). Gender-role conflict scale: College men's fear of femininity. *Sex Roles, 14*(5), 335–350.

Pérez-Gómez, B., Aragonés, N., Gustavsson, P., Lope, V., López-Abente, G., & Pollán, M. (2008). Do sex and site matter? Different age distribution in melanoma of the trunk among Swedish men and women. *British Journal of Dermatology, 158*(4), 766–772.

Reddy, G. (2005). *With respect to sex: Negotiating hijra identity in South India.* Chicago: University of Chicago Press.

Rich, A. C. (1994). *Blood, bread, and poetry: Selected prose, 1979–1985.* New York: Norton.

Schiebinger, L. L. (1999). *Has feminism changed science?* Cambridge, MA: Harvard University Press.

Schippers, M. (2007). Recovering the feminine other: Masculinity, femininity, and gender hegemony. *Theory and Society, 36*(1), 85–102.

Seem, S. R., & Clark, M. D. (2006). Healthy women, healthy men, and healthy adults: An evaluation of gender role stereotypes in the twenty-first century. *Sex Roles, 55*(3), 247–258.

Shilling, C. (2005). *The Body in Culture, Technology & Society.* London: SAGE Publications, Ltd.

Spade, D. (2006). Mutilating gender. In S. Stryker & S. Whittle (Eds.), *The transgender studies reader* (pp. 315–318). New York: Routledge.

West, C., & Zimmerman, D. H. (1987). Doing gender. *Gender & Society, 1*(2), 125–151.

West, C., & Zimmerman, D. H. (2009). Accounting for doing gender. *Gender & Society, 23*(1), 112–122.

Whittle, S. (2006). Foreword. In S. Stryker & S. Whittle (Eds.), *The transgender studies reader* (pp. xi–xvi). New York: Routledge.

Implications of Sex and Gender for Health Research

3

From Concepts to Study Design

Joy L. Johnson

Robin Repta

Shirin Kalyan

The importance of incorporating sex and gender in health research is well established (Annandale & Hunt, 1990; Bird & Rieker, 2008; Wizemann & Pardue, 2001; Lorber, 1996). This approach not only leads to better science by elucidating the specific mechanisms of health and disease but also provides evidence on which interventions can be improved and inequities corrected. The inclusion of sex and gender in research is therefore a matter of ethics, as to deny or overlook the impact of these health determinants can ultimately and dramatically affect the well-being of individuals and groups.

As was emphasized in the previous chapter, the way gender and sex are conceptualized has implications for how they will be operationalized and studied. The concepts of sex and gender must also be considered within broader frameworks that outline their relationship with other key concepts or variables. Sex and gender cannot be studied in a vacuum. All research studies are guided by explicit or implicit theoretical frameworks. Gender, for example, is highly contextual and shaped by other social locations. For example, the gendered experience of being a First Nations woman in

Canadian society can be very different for economically privileged women than for economically disadvantaged women. Social locations intersect with each other in powerful ways, and therefore, when designing studies, we must frequently supplement a gender perspective with additional determinants. Sex is a biological concept that also benefits from theoretical perspectives related to development, function, and understandings of biological systems.

From a design perspective, perhaps the most difficult challenge is to bring the biological and social realms *together* in designing studies that consider how sex and gender connect to create particular outcomes. Investigating the dual influences of sex and gender is important because of the mutually dependent and reinforcing nature of these concepts. Acknowledging the interplay between sex and gender is also key, as these concepts influence each other in important ways. In this chapter, we highlight the multifaceted nature of gender and sex, as well as the need for these concepts to be situated in broader social and biological contexts when incorporated into research plans. We discuss additional biological and social determinants of health that deserve attention in research studies, and we review some analytic considerations that arise when these concepts are included in research plans. We highlight the ways that *all* health determinants, including social and biological determinants, overlap and work together to produce health, acknowledging that this produces both conceptual and analytic challenges. We conclude the chapter by describing some promising models that facilitate the investigation of both biological and social influences in a single study, as a means of bridging the social and biological disciplines to move the field of gender and health forward. In this concluding section we highlight some of the ethical issues that arise when taking gender and sex into account in health research. We acknowledge that additional research is needed, particularly to develop more precise and sensitive measures and models for measuring both sex and gender. Finally, throughout the text, we use examples to illustrate both the effects of sex and gender on health and the ethical importance of including these concepts in health research, as attending to sex and gender influences not only produces better science but also improves the health of populations (Johnson, Greaves, & Repta, 2007).

Gender and Other Social Locations

THE CONTEXTUAL NATURE OF GENDER

It is important to acknowledge the contextual nature of gender when using this concept in health research. Gender does not operate in isolation but instead works together with other social variables to create unique health outcomes. Therefore, while studying the effects of gender on health is productive, consideration of other social determinants is also important. Factors such as ethnicity, social class, sexual identity, age, and culture intersect with gender to impact the distribution of health and illness within and across populations. Researchers need to consider these additional locations in order to fully elucidate the ways that social factors shape health outcomes to affect individuals and populations differently. These are important and necessary steps to thinking theoretically and empirically about the source of health inequities. Investigating the arrangement of social determinants in sex- and gender-focused health research can be viewed as a key to overcoming the methodological "impasses" that have blocked progress in studying gender in its social context (Annandale & Hunt, 1990; Kandrack, Grant, & Segall, 1991). To date, it has been difficult to merge the various frameworks that shape gender-focused research. Expanding our sex and gender perspective to include other social factors will not only move us forward conceptually and theoretically, but will better enable us to explain and address health issues and differences with tangible public health and policy consequences.

SOCIAL DETERMINANTS OF HEALTH

The social determinants of health exist alongside biological and health system determinants and highlight the propensity for health and disease to be patterned by race, class, gender, and other social influences. They emphasize the importance of meso- and macro-level resources and privileges in creating health and disease (e.g., access to health care, safe housing, and transportation) as opposed to the individual-level factors that often dominate biomedical and epidemiological research (e.g., hypertension, obesity) (Benoit & Shumka, 2009). Research frameworks that incorporate the social determinants of health therefore extend beyond health and disease models that focus on strictly biological causes and individual behaviors by directing attention to the ways that social, cultural, and environmental factors affect the health of individuals and communities. The number of social determinants and their descriptions differ according to various research and public health groups, but the following factors are generally perceived to be important: income, education, social status, education, employment, race, ethnicity, place, gender, and culture (Benoit & Shumka, 2009; World Health Organization Commission on Social Determinants of Health, 2008).

WHAT THE SOCIAL DETERMINANTS OFFER

Incorporating the social determinants of health into research frameworks immediately provides a more rigorous appraisal of the factors impacting gender and health and sets the stage for research to identify the specific mechanisms that create health differences and inequities within and across populations. For this reason, a theoretical framework that incorporates gender and other social determinants of health is not only a more rigorous and comprehensive research paradigm but also a promising means of addressing social factors and injustices. In studies of gender and health, additional social determinants can help researchers avoid homogenizing women and men by acknowledging the diversity inherent in each of these groups. As Courtenay (2000) cautions, by reporting research findings in ways that subscribe to binary conceptions of differences, or that report differences in stereotypic ways, we risk affirming the very social structures that we intend to critique. Adding social dimensions to research frameworks follows the growing calls in the literature and across disciplines to move beyond binary understandings of social determinants and to disrupt the static categories by which we organize research findings (Lorber, 1996). Below we highlight some important social dimensions to consider when conducting gender and health research. There are many other aspects of social location that can be examined, and therefore we acknowledge that this list is not exhaustive and that other social determinants of health will be important to consider, depending on the topic. Furthermore, it is important to recognize that certain dimensions might not be relevant for all studies; design choices about the inclusion of concepts always need to be shaped by the particular project at hand and the population being studied.

"RACE" AND ETHNICITY

The meaning of "race"[1] is culturally and historically specific, as physical differences are interpreted in various ways around the world. Currently in many places, including North America, "race" is a social identity that we attribute to ourselves and others, based on physical traits such as skin color, hair texture, and facial features. Ethnicity refers to a person's ancestral, cultural, religious, and linguistic background and is closely related to "race." These terms are often conflated. However, neither "race" nor ethnicity has a valid biological basis: Research has repeatedly shown that human race taxonomies are socially constructed and that observed physical and cultural differences between individuals do not necessarily translate to biological or genetic differences (Collins, 2004; Lee, 2009; Williams, 1997). Geographical origin can shape susceptibility to certain health conditions, due to genetic adaptations over time, but this should not be confused with "race" or given

---

[1]While we recognize that all social determinants are socially constructed, we use quotation marks around "race" to emphasize this point, as "race" is frequently mistaken as a biological construct and incorporated into research frameworks without acknowledgment of its social origin and consequence.

overriding importance as a health determinant. For example, research has shown that women of East Asian ancestry tend to metabolize estrogen more rapidly than women of European descent due to differences in the enzyme CYP3A4; rapid estrogen metabolism affects risk for breast cancer as well as the metabolism of prescription drugs (Lin, Anderson, Kantor, Ojemann, & Wilensky, 1999). The ways these types of findings are described are often problematic as the terminology used can reify racial categories instead of pointing to the genetic and geographical sources of difference. As Williams (2008) asserts, "It is not biologically plausible for genetic differences alone to play a major role in racial/ethnic differences in health. . . . Biology is not static but adapts over time to the conditions of the environment. Thus, for racial/ethnic groups living under different environmental conditions, inter-action between biology and socially determined exposures can lead to adaptations that may contribute to population differences in health" (p. S40). For this reason, it is important to focus on geography or genetics when researching biological sources of health discrepancies and not "race," as this masks the real source of difference.

Unfortunately, the use of "race" in research is rarely defined or operation-alized accurately (Lee, 2009). As Lee (2009) points out, "The very act of doing biomedical research relies on folk taxonomies of race and ethnicity that do not neatly and clearly dissect groups into distinct, mutually exclusive categories for analysis" (p. 1188). This raises questions about the use of static, self-evident racial categories in research and prompts the need for more nuanced measures. However, while complex and lacking biological relevance, "race" is still a central means of social classification with impor-tant consequences for income, education, power, and, relatedly, health (Collins, 2004; Krieger, 2000). "Race" intersects with gender to create health opportunities and disadvantages for certain groups of people. For example, "White" women have a higher incidence of breast cancer than "Black" women, but a lower mortality rate. Part of this discrepancy is due to the fact that "Black" women are more likely than "White" women to have advanced stages of cancer at the time of diagnosis, which has been posited to be the result of poorer socioeconomic status, a delay in seeking treatment, and bar-riers to accessing health care, specifically mammography screening (Bassett & Krieger, 1986; Bradley, Given, & Roberts, 2002; Lannin et al., 1998; Lin et al., 1999). These factors are the result of both gender and "racial" dynam-ics, whereby institutionalized racism, institutionalized gender, gender roles, and socioeconomic status account for differences that biological research cannot (Bassett & Krieger, 1986; Bradley et al., 2002; Lin et al., 1999).

PLACE

Place, or a person's environment, is an important health determinant that can shape the risks people face, the opportunities afforded to them, and the "cultural geography" of their lives (Gesler & Kearns, 2002). Space can be thought of as the reproduction of social relations within particular environments, and as fundamental to the maintenance of societal structures such as capitalism, and social hierarchies like "race" and gender. Space is therefore contingent on place and vice versa.

Spaces and places and the degree to which we feel comfortable within them are gendered; furthermore, the intersection of place and gender manifests to create new conditions and health effects, as opposed to layers of privilege or oppression. In this way, the gendering of space and the spatial arrangement of gender occur simultaneously and impact the way both gender and space exist in certain contexts. As Massey (1994) describes, "This gendering of space and place both reflects *and has effects back on* the ways in which gender is constructed and understood in the societies in which we live" (p. 186, emphasis in original). Place and gender together impact the production of health by shaping, for example, the ways that individuals interact with health care systems; the environments in which they work, live, and enjoy leisure time; and the cultural values to which they are exposed (Macintyre, Ellaway, & Cummins, 2002). A 2007 study by Shoveller, Johnson, Prkachin, and Patrick in a rural Canadian community showed that both place and gender constrain young people's decision making around sexual health. They found that a lack of public transit service and vehicle ownership produced an environment where sexual relationships would often form between older boys and younger girls as means of providing/accessing transportation in this rural area (Shoveller et al., 2007). The interactions between social determinants of health and place are not straightforward and can produce unexpected and important insights into the ways in which spatial and gendered health behaviors are located within and contingent upon social arrangements (e.g., power and privilege).

SOCIOECONOMIC STATUS AND SOCIAL CLASS

The concept of class references a social hierarchy where individuals are arranged according to economic factors and where power and authority are unevenly distributed, resulting in different amounts of control and influence between the higher and lower classes. Class is related to and used as a metaphor for social, cultural, and economic capital and identity. Social class is also related to socioeconomic status (SES), a complex comprisal of education, occupation, and income measures. SES and class form one of the best documented social determinants of health, as low SES and low class have been consistently correlated with poorer health, poorer health behaviors, and greater disease burden (Barbeau, Krieger, & Soobader, 2004; Friestad & Klepp, 2006; Lantz et al., 2001), although the measures used to document SES have been problematized (Annandale & Hunt, 1999; Braveman et al., 2005). For example, the health hazards associated with working-class positions can be missed when occupation is the sole measure of socioeconomic status or class, as many "blue collar" occupations are well paid. This also highlights the problematic conflation of SES and class. Therefore, while it is generally acknowledged that higher SES is associated with better physical and social environments and supports, and better resources and opportunities (Benoit & Shumka, 2009), studies investigating the specific mechanisms behind the SES-health gradient are ongoing and needed, particularly among heterogeneous subpopulations.

The class hierarchy is strongly gendered, as more women than men occupy the lower levels of the socioeconomic ladder and because within any socioeconomic rank, men's health concerns tend to take higher priority within families and communities than do women's. As Iyer, Sen, and Östlin (2008) explain, "Class-related barriers are differentiated by gender. Women tend to have poorer access to, and control over, resources within households, in communities, and in credit markets, and are tied to gendered divisions of labour that leave them with little time or opportunity for health seeking" (p. 18). These examples illustrate the importance of examining SES and class effects on health, and the ways that these concepts interact with gender to alter health outcomes.

AGE

Chronological age acts as a determinant of health by treating individuals differently according to their perceived or actual age. In this way, age acts not only as a signifier of years lived, but as a "relational system of oppression" (Carpenter, 2000, p. 50). The meaning of age, like all health determinants, is strongly shaped by other variables such as gender, ethnicity, and SES. For example, Kosiak, Sangl, and Correa-de-Araujo (2006) showed that health providers are more likely to dismiss older women's concerns as emotional rather than physical issues, and to believe that their conditions are a "normal" part of the aging process, therefore not requiring treatment. Their substandard treatment is attributed to their position as older, female citizens (Kosiak et al., 2006). Furthermore, the literature abounds with examples of young men engaging in "risky" activities and behaviors as a result of masculine ideals that emphasize invincibility, courage, and aggression (Kimmel, 2008). In this example, the intersection of age and gender impacts the health of young men and has been postulated as a contributing factor behind men's greater risk for vehicle accidents, workplace death, and suicide (Byrnes, Miller, & Schafer, 1999; Cleary, 2005; Cleary, Corbett, Galvin, & Wall, 2004). As with much health disparities research, there is a danger of emphasizing differences with respect to age, sex, "race," and so forth while neglecting between-group similarities and within-group differences. Researchers must take care to examine the effects of social variables while also acknowledging the heterogeneous nature of any age-group.

SEXUAL IDENTITY

Sexual identity impacts health in a myriad of ways, from affecting individuals' sexual contact with others to structuring their experiences with health care institutions, within families, and with respect to economic and social life events (Fish, 2006). Discrimination based on sexual identity is a marginalizing force that impacts health in addition to social and economic life and that works in concert with other social determinants to create unique circumstances and, relatedly, inimitable health issues. For example, DeHart (2008) found in her study of 173 lesbian women that perceptions of heterosexism and homophobia in breast health care settings influenced the amount of discussion women had with their health care providers, the care they received, and, for some women, their frequency of service use. DeHart also found that heterosexism and homophobia contributed to the women's breast health behaviors, including their use of both breast exams and complementary/alternative care options. DeHart's study emphasizes that social structures impact individuals' health as well as the need for culturally competent health care.

Sexual identity also operates in conjunction with other social determinants. For example, Hamilton and Armstrong (2009) found that gender, class, and sexual identity intersect to impact how and with whom individuals engage in sexual relationships and practices. Their study found that higher-class heterosexual college women's decision making around short-term sexual relationships (or "hookups") emerged from gendered class beliefs about the importance of higher education over romantic relationships for women and the emphasis placed on male heterosexual privilege and pleasure on college campuses (Hamilton & Armstrong, 2009). These examples illustrate how sexual identity is an important social determinant that affects opportunities for health.

SOCIAL DETERMINANTS AND RESEARCH FRAMEWORKS

The social determinants affect health by structuring and constraining the experiences, choices, and opportunities afforded to individuals (Schulz & Mullings, 2006). Social determinants overlap with one another and operate simultaneously, challenging us to consider the effects of many related factors in research. Choosing a research framework that specifically addresses the ways that multiple social locations manifest to produce privilege or inequity can help to inform the research process and elucidate important health determinants within the data.

Furthermore, incorporating the social determinants of health into research frameworks pushes researchers away from individualistic explanations of health patterns and toward understanding how social forces constrain the health of individuals and populations. This perspective is useful as social impacts can often be amended through public health and policy adjustments.

The Biology of Sex: Broader Biomedical Considerations

THE COMPLEXITY OF SEX

Incorporating sex as a variable in research is necessary as males and females are differentially regulated by endogenous and exogenous factors such that the study of one sex cannot be easily extrapolated to the other. While this basic fact is accepted within many disciplines today and has contributed to a burgeoning research interest in establishing biological sex differences, there are still many areas of study that require additional investigation to understand the mechanisms that produce sex differences. Also, the concept of sexual dimorphism continues to be a powerful framework for examining biological differences between males and females. Yet, research models that only compare differences between males and females obfuscate within- and across-sex variation, limiting the precision and applicability of research results. Health research that does not disaggregate data by sex denies researchers the ability to even start to analyze differences among their study population and limits the applicability of research results to other endeavors such as program, policy, and development.

As mentioned in the previous chapter, sex is a complex biological construct comprising anatomical, physiological, genetic, and hormonal features (Johnson et al., 2007). Sex also refers to sex-based differences at the cellular level, caused by chromosomal differences. Because sex is implicated in the entire human biological system, an understanding of the influence of sex must be complemented by understandings of body functions and systems, developmental processes, and cyclical variation.

DIMORPHISM AND DETERMINISM

The concept of sexual dimorphism is predicated on the belief that differences between sexes of the same species exist, and that these differences are phenotypically distinct. While commonly believed to be obvious at birth, represented by visible (or internal, nonvisible) sex organs and comprising two categories (male/female), sex is actually a complex and ambiguous concept, which also exists as a continuum and represents a range of diversity. In designing research studies, this ambiguity is often not considered. Sexual development is not predetermined at the time of conception. While testosterone and anti-Mullerian hormone (AMH), also called

Mullerian-inhibiting hormone (MIH), begin to guide sexual development at conception, the influence of these hormones does not cease and instead continues to affect sexual development throughout the life span (Jost, 1947). In humans, sexual differentiation is primarily influenced by chromosomal sex at fertilization.

However, while XX and XY are the typical chromosomal arrangements for women and men, respectively, combinations XO (no second chromosome), XXY, XYY, and XXX exist, along with XY women and XX males (see Table 3.1).

Sex differentiation involves more than hormones. In the 1990s, the testis determining factor (TDF) was identified as the sex-determining region Y (SRY) gene on the Y chromosome, which changed our analytic perspective. This perspective continues to evolve; we now know that changes in this gene account for only 15% of XY females (Hawkins, 1993) and 10% of XX males, where SRY is inadvertently "copied" onto the X chromosome (Boucekkine et al., 1994). A number of different genes involved in sex determination have been discovered (reviewed in Haqq & Donahoe, 1998; Rinn & Snyder, 2005), and not all of these sex-determining genes are found on the X and Y chromosomes; nor is their expression restricted to the gonads. This emphasizes the importance of studying the *entire* organism.

Given the variation and complexity of sex, it becomes evident that research frameworks that assume sexual dimorphism are wholly unrepresentative of the diversity that exists and overlook important variation in populations. Incorporating sex as a variable therefore requires an appreciation of the scope of sex and the avoidance of narrow definitions and

Table 3.1   Rare Human Sex-Reversed Conditions That Have Led to a Better Understanding of the Genetic Basis of Sex Determination

Genotype	Phenotype	Characterization
XX	Male	Normal male genitalia, no Mullerian structures, and small azoospermic testes
XY	Female	Pure gonadal dysgenesis with normal female genitalia and well-developed uterus
XXY, XYY, XO	Intersex	Ambiguous genitalia with the persistence of some Mullerian structures with the presence of ovarian and testicular tissue in gonads

conceptualizations. Furthermore, because sex differences develop over time and are multifactorial, researchers need to be cognizant of context when incorporating the influence of sex. Thus, above all, research should not use sex as a proxy for biological difference, unless accompanied by ample justi- fication and a specific analytical strategy. By using more precise measures of sex that are specific to the research topic at hand (e.g., body weight, lung capacity, hormone levels), researchers will be better positioned to identify the source of difference and investigate mechanistic intricacies.

FORM AND FUNCTION

In 2001, the Committee on Understanding the Biology of Sex and Gender Differences of the Institute of Medicine in the United States pub- lished a landmark report that documented, with compelling evidence, the importance of including sex as a variable in basic and clinical health research (Wizemann & Pardue, 2001). One of the key recommendations of the report was to examine and account for the source of cellular and biological material used in research (Wizemann & Pardue, 2001). In basic science research, the issue is not whether sex "matters," but whether research design can adequately capture how much it matters. A more help- ful question for scientists may be "How, when, and why does sex matter?" This question often cannot be answered unless we examine form and function with a systems perspective.

Given the contribution of genotypic sex to phenotypic development, it is not surprising that congruent body parts, tissues, and molecules that share a similar purpose actually diverge in form and function based on sex. Studies have confirmed that there are numerous differences between males and females. Sex-based differences in body fat composition and distribu- tion (Wells, 2007), foot anatomy (Zifchock, Davis, Hillstrom, & Song, 2006), bone architecture and strength (Hogler et al., 2008; Iuliano-Burns, Hopper, & Seeman, 2009; Nguyen et al., 2001), and brain size and organi- zation (Christakou et al., 2009; Gilmore et al., 2007) are examples of some well-characterized discrepancies in biological form and function.

Sex is a variable affected by many covariates. This means it is crucially important to take biological context into consideration when evaluating sex differences. Results derived from petri dishes warrant further investiga- tion at the cellular, molecular, or genetic level to ensure that contextual factors are accounted for. Furthermore, physiological functions must be studied in vivo. Sex difference in the drug- and hormone-metabolizing activity of liver enzymes may not be apparent as easily in a petri dish because many of the differences are embedded in the hormonal milieu of the male and female bodies. For example, the environmental endocrine disruptor bisphenol A (BPA) is metabolized and secreted from men's and women's bodies differently, such that higher serum levels are found in men

(Takeuchi & Tsutsumi, 2002). The mechanism leading to this sex difference would not be found by studying the enzyme UDP-glucuronosyltransferase, which modifies BPA for secretion, in isolation. By creating differential hormonal environments using ovariectomized female mice treated with testosterone, it became evident that UDP-glucuronosyltransferase expression is influenced by androgens (Takeuchi et al., 2006). Finally, as sex differences exist at every level of the human body and persist throughout the life course, it is necessary to conduct research at various points of the life cycle and to extend the research lens to issues and areas that are underresearched, all while acknowledging the range of "sex."

TAKING HORMONAL VARIATION INTO ACCOUNT

While it is now well accepted in the health literature that men and women experience health and illness differently, research has yet to redress the history of clinical health research that has focused primarily on men. The cyclical nature of the female reproductive system and its dynamic relationship with age complicate the study of sex-based factors in biological systems. However, failing to include sex-based differences in study design and analyses has critical consequences. For example, a male bias in drug efficacy and side effect research led to the withdrawal of 8 out of 10 prescription drugs from the U.S. market in 2005 specifically as a result of their ill effects in women (Simon, 2005). Given the divergent developmental and functional trajectories of male and female bodies, health research and clinical practice need to account for the effects of hormonal variation. Accounting for hormonal variation by measuring levels of estrogen, progesterone, and testosterone is important because it ensures that research more directly pinpoints the source of health differences.

Sex and Gender Together: Design Frontiers

As health researchers grapple with challenging discrepancies in health outcomes between men and women, it becomes clear that such discrepancies are the result of both biological and social influences. There is an urgent need for research frameworks to account for the ways that "sexed" biological factors (e.g., body size, weight, height, hormones) *and* "gendered" social dimensions (e.g., socioeconomic status, physical environment, "race") collectively influence health. In this way, health researchers are recognizing the importance of bridging disciplines, research paradigms, and methods to explain the persistence of health disparities. However, it is often difficult to find common ground between biomedical and social research paradigms as they are rooted in different epistemological and methodological traditions. For example, with respect to health disparities, biomedical researchers hold intrinsic biological differences at fault for creating differences between or across groups, whereas social science researchers point to societal conditions as the cause for inequitable health status (Bird & Rieker, 2008). Research that is able to address both biological mechanisms and social processes will be better equipped to deal with some of the perplexing questions arising in the field of gender, sex, and health. As Bird and Rieker (2008) emphasize, "Only through an interdisciplinary approach that brings together both social and biological research can we hope to shed light on how and why gender differences in health occur. Such knowledge will most certainly alter the way we think about health, which in turn will create a new realm of possibilities for intervention and change" (p. 5). We suggest a number of research designs below that hold great promise for the field of gender and sex studies as a means of incorporating both biomedical and social factors together in a single study.

ADDING GENDER TO STUDIES ON SEX

Accounting for the effects of gender in studies focused on biological sex requires an additional layer of design complexity and analysis but can greatly enhance the rigor of a study and can also help to contextualize "sexed" research findings. Figure 3.1 illustrates how biological processes defined by sex combine with gender to influence systemic outcomes that, in turn, reinforce subsequent downstream physiological events. Due to these relationships it is important to acknowledge the impact of gender in studies on sex by including social variables in research designs and analyses.

The complex integration of sex and gender in biological function is manifested in the cardiovascular system. The cardiovascular system and its sex-discrepant performance have challenged our experimental approach to understanding human health and disease. After spending a great deal of time and money studying heart disease and cardiovascular function almost exclusively in men, it has become evident that excluding a sex and gender analysis has resulted in costly oversights and significant gaps in knowledge (Simon, 2005).

Men have almost twice the total incidence of coronary heart disease morbidity and mortality of women (Lerner & Kannel, 1986). For a long time, these observed differences between the sexes were believed to be caused by gender-specific behavior and lifestyle choices, such as smoking, unhealthy diets, work stress, and greater exposure to hazards, and not biology. While "lifestyle" factors were shown to account for some of the discrepancy, subsequent research conducted that compensated for behavioral differences could not fully explain men's greater risk of developing coronary heart disease (Wingard, Suarez, & Barrett-Connor, 1983). Women's more favorable heart and vascular profile was subsequently attributed to the

Figure 3.1   Bidirectional Factors That Modulate the Effect of Sex and
Gender as Continuous Variables in Biological Processes

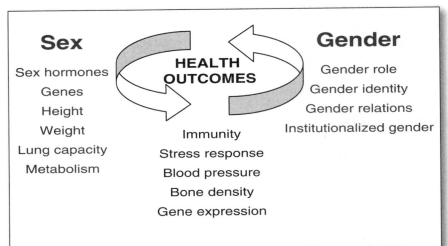

It is difficult to separate physiological processes (shown in the middle) as
being attributed to either sex (i.e., innate, built-in characteristics; shown
in on the left) or gender (i.e., social characteristics that shape exposure
and experience; shown on the right). For example, an individual's genes
are almost entirely attributed to an innate feature; however, we now
realize that regulation of gene expression is often a response to
exposure to both social conditioning (e.g., learning to fear something
would induce gene expression of stress-induced molecules in a
fear-conditioned person, but not in someone who has not been
conditioned to fear the same stimulus) and exogenous stimulants, and
the exposure and influence of these are shaped by both sex and gender.

protective effect of ovarian-sourced sex steroid hormones (estrogen and
progesterone) since postmenopausal women have an increased incidence
of cardiovascular disease (CVD) compared with age-matched premeno-
pausal women (Barrett-Connor, 1995). However, when the effect of
ovarian hormone therapy (estrogen with or without progestin) on a number of cardiovascular end points was tested in large randomized
placebo-controlled trials, the results were disappointing and perplexing.
Not only was there no beneficial effect on coronary artery disease, but
women in the active hormone treatment arm actually had a significant
increase in risk of stroke and thromboembolism (Grady, Hulley, &
Furberg, 1997; Hulley et al., 1998; Hulley & Grady, 2004).

By adding social variables to studies on CVD, researchers have identified lack of social support as an independent risk factor associated with
increased morbidity and mortality among CVD patients (Fischer Aggarwal,
Liao, & Mosca, 2008; Knox & Uvnäs-Moberg, 1998; Wang, Mittleman, &
Orth-Gomer, 2005). Additional research has suggested that the buffering

effect of social support is mediated through mechanisms associated with the release of oxytocin (Knox & Uvnäs-Moberg, 1998) and higher levels of physical activity and wine servings per week (Fischer Aggarwal et al., 2008), among other mechanisms. These findings are gendered, as women have been found to provide and use social support differently than men (Wang et al., 2005). These types of findings, made possible by the addition of psychosocial measures, lead to improved understandings of the mechanisms behind sex differences in CVD. In this way, adding measures of gender to studies on sex can provide a fuller picture of the risk factors and etiology of disease.

Figure 3.2 attempts to summarize the tenacious relationship between sex, biology, and health. The only certainty is that the equation that defines any health variable as a function of gender is unlikely to be a simple linear regression.

INTERSECTIONAL-TYPE ANALYSES

Intersectionality is a research framework that acknowledges a person's membership in multiple social groups and the equal importance and

Figure 3.2   An Attempt to Summarize the Relationship Between Sex, Gender, and Biological Research, Which Is Not a Simple Linear Regression

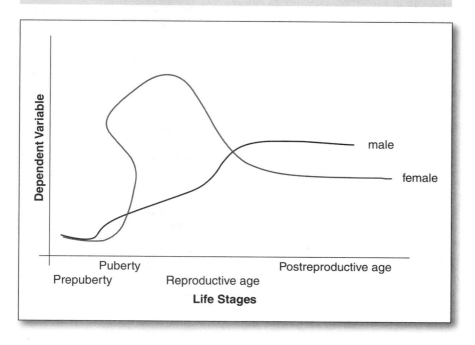

cumulative impact of all social identities in determining a person's life experiences, chances, and opportunities (Crenshaw, 1989, 1991; Hill Collins, 2000). Intersectionality therefore directs attention to the particular social location of individuals, which can be thought of as the intersection of their multiple social group memberships. This unique position therefore incorporates many contextual factors that contribute to health. In this way, while typically used in qualitative and social science research, an intersectional framework can also include biological health variables to provide a more complete picture of the factors that contribute to health in a study.

Intersectional frameworks can help to examine the intersection of biological and social hierarchies on health by highlighting the heterogeneity inherent in individuals and groups. This is achieved by positioning biological variables and social locations as the central focus of analysis, as opposed to single dimensions. Furthermore, with respect to research design, intersectional approaches to research avoid "analytic conflation" whereby categories or variables are assumed to be analogous, or alike in content or form (Dhamoon & Hankivsky, in press). Instead, intersectional frameworks focus on the experiences and patterns that are created at the intersection of multiple health determinants, based on the understanding that intersecting variables and categories create unique health circumstances that are more than the addition of multiple factors, experiences, or roles (Hankivsky & Christoffersen, 2008; Hankivsky & Cormier, 2009). Thus, the goal of intersectional research is not to isolate the effects of particular social locations or biological variables, but rather to illuminate the processes through which health is created and maintained (Schulz & Mullings, 2006). This is done by analyzing at least two categories or variables and acknowledging the interacting nature of these categories or variables, while also highlighting within-category diversity whenever possible. Intersectional studies assume a more inductive position than other types of research, where the categories of investigation are chosen, or at least confirmed, after the investigation has commenced and the relevance of different categories or variables can be appraised. This is a considerable shift from quantitative approaches where variables are chosen from the outset and assumed to always function similarly (e.g., "race" and class as heterogeneous as opposed to constant variables) (Hancock, 2007). Finally, an intersectional framework recognizes the "structure of constraint" within which people make choices about their health (Schulz & Mullings, 2006, p. 4), incorporating structural-level influences of health in analyses. This helps to specifically explore issues of power, and to acknowledge the societal forces that impact health and that are amenable to change.

Intersectionality is beneficial because it moves our attention past categories ("race," class, gender) and directs attention to the overarching context in which health behaviors and processes occur (Clow, Pederson, Haworth-Brockman, & Bernier, 2009). Because we can get lost in binaries of White/Black, rich/poor, and so on, intersectionality is also useful as a means of directing attention to social processes that necessarily move beyond binary descriptions. Progressive arguments and constructive theoretical discussions are taking place about how to incorporate intersectional-type analyses in biomedical research, with basic recommendations and research frameworks emerging from these discussions (Dhamoon & Hankivsky, in press; Dworkin, 2005; Hancock, 2007; Hankivsky et al., 2010; Kelly, 2009; McCall, 2005).

The concept of theoretical sensitivity provides useful insights into how an intersectional approach might be implemented. Theoretical sensitivity, first described by qualitative methodologists Strauss and Corbin (1990), is based on the recognition that researchers bring different degrees of sensitivity to data analysis and acknowledges subtleties in the meaning of data (Strauss & Corbin, 1990). Sensitivity to data grows with experience and by making use of relevant theoretical tenets, enabling researchers to be more aware of data meaning (Orland-Barak, 2002). In this way, thinking back and forth about social categories and the "layers" of an intersectional analysis enhances one's ability to be sensitive toward the data and to acknowledge multiple "layers" of meaning.

Similarly, reflexivity can be considered a useful methodological stance for researchers to adopt to recognize their own positionality. As Hankivsky et al. (2010) describe, "Even the most well-intentioned researchers often fail to recognize the extent to which any research project is a *process* of social construction in which discourses about categories and differences are both produced and reproduced in a way that often causes harm and undermines autonomy and empowerment of those who are vulnerable and marginalized" (p. 11). In this way, using an intersectional approach in research can direct attention to not only the socially constructed nature of categories and labels for participants, but also the positionality of researchers. This also encourages an awareness of the inevitable power dynamics that occur between researchers and the researched (Hankivsky et al., 2010).

The heavy emphasis on social experience and the complexity of theorizing around the historical and cultural aspects of experience can make it daunting for researchers from more biomedical backgrounds to use intersectionality. It can also be challenging to choose which factors to examine within an intersectional framework, particularly for researchers who are used to a hypothesis-testing research approach. Finally, the increasing focus on specific populations raises questions about sample size and saturation, warranting more specific discussion around the application of this theory in quantitative studies. Much more work is needed to provide concrete methodological guidance to researchers to enable the use of intersectional analyses in empirical studies of sex and gender and health.

MULTILEVEL AND SYSTEMS MODELING

Multilevel modeling approaches differ from single-level models in that they are able to investigate the effect of many variables on outcomes of interest, ensuring that the context of processes is accounted for. Multilevel models are therefore good analytic frameworks for the study of many layers of sex and gender as they can simultaneously analyze both individual-level and group-level factors that contribute to health and disease (Johnson et al., 2007). This ensures that contextual factors are included in analyses and provides a rigorous approach to studying sex and gender influences. In this way, multilevel models can provide a means of studying "cells within bodies," as various levels of genetic, cellular, and anatomical factors can be examined alongside social variables such as gender, socioeconomic status, and "race." This type of research will be better able to explain and address health disparities by including multiple "lenses" of sex and gender in single studies. For example, Subramanian, Chen, Rehkopf, Waterman, and Krieger (2005) used a multilevel model to study the simultaneous impact of neighborhood, age, "race," and gender on mortality rates in Massachusetts between 1989 and 1991. By nesting cross-tabulated individual characteristics (age, "race," gender) within census block groups and census tracts (two measures of neighborhood geography), the authors demonstrated that neighborhood heterogeneity is significantly related to morality and "race" in Massachusetts, and related to patterns of poverty at the census tract level (Subramanian et al., 2005). While these types of studies provide a framework for studying sex, gender, and other social variables within a single study, this type of analysis is novel within the field of gender and health. Additional work is needed to more fully develop this analytic approach.

GENE-ENVIRONMENT INTERACTION

Gene-environment, or epigenetic, studies investigate interactions between genetic factors and the environment, typically examining the ways in which environmental and other contextual factors influence gene expression without impacting genetic composition (McCarthy et al., 2009). This type of framework provides a useful model for studying the effects of gender and sex on human health in that it allows researchers to move beyond the nature/nurture debates about the cause of ill health to instead examine the interactions between biological, social, and environmental influences. Epigenetic studies demonstrate that environmental characteristics can add an additional, oftentimes overriding, amount of information to determine health. For example, raising the temperature of laboratory-strain fly embryos can change embryo eye color from red to white, despite identical underlying gene structure (ETH Zurich, 2009).

In this way, gene-environment studies typically observe the influence of environmental factors on phenotypic aspects of health.

Epigenetic research has shown that males and females can respond differently to environmental stimuli. For example, epigenetic research has determined that environmental factors such as early life experience, hormonal exposure, and trauma/injury not only impact gene expression but also contribute to sex differences in the brain (McCarthy et al., 2009). Variations in maternal grooming care among rats (mothers groom male rats more than females) during the early neonatal period are believed to epigenetically modify the DNA, creating effects on sexual behavior that last into adulthood (McCarthy et al., 2009). Also, research on depression in adolescence has found an association between girls and boys carrying the short 5-HTTLPR allele (polymorphism) and responses to environmental stress (Sjöberg et al., 2006). The authors found that boys are more likely to be negatively affected by living in public housing or with separated parents, whereas girls are negatively affected by traumatic family conflicts. Furthermore, the study found that only the girls carrying the polymorphism tended to develop depressive symptoms, which the authors explain as either the use of a gender-insensitive depression measure or a true sex difference related to 5-HTTLPR and hormonal interactions in females (Sjöberg et al., 2006). Establishing that associations exist between genes and environmental factors prepares for additional research to determine the underlying mechanisms behind the association. Gene-environment research frameworks are ideal for investigating sex and gender differences in health, as these types of frameworks acknowledge the inseparable nature of biological and social factors in determining health, and as such use dynamic statistical methods of assessing variance within populations. Overall, gene-environment studies provide a model for the inclusion of biological and social factors in research and are therefore a useful approach for studies focused on gender, sex, and health.

ETHICAL IMPLICATIONS OF DESIGN CONSIDERATIONS

At the beginning of the chapter we put forth the argument that incorporating sex and gender in health research is an ethical matter, in that attending to salient influences can lead to better health interventions and programs. Lawrence and Rieder (2007) remind us that to promote public health, it is necessary to understand the problems confronting different populations. They go on to claim that if public health is concerned with the reduction of social and health inequities, then it is unethical not to include sex and gender considerations in health research, policies, and practices.

As we develop new research approaches that account for gender and sex, there is a need to consider the unanticipated consequences that might arise from a focus on gender and sex. Epstein (2007) cautions that when we valorize certain categories we risk concealing others. He also suggests that we risk the problem of overgeneralization that can lead to sex or gender profiling. Research that focuses on difference can on occasion magnify differences that may not be meaningful or important. Thus, Epstein argues that the "inclusion and difference paradigm" does not adequately address health disparities. One strategy to mitigate these consequences is to remain committed to moving beyond describing differences by looking for ways to move research findings into practice and policy. Another strategy involves incorporating community perspectives in our research in order to ensure that our findings reflect community-relevant issues. It is also important to acknowledge that in some circumstances no relevant gender or sex influences exist, and to recognize that humans share a number of common features and experiences. We must continue to ask the question "What differences make a difference?"

Conclusion

Incorporating *both* sex and gender into research studies on health is challenging. We have discussed the importance of contextualizing our understandings of gender and sex and proposed some models for incorporating sex and gender in single studies. The models provided in this chapter are a promising means to begin moving beyond single-discipline studies of health, but we recognize that more work is needed to reconcile research methods with the theoretical developments that have been made in the field of sex and gender research. Better measures for both gender and sex are needed; measures of gender are needed to capture the inherent complexity of the concept, whereas the more developed measures of sex and gender need to move away from dualistic interpretations of biological or social difference. Comprehensive and valid research models are needed that combine social and biological health variables and the ways in which sex and gender affect each other reciprocally. To develop methods and the field more generally, partnerships need to be established between disciplines. Researchers need to work together to understand and appreciate the epistemological and methodological traditions of other disciplines. Funding bodies can aid in this regard by providing funds for multidisciplinary gender, sex, and health research; confirming their support of this field; and improving the financial climate for this type of research. Progress made with respect to gender, sex, and health research design and measurement techniques will raise new issues, answer questions, and improve our understandings of the impact of these determinants on health. The gender and health research enterprise is thus an exciting area, and an important focus of study. Research on the combined effects of sex and gender on health not only will advance the field of health research, but will help to improve the health and well-being of populations and individual men and women, and girls and boys. For these reasons, attention paid to analytic frameworks is not only good science but also a matter of ethics.

References

Annandale, E., & Hunt, K. (1990). Masculinity, femininity and sex: An exploration of their relative contribution to explaining gender differences in health. *Sociology of Health and Illness, 12*(1), 24–46.

Annandale, E., & Hunt, K. (Eds.). (1999). *Gender inequalities in health: Research at the crossroads.* Buckingham, UK: Open University Press.

Barbeau, E. M., Krieger, N., & Soobader, M. (2004). Working class matters: Socioeconomic disadvantage, race/ethnicity, gender, and smoking in NHIS 2000. *American Journal of Public Health, 94*(2), 269–278.

Barrett-Connor, E. (1995). Postmenopausal estrogen and heart disease. *Atherosclerosis, 118*(Suppl.), S7–S10.

Bassett, M. T., & Krieger, N. (1986). Social class and black-white differences in breast cancer survival. *American Journal of Public Health, 76*(12), 1400–1403.

Benoit, C., & Shumka, L. (2009). *Gendering the health determinants framework: Why girls' and women's health matters.* Vancouver, BC, Canada: Women's Health Research Network.

Bird, C. E., & Rieker, P. P. (2008). *Gender and health: The effects of constrained choices and social policies.* Cambridge, UK: Cambridge University Press.

Boucekkine, C., Toublanc, J. E., Abbas, N., Chaabouni, S., Ouahid, S., Semrouni, M., et al. (1994). Clinical and anatomical spectrum in XX sex reversed patients: Relationship to the presence of Y specific DNA-sequences. *Clinical Endocrinology, 40*(6), 733–742.

Bradley, C. J., Given, C. W., & Roberts, C. (2002). Race, socioeconomic status, and breast cancer treatment and survival. *Journal of the National Cancer Institute, 94*(7), 490–496.

Braveman, P. A., Cubbin, C., Egerter, S., Chideya, S., Marchi, K. S., Metzler, M., et al. (2005). Socioeconomic status in health research: One size does not fit all. *Journal of the American Medical Association, 294*(22), 2879–2888.

Byrnes, J. P., Miller, D. C., & Schafer, W. D. (1999). Gender differences in risk taking: A meta-analysis. *Psychological Bulletin, 125*(3), 367–383.

Carpenter, M. (2000). Reinforcing the pillars: Rethinking gender, social divisions and health. In E. Annandale & K. Hunt (Eds.), *Gender inequalities in health* (pp. 36–63). Buckingham, UK: Open University Press.

Christakou, A., Halari, R., Smith, A. B., Ifkovits, E., Brammer, M., & Rubia, K. (2009). Sex-dependent age modulation of frontostriatal and temporo-parietal activation during cognitive control. *NeuroImage, 48*(1), 223–236.

Cleary, A. (2005). Death rather than disclosure: Struggling to be a real man. *Irish Journal of Sociology, 14*(2), 155.

Cleary, A., Corbett, M., Galvin, M., & Wall, J. (2004). *Young men on the margins*. Dublin, Ireland: Katharine Howard Foundation.

Clow, B., Pederson, A., Haworth-Brockman, M., & Bernier, J. (2009). *Rising to the challenge: Sex- and gender-based analysis for health planning, policy and research in Canada*. Halifax, NS, Canada: Atlantic Centre for Excellence in Women's Health.

Collins, F. S. (2004). What we do and don't know about "race," "ethnicity," genetics and health at the dawn of the genome era. *Nature Genetics Supplement, 36*(11), S13–S15.

Courtenay, W. H. (2000). Constructions of masculinity and their influence on men's well-being: A theory of gender and health. *Social Science & Medicine (1982), 50*(10), 1385–1401.

Crenshaw, K. W. (1989). Demarginalizing the intersections of race and sex: A black feminist critique of antidiscrimination doctrine, feminist theory, and antiracist politics. *University of Chicago Legal Forum,* 139–167.

Crenshaw, K. W. (1991). Mapping the margins: Intersectionality, identity politics and violence against women of colour. *Stanford Law Review, 43*(6), 1241–1299.

Dales, R. E., Mehdizadeh, A., Aaron, S. D., Vandemheen, K. L., & Clinch, J. (2006). Sex differences in the clinical presentation and management of airflow obstruction. *European Respiratory Journal, 28*(2), 319–322.

DeHart, D. D. (2008). Breast health behavior among lesbians: The role of health beliefs, heterosexism, and homophobia. *Women & Health, 48*(4), 409–427.

Dhamoon, R., & Hankivsky, O. (in press). Why the theory and practice of intersectional-type approaches matters to health research and policy. In O. Hankivsky (Ed.), *Intersectionality and health research in Canada*. Vancouver, BC, Canada: UBC Press. It is due for release in May 2011.

Dworkin, S. L. (2005). Who is epidemiologically fathomable in the HIV/AIDS epidemic? Gender, sexuality, and intersectionality in public health. *Culture, Health & Sexuality, 7*(6), 615–623.

Epstein, S. (2007). *Inclusion: The politics of difference in medical research*. Chicago: University of Chicago Press.

ETH Zurich. (2009, April 13). Epigenetics: DNA isn't everything. *ScienceDaily*. Retrieved December 17, 2010, from http://www.sciencedaily.com/releases/2009/04/090412081315.htm

Fischer Aggarwal, B. A., Liao, M., & Mosca, L. (2008). Physical activity as a potential mechanism through which social support may reduce cardiovascular disease risk. *Journal of Cardiovascular Nursing, 23*(2), 90–96.

Fish, J. (2006). *Heterosexism in health and social care*. Houndmills, Basingstoke, Hampshire, UK: Palgrave Macmillan.

Friestad, C., & Klepp, K. (2006). Socioeconomic status and health behaviour patterns through adolescence: Results from a prospective cohort study in Norway. *The European Journal of Public Health, 16*(1), 41–47.

Gesler, W. M., & Kearns, R. A. (2002). *Cultureplacehealth*. London: Routledge.

Gilmore, J. H., Lin, W., Prastawa, M. W., Looney, C. B., Vetsa, Y. S., Knickmeyer, R. C., et al. (2007). Regional gray matter growth, sexual dimorphism, and cerebral asymmetry in the neonatal brain. *The Journal of Neuroscience, 27*(6), 1255–1260.

Grady, D., Hulley, S. B., & Furberg, C. (1997). Venous thromboembolic events associated with hormone replacement therapy. *Journal of the American Medical Association, 278*(6), 477.

Hamilton, L., & Armstrong, E. A. (2009). Gendered sexuality in young adulthood: Double binds and flawed options. *Gender & Society, 23*(5), 589–616.

Hancock, A. (2007). When multiplication doesn't equal quick addition: Examining intersectionality as a research paradigm. *Perspectives on Politics, 5*(1), 63.

Hankivsky, O., & Christoffersen, A. (2008). Intersectionality and the determinants of health: A Canadian perspective. *Critical Public Health, 18*(3), 271.

Hankivsky, O., & Cormier, R. (2009). *Intersectionality: Moving women's health research and policy forward.* Vancouver, BC, Canada: Women's Health Research Network.

Hankivsky, O., Reid, C., Cormier, R., Varcoe, C., Clark, N., Benoit, C., et al. (2010). Exploring the promises of intersectionality for advancing women's health research. *International Journal for Equity in Health, 9*(5), 1–15. doi:10.1186/1475-9276-9-5

Haqq, C. M., & Donahoe, P. K. (1998). Regulation of sexual dimorphism in mammals. *Physiological Reviews, 78*(1), 1–33.

Hawkins, J. R. (1993). Mutational analysis of SRY in XY females. *Human Mutation, 2*(5), 347–350.

Hill Collins, P. (1986). Learning from the outsider within: The sociological significance of Black feminist thought. *Social Problems, 33*(6), S14–S32.

Hill Collins, P. (2000). Gender, Black feminism, and Black political economy. *Annals of the American Academy of Political and Social Science, 568*, 41–53.

Hogler, W., Blimkie, C. J., Cowell, C. T., Inglis, D., Rauch, F., Kemp, A. F., et al. (2008). Sex-specific developmental changes in muscle size and bone geometry at the femoral shaft. *Bone, 42*(5), 982–989.

Holcomb, S. M., & Konigsberg, L. W. (1995). Statistical study of sexual dimorphism in the human fetal sciatic notch. *American Journal of Physical Anthropology, 97*(2), 113–125.

Hulley, S. B., & Grady, D. (2004). The WHI estrogen-alone trial: Do things look any better? *Journal of the American Medical Association, 291*(14), 1769–1771.

Hulley, S., Grady, D., Bush, T., Furberg, C., Herrington, D., Riggs, B., et al. (1998). Randomized trial of estrogen plus progestin for secondary prevention of coronary heart disease in postmenopausal women: Heart and Estrogen/Progestin Replacement Study (HERS) research group. *Journal of the American Medical Association, 280*(7), 605–613.

Iuliano-Burns, S., Hopper, J., & Seeman, E. (2009). The age of puberty determines sexual dimorphism in bone structure: A male/female co-twin control study. *The Journal of Clinical Endocrinology and Metabolism, 94*(5), 1638–1643.

Iyer, A., Sen, G., & Östlin, P. (2008). The intersections of gender and class in health status and health care. *Global Public Health: An International Journal for Research, Policy and Practice, 3*(Suppl. 1), 13–24.

Johnson, J. L., Greaves, L., & Repta, R. (2007). *Better science with sex and gender: A primer for health research.* Vancouver, BC, Canada: Women's Health Research Network.

Jost, A. (1947). Recherches sur la differenciation sexuelle de lembryon de lapin. *Archives d'Anatomie Microscopique et de Morphologie Experimentale, 36*(4), 151–315.

Kandrack, M., Grant, K. R., & Segall, A. (1991). Gender differences in health related behaviour: Some unanswered questions. *Social Science & Medicine, 32*(5), 579–590.

Kelly, U. A. (2009). Integrating intersectionality and biomedicine in health disparities research. *Advances in Nursing Science, 32*(2), E42–E56.

Kimmel, M. (2008). *Guyland: The perilous world where boys become men: Understanding the critical years between 16 and 26.* New York: HarperCollins.

Knox, S. S., & Uvnäs-Moberg, K. (1998). Social isolation and cardiovascular disease: An atherosclerotic pathway? *Psychoneuroendocrinology, 23*(8), 877–890.

Kosiak, B., Sangl, J., & Correa-de-Araujo, R. (2006). Quality of health care for older women: What do we know? *Women's Health Issues, 16*(2), 89–99.

Krieger, N. (2000). Refiguring "race": Epidemiology, racialized biology, and biological expressions of race relations. *International Journal of Health Services: Planning, Administration, Evaluation, 30*(1), 211–216.

Lannin, D. R., Mathews, H. F., Mitchell, J., Swanson, M. S., Swanson, F. H., & Edwards, M. S. (1998). Influence of socioeconomic and cultural factors on racial differences in late-stage presentation of breast cancer. *Journal of the American Medical Association, 279*(22), 1801–1807.

Lantz, P. M., Lynch, J. W., House, J. S., Lepkowski, J. M., Mero, R. P., Musick, M. A., et al. (2001). Socioeconomic disparities in health change in a longitudinal study of US adults: The role of health-risk behaviours. *Social Science & Medicine, 53*(1), 29–40.

Lawrence, K., & Rieder, A. (2007). Methodologic and ethical ramifications of sex and gender differences in public health research. *Gender Medicine, 4*(Suppl. B), S96–S105.

Lee, C. (2009). "Race" and "ethnicity" in biomedical research: How do scientists construct and explain differences in health? *Social Science & Medicine, 68*(6), 1183–1190.

Lerner, D. J., & Kannel, W. B. (1986). Patterns of coronary heart disease morbidity and mortality in the sexes: A 26-year follow-up of the Framingham population. *American Heart Journal, 111*(2), 383–390.

Lin, Y., Anderson, G., Kantor, E., Ojemann, L., & Wilensky, A. (1999). Differences in the urinary excretion of 6-beta-hydroxycortisol/cortisol between Asian and Caucasian women. *The Journal of Clinical Pharmacology, 39*(6), 578–582.

Lorber, J. (1996). Beyond the binaries: Depolarizing the categories of sex, sexuality, and gender. *Sociological Inquiry, 66*(2), 143–160.

Macintyre, S., Ellaway, A., & Cummins, S. (2002). Place effects on health: How can we conceptualise, operationalise and measure them? *Social Science & Medicine, 55*(1), 125–139.

Massey, D. B. (1994). *Space, place, and gender.* Minneapolis: University of Minnesota Press.

McCall, L. (2005). The complexity of intersectionality. *Journal of Women in Culture and Society, 30*(3), 1771–1800.

McCarthy, M. M., Auger, A. P., Bale, T. L., de Vries, G. J., Dunn, G. A., Forger, N. G., et al. (2009). The epigenetics of sex differences in the brain. *Journal of Neuroscience, 29*(41), 12815–12823.

Mollerup, S., Ryberg, D., Hewer, A., Phillips, D. H., & Haugen, A. (1999). Sex differences in lung CYP1A1 expression and DNA adduct levels among lung cancer patients. *Cancer Research, 59*(14), 3317–3320.

Nguyen, T. V., Maynard, L. M., Towne, B., Roche, A. F., Wisemandle, W., Li, J., et al. (2001). Sex differences in bone mass acquisition during growth: The Fels longitudinal study. *Journal of Clinical Densitometry: The Official Journal of the International Society for Clinical Densitometry, 4*(2), 147–157.

Orland-Barak, L. (2002). The theoretical sensitivity of the researcher: Reflections on a complex construct. *Reflective Practice: International and Multidisciplinary Perspectives, 3*(3), 263.

Rinn, J. L., & Snyder, M. (2005). Sexual dimorphism in mammalian gene expression. *Trends in Genetics: TIG, 21*(5), 298–305.

Schulz, A. J., & Mullings, L. (2006). *Gender, race, class, and health: Intersectional approaches.* San Francisco: Jossey-Bass.

Shoveller, J., Johnson, J., Prkachin, K., & Patrick, D. (2007). "Around here, they roll up the sidewalks at night": A qualitative study of youth living in a rural Canadian community. *Health & Place, 13*(4), 826–838.

Simon, V. (2005). Wanted: Women in clinical trials. *Science, 308*(5728), 1517.

Sjöberg, R. L., Nilsson, K. W., Nordquist, N., Öhrvik, J., Leppert, J., Lindström, L., et al. (2006). Development of depression: Sex and the interaction between environment and a promoter polymorphism of the serotonin transporter gene. *The International Journal of Neuropsychopharmacology, 9*(4), 443.

Strauss, A. L., & Corbin, J. M. (1990). *Basics of qualitative research: Grounded theory procedures and techniques.* Newbury Park, CA: SAGE.

Subramanian, S. V., Chen, J. T., Rehkopf, D. H., Waterman, P. D., & Krieger, N. (2005). Racial disparities in context: A multilevel analysis of neighborhood variations in poverty and excess mortality among black populations in Massachusetts. *American Journal of Public Health, 95*(2), 260–265.

Takeuchi, T., & Tsutsumi, O. (2002). Serum bisphenol A concentrations showed gender differences, possibly linked to androgen levels. *Biochemical and Biophysical Research Communications, 291*(1), 76–78.

Takeuchi, T., Tsutsumi, O., Ikezuki, Y., Kamei, Y., Osuga, Y., Fujiwara, T., et al. (2006). Elevated serum bisphenol A levels under hyperandrogenic conditions may be caused by decreased UDP-glucuronosyltransferase activity. *Endocrine Journal, 53*(4), 485–491.

Wang, H., Mittleman, M. A., & Orth-Gomer, K. (2005). Influence of social support on progression of coronary artery disease in women. *Social Science & Medicine, 60*(3), 599–607.

Wells, J. C. (2007). Sexual dimorphism of body composition. *Best Practice & Research: Clinical Endocrinology & Metabolism, 21*(3), 415–430.

Williams, D. R. (1997). Race and health: Basic questions, emerging directions. *Annals of Epidemiology, 7*(5), 322–333.

Williams, D. R. (2008). Racial/ethnic variations in women's health: The social embeddedness of health. *American Journal of Public Health, 98*(Suppl. 1), S38–S47.

Wingard, D. L., Suarez, L., & Barrett-Connor, E. (1983). The sex differential in mortality from all causes and ischemic heart disease. *American Journal of Epidemiology, 117*(2), 165–172.

Wizemann, T. M., & Pardue, M. (Eds.). (2001). *Exploring the biological contributions to human health: Does sex matter?* Washington, DC: National Academy Press.

World Health Organization Commission on Social Determinants of Health. (2008). *Closing the gap in a generation: Health equity through action on the social determinants of health: Commission on social determinants of health final report: Executive summary.* Geneva, Switzerland: Author.

Zifchock, R. A., Davis, I., Hillstrom, H., & Song, J. (2006). The effect of gender, age, and lateral dominance on arch height and arch stiffness. *Foot & Ankle International/American Orthopaedic Foot and Ankle Society [and] Swiss Foot and Ankle Society, 27*(5), 367–372.

Approaches to the Measurement of Gender

Pamela A. Ratner

Richard G. Sawatzky

A re there gender differences in the likelihood of being admitted to an intensive care unit following a stroke (Saposnik et al., 2008)? Is gender associated with the percentage of daily caloric intake that rural adolescents consume from snacking (Townsend, 2002)? Are there "gender differences in . . . long-term outcomes [mortality] after acute NSTEMI [non-ST-elevation myocardial infarction]" (Heer et al., 2006, p. 160)? Do "demography, intellectual background, parental environment, and parental education and employment" predict "a person's gender role orientation" (Judge & Livingston, 2008, p. 995)? Do observed gender disparities in prevalence rates of depressive symptoms "actually reflect higher rates of depressive disorders among women, [and] a greater tendency of women to express their feelings, or [are they] simply an artifact of measurement procedures" (Stommel et al., 1993, p. 240)? Is impulsivity "associated with health-risk behaviours in the same ways for men and women" (Stoltenberg, Batien, & Birgenheir, 2008, p. 252)? Have the "perceptions of the gender associations of instrumentality and expressiveness" as measured with the Bem Sex Role Inventory (Bem, 1974) changed as gender roles have changed (Colley, Mulhern, Maltby, & Wood, 2009, p. 384)?

The researchers who addressed these questions have all studied aspects of gender. At first blush, several if not all of these questions appear to be similar in nature. Yet, each study cited in this introduction applied a different model to address the question of interest. It is noteworthy that the authors were not explicit in their conceptualizations of gender. For the most part, we have interpreted their work as being related to social, rather than biological, processes and hence related to gender, rather than sex. In some instances, however, the examples provided may be related to both sex and gender. The distinction is important but often obscured because of a lack of explicit theoretical proposition and the interchangeable use of the terms *gender* and *sex* by many researchers. This observation is highly relevant because the measures typically employed (how the concept is operationalized) are identical (e.g., self-reported female or male) for two very different concepts (sex and gender). The concept can only be defined, as a result, by its theoretical context.

In this chapter, we seek to clarify what is meant when we discuss approaches to the measurement of gender. Implicit in this discussion is the notion that, in addition to the need for precise, unequivocal, and unambiguous definitions of the phenomenon or characteristic we are interested in, we must consider how the measure is embedded within the research design. That is, we must consider the models that embed notions of gender. Measurement is commonly defined as "the assignment of numerals to objects or events according to rules" (Stevens, 1946, p. 677), although it also has been said, more expansively, to be "a process by which an attempt is made to understand the nature of a variable" (De Ayala, 2009, p. 1). Bridgman (1927) argued that "the proper definition of a concept is not in terms of its properties but in terms of actual operations" (p. 37). It is in the latter sense that we are most interested. We must understand the types of explanation pursued, and the strengths and limitations of the various models used to provide such explanation. Some readers might question whether we have conflated conceptualization (the process of defining concepts and specifying how they are related) and operationalization (moving from the abstract to the empirical level). We are of the opinion that these two considerations are inextricably linked such that there must be correspondence between a set of measures and the relations between them (Suppes & Zinnes, 1963). Before we further discuss models that contain constructs or concepts and their measures, we offer some definitions. We define a *measure* as an observable form of data obtained through interview, self-report, or direct observation that is quantified through a set of rules and that serves as an "empirical analog" (Stine, 1989, p. 152) of a construct or concept, which is an unobservable, abstract notion or phenomenon that holds some theoretical interest or purpose (Viswanathan, 2005).

Some may argue that there is a vast difference between addressing the measurement of well-defined concepts or constructs and the measurement of associations or relationships among those concepts or constructs. Blalock (1986), however, aptly argued that, especially in the presence of multiple factors (e.g., complex social contexts), concepts are defined in ways that permit notions of causality to slip "into the picture via the back door" (p. 21). That is, causal assumptions, or claims about causes or effects, may be embedded in the definitions themselves. For example, if gender, as a social process, is the focus of a study, then an implicit assumption is that there are social variables that produce it (cause it). Conversely, if the male/female indicator is intended to represent sex, then the variables that produce it, although not necessarily specified in a model, include such things as hormones, genitalia, chromosomes, and so forth. In our case, gender may be defined by some antecedents such as socialization practices or societal norms and by its outcomes, such as behavior, attitudes, roles, or health outcomes. All this is to say that theory and measurement are inextricably linked and that all measurement is theory laden.

We intend to make explicit some of the sorts of models that researchers specify either formally or otherwise as they apply their measures and undertake their analyses of gender. In the examples provided at the beginning of this chapter, the researchers putatively measured gender-related or -specific rates, differences, associations, consequences, and antecedents, and the effects of gender on other measures, as well as having attempted to measure gender itself (i.e., gender can be measured directly and independently of other concepts or constructs). We explore each model, in turn, as we elicit some sharp distinctions. We examine these attempts at measurement, with gender implicated, to highlight the various substantive influences of gender, including its differences or impacts, its effects on the measurement of other concepts as artifact or bias, and the combination of these influences such that differences and associations can be minimized or exaggerated by sensitivity to such artifacts. We explore models of the antecedents and outcomes of gender, the effects of gender on other associations, and finally gender itself: gender qua gender.

Before we proceed, however, we acknowledge the discomfort that arises when notions of causality are presented. Readers will very likely have been influenced by the philosophy of David Hume (1739/2003, 1748/2007), who argued that we have no logical means by which to establish or prove that relationships are causal in nature. We take the philosophical stance that causality is only one of many possible explanations of the associations or relationships that we observe. The data researchers collect may correspond with a causal explanation, yet their findings cannot confirm or prove a causal inference because there will be alternative explanations or competing models that also will be consistent with their data (Lanes, 1988). Consequently, the goal of science is to develop and test alternative or competing models to explain the associations that we observe and to attempt to reject or refute some of those models; the establishment of causality is illusory (Popper, 1959/1992). Illusory as it may be, we are not arguing that we can never make causal claims. Surely we can, but only when all other explanations (noncausal) have been postulated and refuted or rejected. It is in this spirit that we present the following models as examples that researchers have specified in their quest to understand gender and health. The models that we pose are offered as a means of articulating their limitations and some competing explanations. We have not intended to offer specific criticisms of the published works; indeed, some of the models that we have drawn from these works have been inferred, were not necessarily the primary interest of the researchers, and may not incorporate all elements of the researchers' study designs. Our intention is to draw attention to the analytical models that ostensibly address similar questions about gender and that, upon further examination, are found to have fundamentally different theoretical meanings and implications.

Gender Effects or Consequences

Perhaps the simplest model that researchers have applied is that which specifies the health effects or outcomes of gender. These are typically expressed in two ways: (a) as differences in the health status or outcomes of the genders and (b) as associations or correlations between gender and health outcomes. In these models, the researcher aims to demonstrate whether the probability of an event, or the quantity of a variable, depends on the quantity of another variable—in this case, gender. We have expressed these hypothesized structures or models in schematic diagrams, which have, by convention, become useful means of portraying relationships assumed to hold among the variables of interest (Byrne, 2006).

As an example, Saposnik et al. (2008) explored whether there was a gender difference in Canadian men's and women's likelihood of being admitted to an intensive care unit (ICU) following a stroke (they studied 26,676 patients, in 606 Canadian hospitals, in 2003–2004). Their model can be represented as shown in Figure 4.1. This type of analysis is typically presented as a cross-tabulation of gender with another categorical variable. Rarely is this analysis recognized as a direct effects model. The idea is that the measurement or classification of *gender* can have a symbol or value assigned to it, at a given time, and that the symbol or numeric value will vary across individuals; that is, people can be differentiated by the symbol or value assigned to them (e.g., in the Saposnik et al., 2008, case, *man* or *woman*). Further, a second variable, *ICU admission following stroke*, which has the attributes "yes, admitted" and "no, not admitted" (measured categorically), is shown to be an effect or outcome of gender. The researchers concluded that gender was associated with the probability of the event of interest, admission to an ICU, because relatively more men than women were admitted after a stroke. They reported that 16.2% of Canadian men with strokes and 14.0% of Canadian women with strokes, under the age of 80 years, were admitted to ICUs and that, similarly, 9.4% of Canadian men versus 6.5% of Canadian women over the age of 80 years were admitted. These differences were observed although the men and women in the sample did not differ in terms of their comorbidities (additional disorders), medical complications, or stroke fatality rates (the proportion of patients that died).

Whereas the previous study compared two categorical variables, gender also has been studied in relation to continuous variables as is shown in this second example of a simple gender effects model. In this example, Townsend (2002) explored an association between gender and a health behavior (measured on a continuum). She reported that a small part of the variance in the percentage of total calories that rural adolescents consume from eating snacks (foods eaten between meals) can be explained by gender (see Figure 4.2). Girls were noted to consume a "significantly higher percent[age] of calories from snacks even though . . . [boys] consumed significantly more total daily calories" (Townsend, 2002, p. 137).

How was the gender of the study participants determined in these two instances? Both studies relied on a simple binary categorical variable, where individuals were mutually exclusively coded as being "female" or "male"; in the Saposnik et al. (2008) study the data were obtained from a national database of patients' hospital discharge information. Typically, patients' gender is assigned by a clerk's or nurse's "reading" of a person's gender. In Townsend's (2002) study, it is not apparent how gender was

Figure 4.1   A Schematic Diagram of a Direct Effect of Gender: A Gender Difference

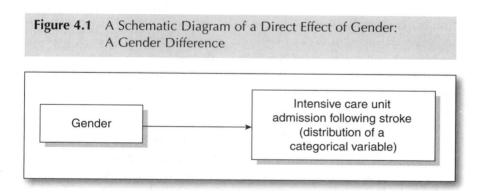

Figure 4.2   A Schematic Diagram of a Direct Effect of Gender: A Gender Association

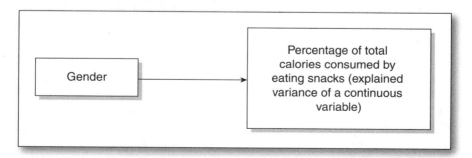

determined; the participating students may have completed a questionnaire and self-reported their gender, their teachers may have "assigned"
gender, or the researcher, in an interview, may have "read" the students'
genders. Additionally, although not explicit in the study reports, notions
of gender are embedded in the associations or relationships studied. In the
first instance, Saposnik et al. may have hypothesized that gender is a social
construction that ascribes qualities and value to people and creates
inequalities, including the unequal distribution of social resources and
unequal treatment in health care. Townsend, on the other hand, took a
psychological approach, and may have hypothesized that gender manifests
its properties in specific behavior and forms of coping with vulnerabilities
and social circumstances, or that it results from socialization processes
(Bird & Rieker, 2008; Geiger, 2006).

Are there other explanations of the associations observed in these two
studies? Is gender associated with or causally linked to health service access
and to diet? Or are these simple, direct effect models inadequate? One
ever-present alternative explanation of an observed association is chance
or random error. Unless one is studying every member of an entire population, there is always the possibility that sampling variability will produce
results that are imprecise or inaccurate. This possibility can never be
eliminated entirely. Another alternative explanation to a causal explanation is bias; that is, there is some type of systematic error that resulted in
incorrect estimates of the associations. Various sources of error or bias can
be present and range from researchers' decisions about who should be
included in their studies, to participants not completing all aspects of a
study and thus not contributing full information, to the introduction of
errors in measurement or classification, broadly defined, such that participants do not respond in comparable manners or entirely honestly or
researchers use inappropriate measurement tools or methods of classification. Study designs can be strengthened to avoid or minimize some of
these sources of bias, but nonetheless, bias should always be considered as
a possible alternative explanation (Fletcher & Fletcher, 2005). Given that
chance and bias are always possibilities, skepticism is a recommended
stance at least until an association appears consistently in publication after
publication and in sample after sample (Taveggia, 1974).

A third and particularly relevant alternative explanation for a model is
confounding. In this case, the research finding may be due to the influence
of another, unstudied factor. In some cases, an association arises because
of the influence of another variable, what statisticians often refer to as a
"lurking variable" (Moore, McCabe, & Craig, 2009). Confounding is present when the effects of the study variable (gender) and the lurking variable
cannot be distinguished from each other. For example, is it possible that
the men and women in Saposnik et al.'s (2008) study differed on the basis
of socioeconomic status (SES) and that SES was also associated with ICU

admission? When variables are interrelated, we may not be able to make reasonable inferences about causation. In the presence of confounding, we cannot distinguish the influence of the variables (e.g., gender and SES), we cannot determine how strong the influence of gender may be if there is an effect (the relationship is partially confounded), and indeed, we cannot determine whether gender has an effect at all (the relationship is completely confounded).

An example of confounding is apparent in the work of Heer et al. (2006), who analyzed data from a German registry of patients with acute coronary syndrome and compared the outcomes of 6,358 men and women who had had non-ST-elevation myocardial infarctions (NSTEMIs) between 2000 and 2002. (Here, too, it is not explicit how the classification categories *women* and *men* were assigned.) Acute coronary syndrome has the features of unstable angina but also is associated with myocardial necrosis or heart damage, and is a major cause of morbidity and mortality; patients with this type of myocardial infarction (MI) may have a higher long-term risk of death than patients with ST-segment elevation MIs (Grech & Ramsdale, 2003). Heer et al. (2006) reported that women had a greater risk of dying, compared with men (13.6% vs. 9.7%), within the first year of hospital discharge (odds ratio [OR] = 1.47; 95% confidence interval [CI]: 1.25–1.72). Some have hypothesized that this increased risk of death arises because women are treated less aggressively following discharge with appropriate cardiac medications. This model is similar to the direct effects described above as shown in Figure 4.1. However, Heer et al. considered the potential for confounding in their design and subsequently learned that there is no difference in the risk of mortality, once one considers the differences in age between the affected men and women. The age-adjusted odds ratio of mortality was 0.92 (95% CI: 0.76–1.11); it was not statistically significant. This occurred because the female patients were older than the male patients (average age was 72.8 years vs. 65.3 years) when they were admitted to the hospital at the time of their NSTEMI, and older people were more likely to succumb to the disorder. The model that represents the influence of this "lurking" variable, age, is provided in Figure 4.3.

It is readily apparent that if confounding factors are not measured or considered, a spurious explanation will be provided. Consequently, it is an epistemic reality that some important questions about gender and causality may not be answerable, especially in observational studies and at least not without the assumption that there is no residual confounding lurking outside one's model (Greenland & Morgenstern, 2001). This is a significant challenge to researchers who must specify models that encompass relevant factors yet maintain some degree of parsimony in their explanations both for practical and for theoretical reasons. Readers are cautioned,

Figure 4.3 A Schematic Diagram of a Direct Effect of Gender Adjusted for Confounding

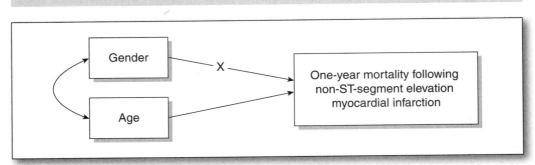

however, that "intellectual blinders" or "ideological biases" may lead to the omission of factors in our models, and thus alternative explanations may be ignored or left unaddressed.

Antecedents of Gender

In the examples provided above, the researchers all studied gender *effects* or *outcomes*. Gender was treated as an observable *binary* variable, albeit none of the researchers explained how the observations of gender were made, what criteria were applied to provide a binary classification, or why a binary classification was more suitable than a more complex classification or continuous measure of gender. Indeed, it is not clear, in all cases, whether *gender* could have been used synonymously with *sex* or whether a theoretical distinction between the social and the biological had been made, and whether one, the other, or both were at work (see Moore, 1994). Other researchers have been more explicit about their conceptualizations of gender and have applied very different sorts of models. Taking a different view of its actual operations, gender is treated as the outcome, not the antecedent or cause. That is, these researchers are in search of what produces gender, or at least some aspect of it.

As an example, Judge and Livingston (2008) were interested in those factors that shape *gender role orientation* and what it subsequently produces (economic consequences or earnings, in their case). We focus on only part of their model. In this case, the aspect of gender that is of interest is beliefs about the "proper roles for men and women at work and at home" (p. 995), as Judge and Livingston (2008) defined the concept. They inferred gender role orientation by summing the responses to five attitudinal items that were scored on a 4-point disagree-agree scale. The total score was their operationalization of gender role orientation, which was theorized to be a continuum of egalitarian (lower scores) to traditional (higher scores) views of men's and women's roles in work and family life.

They suggested that relatively stronger egalitarian or traditional gender role orientations are determined, in part, by demography, intellectual background, parental environment, parental education, and parental employment. They acknowledged that there are other conceptualizations labeled "gender role orientation," including the notion of *trait*-based masculinity and femininity (see Rammsayer & Troche, 2007), although they conceived of the construct as a *state*-like characteristic (i.e., it is amenable to change). The model is represented in Figure 4.4. Their analyses were based on interview data collected for the U.S. National Longitudinal Survey of Youth, which enrolled 12,686 youths aged 14 to 22 years in 1979 and followed them annually or biennially until they were 42 to 50 years of age.

What we have here is a slightly more complex approach to measurement. The researchers took the participants' responses to five statements about traditional and egalitarian views regarding women's roles in the workforce and gender role balance at work and home and summed the responses. Gender role orientation, in this case, was not directly observed, but rather was inferred from the direct observations of the participants' self-reported attitudes or opinions. It was held that there was some consistency to the attitudes espoused, which corresponded to an abstract concept or construct, and thus it was reasonable to sum the item scores (the extent of agreement or disagreement). Indeed, inherent in the design is a causal inference; that is, the construct, gender role orientation, was assumed to be the only "cause" of the participants' responses to the survey items (Wilson, 2005).

Blalock (1982), many years ago, emphasized that measurement has a set of theoretical assumptions as does substantive theory development. The two exercises are not separable, and in many models the measurement and theoretical components are conflated (Blalock, 1982). Consequently, it cannot be determined whether it is the substantive theory, the measurement structure, or both that are refutable. Judge and Livingston (2008) concluded that gender (perhaps it was sex they intended), ethnicity/race, marital status, education, and general mental ability were antecedents of gender role orientation, which was conceived as a psychological state. Women, African Americans, individuals who were more educated and more intelligent, and those who lived in cities, outside the U.S. South, and in the U.S. Northeast were more egalitarian, while those who were married, who were religious, whose fathers were relatively less educated, and whose mothers did not work outside the home were more traditional in their gender role orientation. The researchers concluded that gender role orientation is shaped by one's

Figure 4.4 A Schematic Diagram of Antecedents of Gender

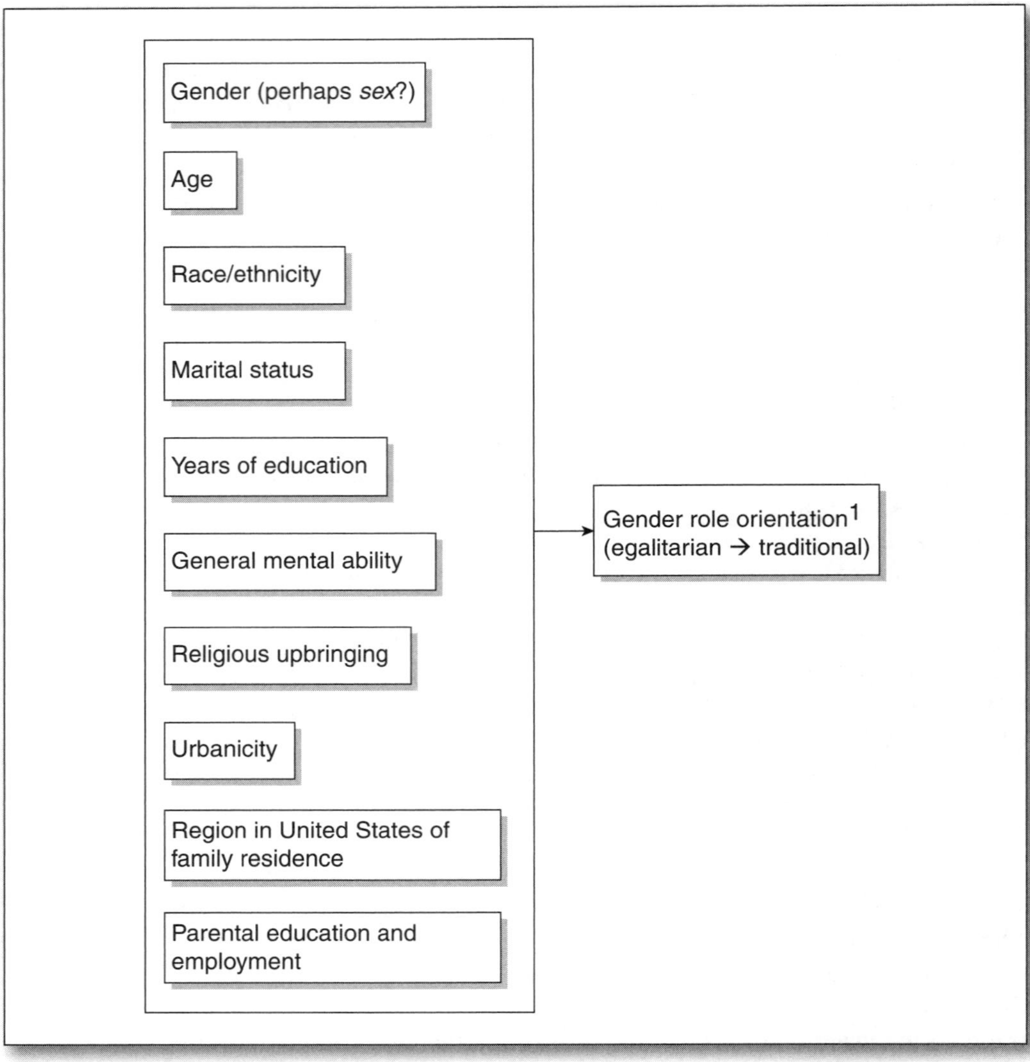

Source: Judge, T. A., & Livingston, B. A. (2008). Is the gap more than gender? A longitudinal analysis of gender, gender role orientation, and earnings. *Journal of Applied Psychology, 93,* 994–1012. Published by the American Psychological Association. Adapted with permission.

[1]Operationalized as the sum of the following on a scale from 1 to 4 (*strongly disagree* to *strongly agree*):

1. A woman's place is in the home, not the office or shop.

2. A wife with a family has no time for outside employment.

3. Employment of wives leads to more juvenile delinquency.

4. It is much better if the man is the achiever outside the home and the woman takes care of the home and family.

5. Women are much happier if they stay home and take care of children.

experiences in childhood, in addition to one's education, marital status, and general intelligence. Did they get it right? In addition to the possibility of random chance findings and confounding (they acknowledged that personality or disposition was omitted and may have been "lurking"), they may have been subject to a particular form of bias especially because their modeling approach assumed the perfect measurement of gender role orientation. Did summing the five opinion items result in a valid measure? It is readily apparent that proper measurement is a necessary condition before one can apply any meaning to a substantive model. Yet, in the model characterized here, the measurement model is implicit and likely contains error, both random and systematic. Although these sources of error were not explicitly addressed by Judge and Livingston, there are mechanisms to incorporate such error in one's models.

Gender Differences in the Measurement of Other Concepts

Whereas the previous model raised questions about potential biases in the interpretation of findings, which may result because of error in the measurement of gender, other models have been applied to examine how gender may bias the measurement of other concepts. This concern applies in particular to the measurement of concepts that are inferred from individuals' self-reports, which may be the only way to apprehend salient aspects of people's expressions of their gender. This source of bias, referred to as differential item functioning (DIF), is apparent when differences in people's scores are not associated with "real" between-group differences (as inferred in the Judge and Livingston, 2008, example), but rather are associated with differences in responses to the items posed (i.e., a set of questions that operationalize a concept) because the items hold significantly different meanings for the groups being compared (Bond & Fox, 2007; Hambleton, Swaminathan, & Rogers, 1991). For example, Stommel et al. (1993) demonstrated a good example of this problem when they explored whether men's and women's apparent differences in their reported symptoms of depression were due to "real" differences in levels of depression or differences in the way they interpreted and responded to a commonly used measurement scale, the Center for Epidemiological Studies–Depression (CES-D) scale (Radloff, 1977) (708 cancer patients were studied; 49% were male). The measure consists of 20 items that assess the frequency at which respondents experience symptoms suggestive of depression (e.g., having crying spells, talking less than usual, having a poor appetite). Stommel et al. (1993) limited their analysis to 18 items that were grouped into three dimensions (factors) of depression: depressive mood, well-being, and somatic symptoms; the measurement structure is represented in Figure 4.5A.

Figure 4.5B poses the question they asked, schematically: Is gender associated with depressive symptomatology (effect A), does this measurement tool exhibit signs of bias because some of the indicators evoke different types of responses in men and women (effect B), or both? Another way of putting this is that the content of the scale's items may not be interpreted equivalently by men and women with respect to their level of depression. Yet another way of putting this is that any gender differences in depression may be confounded by the way in which depression is measured.

Stommel et al. (1993) concluded that two items (i.e., "talking less than usual" and "having crying spells") functioned differently based on the respondent's gender (i.e., were biased). This means that, in the presence of equivalent levels of depressive symptomatology, women's and men's scores would differ because women would be more inclined to endorse the "crying spells" item and men would be more inclined to endorse the "talking less" item. Consequently, use of the scale to determine whether men and women have any notable differences would be exaggerated by this measurement artifact. This type of measurement bias is not the same as gender bias. One has to be sure, when making a gender bias claim, that the genders are being assessed in an equivalent fashion, or the advantage or disadvantage identified is merely an artifact of the measurement tool and is not of substantive interest.

Figure 4.5A   A Schematic Diagram of a Modified Version of the Center for Epidemiological Studies–Depression (CES-D) Scale (Radloff, 1977; Stommel et al., 1993)

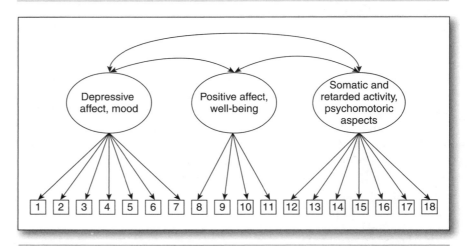

Note: Ovals represent the latent concepts (the dimensions or factors of depression) that are inferred from people's actual responses to the 18 CES-D questions, which are represented as squares.

Figure 4.5B A Schematic Diagram of a Modified Version of the Center for Epidemiological Studies–Depression (CES-D) Scale With Gender Hypothesized as a Substantive and a Methodological Effect (Radloff, 1977; Stommel et al., 1993)

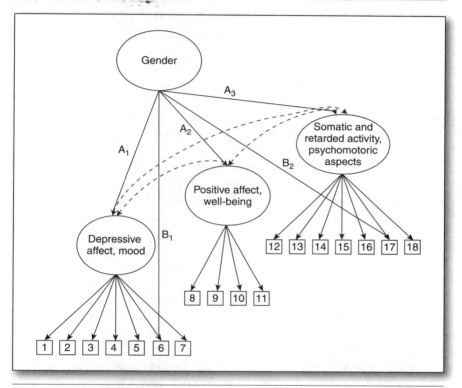

Note: Lines A_1 to A_3 represent direct effects of gender on the corresponding concepts (substantive effects). Lines B_1 and B_2 represent the effect of gender on the item response that is an artifact of a bias in measurement (differential item functioning). The dashed, curved lines are correlations.

Gendered Effects

Some scholars have used the term *gendered effects* in their discussions of gender and health. For example, van Praag, Bracke, Christiaens, Levecque, and Pattyn (2009) explored whether there are *gendered* contextual or community effects associated with problematic alcohol consumption and depression. Davidson, Trudeau, van Roosmalen, Stewart, and Kirkland (2006) argued that several *gendered* values and attitudes affect health, including the meaning people assign to health, which may affect their general health satisfaction, their interactions with health professionals, and their use of unconventional health services. Similarly, Teghtsoonian (2009) posited that the neoliberal policies and reforms of governments have produced *gendered* effects on people's mental health. Although none of these authors explicitly defined what was meant by a *gendered* effect, we suggest that some, if not all, were postulating gender interaction or moderation models; that is, gender serves as a qualifier. There is considerable variation across disciplines in how this idea is expressed; researchers have used the terms *interaction, modification, moderation, modulation, nonsymmetrical effects, variations by gender,* and (possibly) *intersectionality.* Regardless of the term used, the underlying model suggests that gender affects (influences, changes, or modifies) the effect of another factor on an outcome. Technically, "an interaction exists if the magnitude of the effect of one variable on another differs, depending on the particular value possessed by some third variable (often some special condition describing the situation or environment)" (Hayduk, 1987, p. 52).

To differentiate this model from those above, consider the work of Stoltenberg et al. (2008), who sought to determine whether impulsivity (e.g., lack of planning, poor inhibitory control, or difficulty delaying gratification) interacted with gender (was *gendered*) in its influence on young adults' health-risk behavior, including tobacco use, alcohol consumption, and gambling problems. They had 200 university students (62% were female) complete gambling, alcoholism, tobacco use, and impulsivity self-assessments with standardized measurement tools, as well as completing the "Stop Task," a computerized task that provides an index of response inhibition with higher scores indicative of higher levels of impulsivity (Logan, Schachar, & Tannock, 1997). We have represented part of their analyses schematically in Figure 4.6.

What Figure 4.6 indicates, and what Stoltenberg et al. (2008) found, is that gender is associated with having alcohol problems; men are more likely to have alcohol problems. Impulsivity, too, is associated with having alcohol problems; people with higher levels of impulsivity are more likely

Figure 4.6 A Schematic Diagram of a Gendered Effect

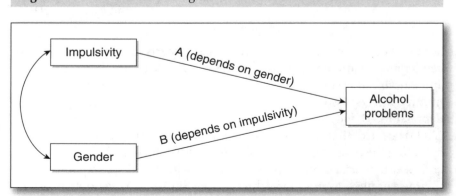

to have alcohol problems. How then is this *gendered?* One cannot indicate the extent to which impulsivity influences alcohol consumption without knowing the gender of the people of interest because the extent to which impulsivity is important as a risk factor varies across the impulsivity continuum, depending on gender. Specifically, when men and women are highly impulsive, there are no apparent gender differences in their risk of having alcohol problems—their risk is equivalent. When men and women have average levels of impulsivity, men have a greater probability of being categorized as having an alcohol problem (probability = .53) compared with women (probability = .37). At the low end of the impulsivity continuum, men are far more likely than women to have alcohol problems (probability = .81 vs. .47). Consequently, we can say that the relationship between impulsivity and alcohol problems is *gendered* in that we must know the gender of the research participants before we can describe the effect of impulsivity. Conversely, and equivalently, we must know something about individuals' impulsivity before we can describe the effect of gender on alcohol consumption; these researchers found that at some levels of impulsivity there were no gender differences.

Gender Qua Gender

Is it possible to *measure* gender, rather than attempting to apprehend it through the study of its operations? About the models described above it can be said that they represent attempts to *understand* gender through its effects or consequences, its antecedents, its effects on the measurement of other constructs, and its effects on the magnitude of other constructs' effects. In most instances, the researchers' work that motivated the provided examples treated gender analytically as a binary variable (male vs. female) with no mention of how it was actually determined (operationalized) or conceptualized. Presumably, the researchers conceptualized gender as existing in the form of two mutually exclusive categories, or they possibly viewed the binary variable as an imperfect measure of an underlying continuum or of several categories. In either case, this approach to the measurement of gender does not take into account any degree of measurement error. This is problematic because the sensitivity, or power, to observe significant study results is reduced when measurement error is ignored or when a concept that exists as a continuum or as several categories is operationalized as a binary. It is therefore useful to find ways of measuring gender that account for measurement error and that allow for some degree of gradation in the measurement, assuming that gender is indeed more than two discrete categories.

Is it possible to measure gender as manifesting as a continuum of expression or as multiple categories? At the risk of being overly simplistic by not differentiating various gender-related concepts such as *gender identity* (e.g., the gender(s) an individual identifies with or the degree to which a person identifies with masculine and feminine personality traits), *gender roles* (e.g., shared expectations of behavior given one's gender), *gender stereotypes* (e.g., shared views of personality traits often tied to gender such as instrumentality in men and expressiveness in women), and *gender attitudes* (e.g., views of others or situations associated with gender such as men thinking in terms of justice and women in terms of care), we present this final model to illustrate the potential to measure gender and to go beyond a simple binary classification; it also represents the capacity to include measurement error within the model.

The Bem Sex Role Inventory (BSRI; Bem, 1981) is based on the notion that varying degrees of masculinity and femininity may coexist within a person. The theory underlying the measurement tool posits that people acquire and display traits, behaviors, and attitudes that complement their gender identity (the manifestations of their gender identity). In the model, gender identity is inferred from the latent concepts of femininity and masculinity based on the observed item responses. The scale consists of 60 adjectives (e.g., *self-reliant, affectionate,* and *gentle*) (20 are believed to be feminine characteristics, 20 are masculine, and 20 are neutral and not scored); a shorter version with 30 items is also available. Respondents describe themselves by providing ratings for each item on a scale from 1 (*never or almost never true*) to 7 (*always or almost always true*). The summed scores indicate degrees of masculinity and femininity held by respondents, which are used to classify them as "feminine," "masculine," "androgynous," or "undifferentiated"—their gender identity (see Figure 4.7).

Colley et al. (2009) asked whether the BSRI actually measures individuals' global self-concepts of their masculinity and femininity, especially because gender roles and stereotypes have changed since the BSRI was developed in the mid-1970s. They analyzed the responses of 761 male (44%) and female (56%) students in the United Kingdom to determine whether the postulated measurement structure was supported—that is, whether responses to the putative masculinity and femininity BSRI items are adequately represented by the two corresponding factors.

Colley et al. (2009) concluded that the postulated measurement structure does not adequately represent the responses of the students they studied. It is not known why their results did not support the validity of the BSRI; they speculated that there may be sufficient sociocultural differences between young people in the United Kingdom and the United States to limit the generalizability of the tool or that there have been sufficient changes in gender identity conceptions over the past three decades to render the BSRI no longer valid. What is relevant to the discussion here is that this model is an attempt to measure gender, to extend the concept beyond a simple binary classification, and has the potential to account for measurement error.

Figure 4.7   A Schematic Diagram of the Bem Sex Role Inventory
(Short-Form) Masculinity and Femininity Dimensions and
the Inferred Gender Identities

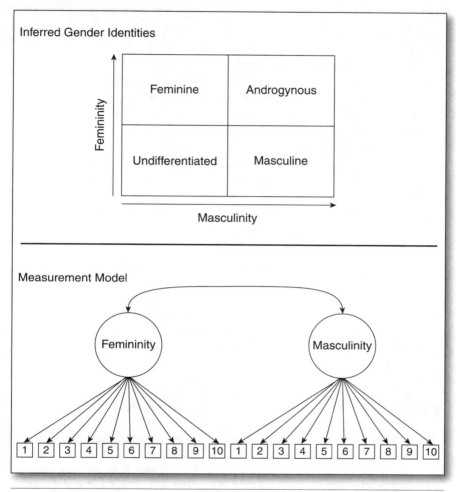

Source: Colley, A., Mulhern, G., Maltby, J., & Wood, A. M. (2009). The short form
BSRI: Instrumentality, expressiveness and gender associations among a United Kingdom
sample. *Personality and Individual Differences, 46,* 384–387. Published by Elsevier.

Conclusion

All the models presented here, which are not representative of all modeling
approaches, contain elements or aspects of gender. The questions that the
researchers posed that motivated our representations of these models all
appeared rather similar in nature, yet the implications of the models in
which gender was embedded are markedly different. They all attempt to
tell us something about gender although it may not have been explicit.

Indeed, whether the concept of gender carried the same meaning in each of these research contexts is uncertain and unlikely. What seems to be required is that health researchers recognize the interplay between theory and research and more strenuously grapple with the untested and implicit assumptions of their models. The important point here is that gender must be understood in context; gender is merely a mental representation that must acquire its content or meaning from context.

What are the arrows in the schematic diagrams included in this chapter? They are the processes that explain how gender arises, manifests, and operates. These are descriptive inferences and the building blocks of causal arguments, yet they are not typically made explicit. If we were to understand better the means by which an effect is produced by gender, how gender influences other effects and measures, and how gender is produced, then we would begin to approach the disambiguation of gender as a concept such that it can provide analytic or theoretic utility. After all, we want to know not only what gender is in the abstract, but how it enters into questions of health status, health behavior, and health service delivery.

References

Bem, S. L. (1974). The measurement of psychological androgyny. *Journal of Consulting and Clinical Psychology, 42,* 155–162. doi:10.1037/h0036215

Bem, S. L. (1981). *Bem Sex-Role Inventory: Professional manual.* Palo Alto, CA: Consulting Psychologists Press.

Bird, C. E., & Rieker, P. P. (2008). *Gender and health: The effects of constrained choices and social policies.* Cambridge, UK: Cambridge University Press.

Blalock, H. M. (1982). *Conceptualization and measurement in the social sciences.* Beverly Hills, CA: SAGE.

Blalock, H. M. (1986). Multiple causation, indirect measurement and generalizability in the social sciences. *Synthese, 68,* 13–36.

Bond, T. G., & Fox, C. M. (2007). *Applying the Rasch model: Fundamental measurement in the human sciences* (2nd ed.). Mahwah, NJ: Lawrence Erlbaum Associates.

Bridgman, P. W. (1927). *The logic of modern physics.* New York: Macmillan.

Byrne, B. M. (2006). *Structural equation modeling with EQS: Basic concepts, applications, and programming* (2nd ed.). Mahwah, NJ: Lawrence Erlbaum Associates.

Colley, A., Mulhern, G., Maltby, J., & Wood, A. M. (2009). The short form BSRI: Instrumentality, expressiveness and gender associations among a United Kingdom sample. *Personality and Individual Differences, 46,* 384–387. doi:10.1016/j.paid.2008.11.005

Davidson, K. W., Trudeau, K. J., van Roosmalen, E., Stewart, M., & Kirkland, S. (2006). Perspective: Gender as a health determinant and implications for health education. *Health Education & Behaviour, 33,* 731–743.

De Ayala, R. J. (2009). *The theory and practice of item response theory.* New York: Guilford Press.

Fletcher, R. H., & Fletcher, S. W. (2005). *Clinical epidemiology: The essentials* (4th ed.). Philadelphia: Lippincott Williams & Wilkins.

Geiger, H. J. (2006). Health disparities: What do we know? What do we need to know? What should we do? In A. J. Schulz & L. Mullings (Eds.), *Gender, race, class, and health: Intersectional approaches* (pp. 261–288). San Francisco: Jossey-Bass.

Grech, E. D., & Ramsdale, D. R. (2003). Acute coronary syndrome: Unstable angina and non-ST segment elevation myocardial infarction. *British Medical Journal (Clinical Research Ed.), 326*(7401), 1259–1261. doi:10.1136/bmj.326.7401.1259

Greenland, S., & Morgenstern, H. (2001). Confounding in health research. *Annual Review of Public Health, 22,* 189–212. doi:10.1146/annurev.publhealth.22.1.189

Hambleton, R. K., Swaminathan, H., & Rogers, H. J. (1991). *Fundamentals of item response theory.* Newbury Park, CA: SAGE.

Hayduk, L. A. (1987). *Structural equation modeling with LISREL: Essentials and advances.* Baltimore: Johns Hopkins University Press.

Heer, T., Gitt, A. K., Juenger, C., Schiele, R., Wienbergen, H., Towae, F., et al. (2006). Gender differences in acute non-ST-segment elevation myocardial infarction. *American Journal of Cardiology, 98,* 160–166. doi:10.1016/j.amjcard.2006.01.072

Hume, D. (2003). *A treatise of human nature* (J. P. Wright, R. Stecker, & G. Fuller, Eds.). London: Everyman. (Original work published 1739)

Hume, D. (2007). *An enquiry concerning human understanding* (P. J. R. Millican, Ed.). Oxford, UK: Oxford University Press. (Original work published 1748)

Judge, T. A., & Livingston, B. A. (2008). Is the gap more than gender? A longitudinal analysis of gender, gender role orientation, and earnings. *Journal of Applied Psychology, 93,* 994–1012. doi:10.1037/0021-9010.93.5.994

Lanes, S. F. (1988). The logic of causal inference in medicine. In K. J. Rothman (Ed.), *Causal inference* (pp. 59–75). Chestnut Hill, MA: Epidemiology Resources.

Logan, G. D., Schachar, R. J., & Tannock, R. (1997). Impulsivity and inhibitory control. *Psychological Science, 8,* 60–64.

Moore, D. S., McCabe, G. P., & Craig, B. A. (2009). *Introduction to the practice of statistics* (6th extended version ed.). New York: W. H. Freeman.

Moore, H. L. (1994). *A passion for difference: Essays in anthropology and gender.* Bloomington: Indiana University Press.

Popper, K. R. (1992). *The logic of scientific discovery.* London: Routledge. (Original work published 1959)

Radloff, L. S. (1977). The CES-D scale: A self-report depression scale for research in the general population. *Applied Psychological Measurement, 1,* 385–401.

Rammsayer, T. H., & Troche, S. J. (2007). Sexual dimorphism in second-to-fourth digit ratio and its relation to gender-role orientation in males and females. *Personality and Individual Differences, 42,* 911–920. doi:10.1016/j.paid.2006.09.002

Saposnik, G., Cote, R., Phillips, S., Gubitz, G., Bayer, N., Minuk, J., et al. (2008). Stroke outcome in those over 80: A multicenter cohort study across Canada. *Stroke, 39,* 2. doi:10.1161/STROKEAHA.107.511402

Stevens, S. S. (1946). On the theory of scales of measurement. *Science, 103*(2684), 677–680.

Stine, W. W. (1989). Meaningful inference: The role of measurement in statistics. *Psychological Bulletin, 105,* 147–155. doi:10.1037/0033-2909.105.1.147

Stoltenberg, S. F., Batien, B. D., & Birgenheir, D. G. (2008). Does gender moderate associations among impulsivity and health-risk behaviours? *Addictive Behaviours, 33,* 252–265.

Stommel, M., Given, B. A., Given, C. W., Kalaian, H. A., Schulz, R., & McCorkle, R. (1993). Gender bias in the measurement properties of the Center for Epidemiologic Studies Depression Scale (CES-D). *Psychiatry Research, 49,* 239–250.

Suppes, P., & Zinnes, J. L. (1963). Basic measurement theory. In R. D. Luce, R. Bush, & E. Galanter (Eds.), *Handbook of mathematical psychology* (pp. 1–76). New York: Wiley.

Taveggia, T. C. (1974). Resolving research controversy through empirical cumulation: Toward reliable sociological knowledge. *Sociological Methods & Research, 2,* 395–407.

Teghtsoonian, K. (2009). Depression and mental health in neoliberal times: A critical analysis of policy and discourse. *Social Science & Medicine, 69,* 28–35.

Townsend, C. O. (2002). *Perceived stress, coping and dietary fat intake in rural adolescents: Gender and ethnic differences* (Doctoral dissertation). Available from ProQuest Dissertations and Theses database. (UMI No. 3042815)

van Praag, L., Bracke, P., Christiaens, W., Levecque, K., & Pattyn, E. (2009). Mental health in a gendered context: Gendered community effect on depression and problem drinking. *Health and Place, 15,* 990–998.

Viswanathan, M. (2005). *Measurement error and research design.* Thousand Oaks, CA: SAGE.

Wilson, M. (2005). *Constructing measures: An item response modeling approach.* Mahwah, NJ: Lawrence Erlbaum Associates.

Measuring Biological Sex 5

Gillian Einstein

> *One's sex cannot be simply reduced to and contained by one's primary and secondary sexual characteristics, because one's sex makes a difference to every function, biological, social, cultural, if not in their operations then certainly in significance. (Grosz, 1994, p. 22)*

Measuring biological sex is a broad topic encompassing studies of the physiology of the reproductive system, the role of the brain and endocrine organs in reproduction, chromosomal and phenotypic differences between sexes, and the effects of gendered experience on the corporeal body. This chapter outlines each of these aspects, briefly citing examples and describing traditional and new paradigms for the design of experiments to measure biological sex. It first defines what is meant (for purposes of this chapter) by biological sex. It then describes the traditional research paradigms including experiments measuring the effects of reproductive hormones on behavior and brain and newer models of genetically modified animals. The comparative approach known as "sex differences" research is described, as are mechanisms that might underlie a reciprocal relationship between biological sex and gender.

What Is Biological Sex?

Biological sex is usually considered one's primary or secondary sex characteristics (phenotype) as well as any effects of carrying two X chromosomes or an X and a Y chromosome (genotype) (Johnson,

Greaves, & Repta, 2007; Pardue & Wizemann, 2001). Measuring these would encompass any methods used in biology: genetic, biochemical, anatomical, functional, and behavioral assays. Usually these are measured on the body of interest and are viewed as residing within that body. Thus, biological sex has something important to do with the corporeal body.

Evolutionarily speaking, biological sex is about reproduction. Females and males each have a role to play in the production of offspring, and sex encompasses the behaviors and biological mechanisms that make that possible. On this view, measuring biological sex is not a new endeavor. From time immemorial reproductive behaviors and the genes, hormones, and physiologies associated with those behaviors have been studied up and down the phylogenetic scale (Becker et al., 2008; McEwen & Goy, 1980; Short & Balaban, 1994). Psychologists, botanists, zoologists, veterinarians, endocrinologists, and neuroscientists have long been trying to understand mating, fecundity, and reproductive behaviors.

From the moment Geoff Harris elucidated the connection between the anterior pituitary and the brain by transplanting or electrically stimulating hypothalamic tissue and finding that those manipulations could effect ovulation, it became clear that there was an intimate connection between the nervous and the reproductive systems (Harris, 1937; Raisman, 1997), and hence studying the nervous system became a part of measuring biological sex. Subsequent research focused on understanding the effects of reproductive hormones (estrogens, androgens, and progestins) on what were defined as "female- and male-typical" reproductive behaviors (lordosis and mounting, respectively). This consisted of removing and/or replenishing these hormones to female and male rodents and measuring the effect by determining how often females assumed a receptive position, called lordosis, and males assumed a position facilitating intromission, called mounting (Beach, 1941; Beach & Rasquin, 1942). Because these behaviors were shown to depend on "sex" hormones and therefore were of biological origin, they became a part of the panoply of secondary sex characteristics and, thus, important end points in measuring biological sex.

These early experiments linking the effect of hormones to sexual behavior led to further experiments testing whether these same hormones affected brain development in regions critical for hormone production and secretion (Raisman & Field, 1973; also see Einstein, 2007). This paradigm—removing or replenishing reproductive hormones and measuring sex-typical behavior and/or measuring brain regions—became the preeminent set of methods for studying biological sex in the nervous system. The songbird—canary and zebra finch—served as the clearest model for measuring biological sex because song appeared during the mating season and males sang while females did not. In a series of experiments modifying hormones in the developing canary and zebra finch, Nottebohm and his colleagues used neuroanatomical and behavioral measures (song or no song) to determine that reproductive hormones were correlated with the expression of brain cell groupings without which the males did not sing (Nottebohm, 1980; Nottebohm & Arnold, 1976).[1]

Paradigms for Research on Biological Sex

Models undergirding experimental design will affect the results and interpretation of any experiment designed to measure biological sex. Often implicit in these models are expectations of what is "sex typical" and a binary outcome. All influence the reported results of any measure of biological sex, and it is worthwhile knowing what these assumptions are when developing or interpreting experiments.

Developmental Organization by Reproductive Hormones

The experiments of Goy and Phoenix established a developmental "critical period" during which the removal or replacement of reproductive hormones could alter the sexual template both in behavior and in brain (Phoenix, Goy, Gerall, & Young, 1959). By manipulating reproductive hormones during this critical period the reproductive behavior of females could be "masculinized" and the reproductive behavior of males "feminized" (see Einstein, 2007).

This is currently the paradigm underlying virtually every experiment to explore biological sex in the central nervous system as well as informing the interpretation of sex, gender, and sexual preference differences in humans (Becker et al., 2008; Einstein, 2007). Thus, if an adult female found to have a group of neurons that is different from a male's in size, density, or affinity for hormones or neurotransmitters, the first question is to ask is whether this difference can be altered during the perinatal period. If the homologous difference is found in the human central nervous system, it is then assumed to be influenced by hormones during either the pre- or the perinatal period. Because this paradigm is based on a binary notion of sex—human and nonhuman animals are either XX or XY—the interpretation is that the region is either male-like or female-like. This has led to the interpretation that gay males have a "feminized" brain and to rodent models of sexuality using the display of "female-typical" behavior in males as a model of gay behavior. The simplicity and perhaps even wrongheadedness of this paradigm is highlighted by the fact that many

---

[1]It is worthwhile noting that in mammalian models, differences in neural structures have rarely been associated with functional differences (de Vries, 2004).

gay males engage in what would be defined as a "male typical" role in sex, many humans self-identify as bisexual, and the phenotype of one's sexual partner may be very different from the phenotype about which one fantasizes while having sex (Fausto-Sterling, 2000).

Frank Beach, one of the first scientists to define biological sex for purposes of measurement, was strongly aware that even the cagè environment influenced rodent reproductive behavior (Einstein, 2007). Beach had a broad view of rodent sexuality encompassing bi- as well as hetero- as well as homosexual behavior. In fact, Beach believed that female and male rodents each had the sexual template of the other with the expression of that template driven by social conditions and reproductive hormones (see Beach, 1941; Beach & Rasquin, 1942). As research continued throughout the 20th century, however, eventually the only sexes possible became female and male, and the only types of sexual identification and behavior became gay and straight (Fausto-Sterling, 2000).

Factors Other Than Reproductive Hormones

In addition to measuring reproductive hormones, measuring biological sex requires elucidating (a) the distribution of receptors for those hormones, (b) chromosomal differences that are not on either the X or the Y chromosome, and (c) whether an individual has one or two copies of a gene (called *gene dosage*).

DISTRIBUTION OF HORMONE RECEPTORS

Steroid hormones (estrogens and androgens) traveling around the body in the blood pass directly through cell membranes. Once inside the cell, hormones couple with proteins called hormone receptors. The hormone-receptor complex travels to the nucleus where it initiates gene transcription leading to the production of new proteins. Thus the distribution of steroid receptors reveals where and how strongly estrogens and androgens will affect cell physiology (McEwen, Davis, Parsons, & Pfaff, 1979). For example, XY individuals who are born without androgen receptors have the phenotype of XX individuals. Without the androgen receptor the hormone cannot have its effect on secondary sex characteristics. Estrogen receptors are also critical for the action of estrogens. The admission to an endocrinology clinic of a human male whose growth hadn't ceased occurring resulted in the discovery of the first human who didn't make receptors to estrogens (Smith et al., 1994). His biological sex revealed that the action of estrogens via the estrogen receptor is essential for the cessation of the growth of the long bones and the motility of sperm in males—the former not necessarily linked to the reproductive system and the latter startlingly inexorably bound to our considerations of the male reproductive system (Smith et al., 1994).

In order to study the role of hormone receptors in biological sex it has been important to develop methods to visualize where the hormone receptors are located. One such method uses the immune system to generate molecules called antibodies that can bind strongly to the receptors and deactivate them. The discovery of a second estrogen receptor (ER) led to the development of antibodies to both receptors, ERalpha and ERbeta, as well as to mice in which the genes that make ERalpha or ERbeta or both have been eliminated (ER knockouts). These transgenic animal models have made it possible to study the effects of estrogens on every body system including, ironically enough, the male reproductive system.

GENETICS

Not all of biological sex is mediated by hormones. Finding that, in the rodent, sex differences in certain neurotransmitter systems occurred before the critical period for brain sexual differentiation led to the proposal that some sex differences are genetic and independent of steroid hormone action (Beyer, Eusterschulte, Pilgrim, & Reisert, 1992). In order to understand this more fully, genetic modification methods have been used to "make" mice that carry the Y chromosome with and without the chromosomal region that codes for testicular development and hence the production of testosterone. In this way, hormone production and genes coding for other sex differences on the Y chromosome can be dissociated (de Vries et al., 2002). Such biological models have revealed that in addition to sex-determining genes, the Y chromosome carries genes related to cardiovascular function and blood pressure regulation, potentially predisposing males to earlier onset of cardiovascular disease compared with women (Charchar, Tomaszewski, Strahorn, Champagne, & Dominiczak, 2003). Interestingly, the discovery of a bird (zebra finch) whose right body half was genetically and morphologically male and whose left body was female revealed that even though both sides of the body were exposed in utero to the same hormones, both body and brain phenotypes were independent of those circulating hormones, supporting the importance of genes *other than those that code for reproductive hormones* in establishing biological sex (Agate et al., 2003).

While current genetic methods for measuring biological sex have focused on modifying or eliminating the sex-determining region of the Y chromosome, in animal models the X chromosome is also important. One obvious genetic difference between females and males is that females have two X chromosomes while males have only one. This means that in XY individuals the X-linked genes will all come from the same X chromosome and there will be uniform expression of those genes. However, in XX individuals, some X-linked genes will come from one X chromosome while others will come from the other X chromosome. It is most often the case that genes from both X chromosomes will not be expressed, or one will be "inactivated." Whether it is the mother's or the father's X that is inactivated in a given cell is random. Thus XX individuals are a mosaic of X expression with the genes of one X chromosome being expressed in some cells and the genes of the other X being expressed in neighboring cells *in the same tissue*. Methods for identifying which gene products are from which X chromosome have been developed and used to show a differential distribution of X-linked mRNAs across the mammalian brain (Xu, Watkins, & Arnold, 2006). Differential expression of the two versions of X-linked genes can have repercussions for any body tissue. For example, Simpson-Golabi-Behmel syndrome is an X-linked condition with repercussions for cardiac tissues resulting in a high frequency of cardiac abnormalities (Lin, Neri, Hughes-Benzie, & Weksberg, 1999).

Furthermore, even for the "inactivated" X, not all the genes are actually inactivated. This can lead to a double expression of some X-linked genes in XX individuals. Models and methods have been developed for identifying the origin of X-linked genes because the double expression of a given gene may be important for the development of brain phenotype (Xu, Taya, Kaibuchi, & Arnold, 2005). For example, XO individuals have short stature, webbed necks, and what is described as an "emotional distance." While this phenotype would be categorized as biological sex, emotional distance and a particular body type may engender certain societal reactions that, in turn, may exacerbate emotional distance and physical awkwardness. Just as Kitwood and Bredin (1992) posited that simply being diagnosed with Alzheimer's disease leads to negative interactions that exacerbate the process of neuronal death, how XO individuals are treated or "gendered" by society could influence the severity of "biological" characteristics associated with the genetics.

Studying Biological Sex in Humans

Measuring the role of reproductive hormones, hormone receptors, and genes in making biological sex in humans requires taking tissue or blood during life, gathering tissues after death (autopsy), or "experiments of nature" such as the male without estrogen receptors (described above). An often used human model for studying the development of female-typical behaviors in males involves XY individuals who do not make androgen receptors. These individuals most often identify as female. An often used human model for studying the development of male-typical behavior in XX individuals involves females born with overactive adrenal glands, which leads to producing high levels of androgens (known as congenital adrenal hyperplasia, or CAH). There is also the famous "experiment of nature," or the case of John/Joan, in which one male twin was raised as a female because of a botched circumcision. The first interpretation of the "results" was that sexual identity was socially constructed. Later understandings of John's (David Reimer) sexuality supported a biological model of sexual identity. However, now it is clear that the "experiment" was so confounded by the circumstances of Reimer's life that it is impossible to tease apart what is social and what biological (Diamond & Sigmundson, 1997).

Comparing Female and Male: Sex Differences Research

Sex differences research emerged with the expansion of the definition of biological sex from reproduction to precopulatory behaviors to the nervous system biological sex—that is, when biological sexes became loosened from the bounds of reproduction. The beginnings of this can be seen in McEwen and Goy's (1980) volume on sexual differentiation of the brain with the codification coming 20 years later with the publication of the Institute of Medicine's report, *Exploring the Biological Contributions to Human Health: Does Sex Matter?* (Pardue & Wizemann, 2001). Subsequently, any aspect of the body where difference was found, whether or not it was linked to reproduction, has become known as a "sex difference." Sex differences have been found in body systems as diverse as the nervous, musculoskeletal, cardiovascular, and immune systems (Miller & Hay, 2004). The notion that every cell in the body is "sexed" (perhaps) by virtue of the developmental mechanisms that lay the groundwork for reproductive success is one that is gaining ground (Becker et al., 2008). In humans, there is a growing acknowledgment that the sexing of cells and tissues independent of their role in reproduction has important consequences for health and disease (Becker et al., 2008; Johnson et al., 2007; Pardue & Wizemann, 2001). Thus, in comparative studies of female and male/XX and XY organisms *of whatever body system,* whenever a biological difference exists between female and male it is simply called a "sex difference." Supporting and carrying this comparative approach forward are such scientific societies as the Organization for the Study of Sex Differences and the International Society of Gender Medicine, and there is now a field called "sex differences research" (Becker et al., 2005).

On this view, studies are either designed to include females and males, separating sexes in the data analyses (disaggregating by sex), or carried out in one sex but comparing the results to another study of the same design that was carried out in the other sex. Ultimately such studies aim to reveal significant differences between the means in female and male, gay and straight. Tellingly, in one genetic study in which data from both females and males from 120 French Canadian families from the Saguenay–Lac-Saint-Jean region of Quebec, Canada, were collected and analyzed together, no significant differences in the heritability or linkage of genetic traits associated with cardiovascular disease in the population as a whole were found. However, when the data were disaggregated by sex, of 539 hemodynamic, metabolic, anthropometric, and humoral traits a full one eighth were present *either* in females *or* in males. Most of these were involved with heart rate and blood pressure categories, suggesting that genetic expression plays a role in the observed sex differences in cardiovascular disease (Seda et al., 2008). Even if one is not interested in sex differences, per se, before designing an empirical study it is worthwhile considering which biological system one is going to study and the variables within that system that might affect the condition under study.

Methods measuring sex differences assume that there are two groups that are going to be compared and that a difference is a significant difference of the mean. Much of importance can be learned about biological sex by taking this approach. For example, the clinical trials of d-sotalol neglected to consider sex differences in the open time of the potassium channels in the heart (and probably elsewhere, but it's not been studied), resulting in producing rather than stopping arrhythmias (Woolsey & Singh, 2000). From this unfortunate event, it is now understood that any drug designed to have its effect by prolonging the open time of potassium channels with the standard open time being drawn from males may actually induce arrhythmia in women. This is not an arcane difference since therapeutics including antibiotics, antipsychotics, and antiarrhythmia drugs prolong potassium channel open time and have well-documented adverse effects in women (Arizona Center for Education and Research on Therapeutics, 2009). For lack of comparing female and male responses to drugs in trial, 8 out of 10 drugs were withdrawn from the market between January 1, 1997, and January 1, 2001, because they had greater adverse effects in women than in men (Harkin, Snowe, Mikulski, & Waxman, 2001). Interestingly, the lack of development and testing of treatments in both female and male animals and humans affects both females and males because drugs that have adverse effects in females are removed from the market to the detriment of males (Hayden, 2010).

The comparative approach has also revealed that men and women indeed have different levels of risk for various disorders and experience these conditions in often dramatically dissimilar ways. For example, some autoimmune disorders, such as lupus, are nine times as likely to present in women as in men (Fish, 2008; Pardue & Wizemann, 2001). Myocardial oxygen and glucose metabolism differs between the sexes (Peterson et al., 2007), and there are numerous critical sex differences in the experience of heart disease and myocardial infarction including age at first attack, symptoms, and likelihood of death postattack (Roberts, 2008). It has been proposed that differences in androgen exposure in early development may be one important factor in the earlier onset of atherosclerosis in males (Liu, Death, & Handelsman, 2003). There are sex differences in the etiology, course, and symptoms in patients admitted to the hospital for acute heart failure (AHF), with more women presenting with new-onset AHF and comorbidity with diabetes and anemia than men (Nieminen et al., 2008). Moreover, sex differences have been reported in the outcome of stroke (Bushnell, 2008), the experience of angina with normal coronary arteries (Humphries, Pu, Gao, Carere, & Pilote, 2008), and generalized pain

(Quiton & Greenspan, 2007). Autoimmune diseases have a higher prevalence in females than males. Systemic lupus erythematosus, Graves' disease, Hashimoto's thyroiditis, and Sjögren's syndrome exhibit a 7–10:1 female-to-male predominance; multiple sclerosis, rheumatoid arthritis, and scleroderma exhibit a 2–3:1 female-to-male ratio. However, ankylosing spondylitis, Goodpasture syndrome, Reiter syndrome, and vasculitis all predominate in males (Pardue & Wizemann, 2001).

Ovarian Cycle

When using the comparative approach it is important to take into account different expressions of hormones and patterns of hormonal release between females and males. These differences are important variables even within a given sex depending on age, time of day, and phase of the ovarian cycle. When studying males, varying androgen levels over the course of the day may affect the results of the study; likewise, time point in the ovarian cycle may affect results for females. Determining the circulating levels of hormones is a challenge. There are indirect methods such as counting back- or forward from the first or last day of menstruation and then assuming a mean level of estrogens and progestins. However, assuming an average length of ovarian cycle is highly inaccurate since cycle length can vary by as many as 4 days between women as well as for a given woman (Becker et al., 2008, Chapter 4). There are numerous methods for measuring circulating hormones directly, but each one has its strengths and its weaknesses. One can choose to measure hormones in saliva, serum, or urine using bioassays, antibody-binding assays, or mass spectrophotometry (Bellem, Meiyappan, Romans, & Einstein, 2011).

Nowhere have the effects of differing levels of steroid hormones been more studied than in the brain, where circulating steroid hormones shape brain regions differentially in women and men (Becker et al., 2005; Belcher, 2008; Herzog, 2007; Spencer et al., 2008). These well-established developmental differences are implicated in differences in cognition, mood, and mental health (Becker et al., 2005; Belcher, 2008; Herzog, 2007; Lupien, Maheu, Tu, Fiocco, & Schramek, 2007; Spencer et al., 2008). While this is yet to be established definitively (Clarkson, Petrovic, Einstein, & Stewart, 2009), many studies have reported a positive relationship between menstrual cycle changes and premenstrual, postpartum, and perimenopausal disorders (Rapkin, Moatakef-Imani, & Rasgon, 2002; Rubinow & Schmidt, 2006); major depression and bipolar disorder (Payne et al., 2007); insomnia (Krystal, 2004); catamenial epilepsy (El-Khayat et al., 2008); and obsessive-compulsive disorder (Labad et al., 2005; Vulink, Denys, Bus, & Westenberg, 2006). With respect to brain sex differences in general, depression is twice as prevalent in women as in men (Gorman, 2006). Moreover, 17β-estradiol and testosterone play a major role in modulating sensitivity to pain and analgesia (Craft, Mogil, & Aloisi, 2004), creating sex differences in endogenous pain modulation.

Gender and Biological Sex

While sex difference research often compares only two categories, XX/XY, female/male, it may still be used effectively to pinpoint where the social world—gender—makes its mark on biological sex. Since the world treats females and males differently, the world will have different effects on female and male biologies. This point is spectacularly made by Borkhoff and colleagues (2008) in their exploration of the relative ease with which women and men with the same type and severity of knee problems are recommended for total knee arthroplasty by Ontario practitioners. Interestingly, while the doctors studied stated that the sex of the patient did not enter into their decision to refer, the study revealed that the odds of recommending total knee arthroplasty for a male patient were 22 times greater than those for a female (Borkhoff et al., 2008). One can only speculate on the kinds of biological sex differences that might develop downstream of gendered treatment as the males go through life with knees repaired and the women do not.

Gender Affects Biological Sex

Hormones, anatomy, behavior, and gene expression do not exist in a vacuum. For example, human studies correlating an excess or paucity of one reproductive hormone to a gendered behavior as in CAH females fails to take into account that often these individuals are quite ill. They are in and out of the hospital from birth and exposed to many tests and procedures. Might these circumstances affect their behavior? As well, gender identification might be an important factor influencing differing disease incidence in females and males. Males carry a disproportionate burden (both prevalence and severity) of viral, bacterial, fungal, and parasitic diseases (Fish, 2008). Is this because of a sex difference in the immune system or because gendered behaviors expose each body differentially? Females carry the burden of sexually transmitted infections such as HIV and herpes simplex virus 2 (Fish, 2008). Is this a result of biology or society?

What are some of the mechanisms by which gender might affect biology, and how are these measured?

Experience

It has long been understood that the adult brain can undergo synaptic remodeling and expansion/retraction of somatic representation based on experience (Buonomano & Merzenich, 1998). Particularly pertinent to the interaction of gender and biological sex is a study using single-unit physiology in which the size of the representation of the ventrum in nursing female rodents' brains was compared with that in non-nursing rodents. Nursing rodents were found to have a significantly expanded cortical region representing the ventrum presumably induced by the constant touching and suckling of their pups (Xerri, Stern, & Merzenich, 1994). One can only speculate on the effects of pregnancy and lactation on the human somatosensory cortex or of repeated rape as many women experience in war. Of particular interest to an understanding of female sexuality in general would be a map of the female somatosensory cortex in order to understand the expansions and contractions that might occur with pregnancy, surgeries like mastectomies, and genital cutting as in female circumcision and cosmetic labia reductions (Einstein, 2008). We are currently studying pain and altered sensation in Somali women with female genital cutting and finding altered patterns of sensitivity in the vulvar region, which may be indicative of neural changes to regions critical for biological sex such as Onuf's nucleus in the spinal cord and the representation of the clitoris in the somatosensory cortex (Einstein, 2011).

In addition, experience can alter gene expression, particularly for neurotransmitter receptors implicated in stress and mood. Methyl groups can attach to or remove themselves from DNA coding for neurotransmitter receptors, thereby changing an animal's reactivity to stress throughout life. In a paradigm using cross-fostering of rat pups to high-licking/-grooming or low-licking/-grooming dams, Weaver and colleagues (2004) used molecular genetics to identify a difference in DNA methylation and, hence, gene expression, as a function of a maternal behavior over the first week of life, supporting an earlier finding that the first week of postnatal life is a "critical period" for the effects of early experience on glucocorticoid receptor expression. This in turn can change mothering behavior in the offspring. However, treatment with trichostatin A (histone deacetylase inhibitor) reverses the hypermethylation of portions of the glucocorticoid receptor coding region in the pups of low-licking moms. Thus, genetic effects of early experience can be reversed (Weaver et al., 2004). If female pups are, by nature of simply being XX, licked and groomed less, what might be the effect on the expression of their glucocorticoid receptors and, hence, their response to stress throughout life? We currently do not know whether there are sex differences in epigenetic regulation.

Environment

A close look at biological systems and their sexual components convinces us that there are mechanisms outside of as well as inside the body that work together to form this biological category we call "sex." For example, environmental factors such as temperature may be the key determinant for biological sex for amphibians. Social factors such as lack of one sex or the other may also be a key determinant in "making sex." Female protogynous fish can morph both their social behavior and their reproductive body into that of a male upon recognition that the male fish of the group is gone (Gilbert, 2006). In mammals, smell is an important external cue guiding the expression of biological sex. For example, pheromones not only attract us to potential mates but, as revealed by anatomical methods, have been known for some time to affect synaptic connectivity in the nursing female rodent (Modney & Hatton, 1990). Dulac and Kimchi (2008) have recently found that "sex-typical" behavior in rodents can be reversed by the removal of one of the important olfactory entrants to the brain, the vomeronasal organ (VNO). When the VNO is removed from the female mouse, she attempts to copulate like a male with other mice, emits male courtship vocalizations, solicits by sniffing and chasing intruding mice, and carries out pelvic thrusting in the manner of control males. Here we see that smell can completely reverse "sex-typical" behavior, which had previously been shown (see section on *paradigms*) to be irreversible by hormones after the critical period (Kimchi, Xu, & Dulac, 2007).

Going Forward

What do these various approaches and experimental paradigms reveal about biological sex that is useful for the practicing biologist, the social scientist, and the clinician? For the practicing biologist it means that biology—even adult biology—is not static and impervious to the milieu in which it lives. Using methods that take into account the experience of each experimental subject, be it rodent or human, is critical to understanding any biological system and for human research may signal the necessity of incorporating first-person reports in order to guide experimental design and the interpretation of any findings.

For the social scientist it requires understanding that what they are learning is never happening independently of biology—that, indeed, the social milieu will affect as well as be affected by interactions with the corporeal body. This means that it might be worthwhile to use physiological measures to further understand the effect of the social on the body.

Perhaps most important for the clinician to remember as we enter the era of *evidence-based, personalized,* and *translational medicine*—terms that naturally raise questions about differences and similarities—is that there is not just one biology that provides a standard against which wellness and illness can be measured. Given demonstrated differences in the cellular responses of XX and XY organisms irrespective of what mechanism creates them, if most clinical trials are carried out in males, whose evidence is being used to determine the treatment of females? If gene arrays are capturing individualized genomes, don't we want to understand how the expression of these different genes might vary depending on whether we carry one or two X chromosomes as well as how the expression varies with experience? Will the findings of basic science translate successfully to the clinic if they are not understood in the context of female and male biology?

Measuring biological sex can lead to understanding differences both person-to-person and moment-to-moment, leading to a better understanding of not only an individual's reproductive capacity but also his or her health/illness as well as sense/presentation of self. Some biological sex differences will make a difference; others may exist to ensure that there is no difference (de Vries, 2004).

From studying biological sex we are learning that perhaps the most important shaper of biology is not biological—rather it is experience external to the body that in turn shapes the corporeal body. Thus using these methods and paradigms to elucidate the role that biological sex plays in behavior, health, and disease, it is critical to take into account that the lives and biologies of females and males are different. Chromosomes, developmental history, the expectations of oneself and of others, and life experience can literally produce and sculpt the body's biology and thus belie the simplicity of taking sex to mean only phenotype and/or genotype—female or male. In order to measure biological sex, it may be necessary to use methods aimed at understanding the social in tandem with the biological. Quantitative pain questionnaires given without an understanding of social meanings of pain may not capture an understanding of an individual's pain experience (Dworkin et al., 2009). Thus there really is no "pure" measure of biological sex. Much biological sex is often the *bodily manifestation of environmental/social influences.*[2]

Finally, all of these measures reveal that even biological sex is mutable.

To the great relief of many of us, early experience is not necessarily destiny, and understanding the [neuro]biological mechanisms of intervention remains a vital challenge. (Sapolsky, 2004, p. 792)

References

Agate, R. J., Grisham, W., Wade, J., Mann, S., Wingfield, J., Schanen, C., et al. (2003). Neural, not gonadal, origin of brain sex differences in a gynandromorphic finch. *Proceedings of the National Academy of Sciences, 100*(8), 4873–4878.

Arizona Center for Education and Research on Therapeutics. (2009). *QT drug lists by risk groups.* Retrieved December 15, 2010, from http://www.azcert.org/medical-pros/drug-lists/drug-lists.cfm

Beach, F. A. (1941). Female mating behaviour shown by male rats after administration of testosterone propionate. *Endocrinology, 29*(3), 409–412.

Beach, F. A., & Rasquin, P. (1942). Masculine copulatory behaviour in intact and castrated female rats. *Endocrinology, 31*(4), 393–409.

Becker, J. B., Arnold, A. P., Berkley, K. J., Blaustein, J. D., Eckel, L. A., Hampson, E., et al. (2005). Strategies and methods for research on sex differences in brain and behaviour. *Endocrinology, 146*(4), 1650–1673.

---

[2]This is a point well covered in Chapter 3 of this volume by the discussion of how stress affects the body in general, and how environment affects the strength of bones in particular.

Becker, J. B., Bweklwy, K. J., Geary, N., Hampson, E., Herman, J. P., & Young, E. A. (2008). *Sex differences in the brain: From genes to behaviour.* Oxford, UK: Oxford University Press.

Belcher, S. M. (2008). Rapid signaling mechanisms of estrogens in the developing cerebellum. *Brain Research Reviews, 57*(2), 481–492.

Bellem, A., Meiyappan, S., Romans, S., & Einstein, G. (2011). *Measuring estrogens and progestins in humans: An overview of methods.* Manuscript in preparation.

Beyer, C., Eusterschulte, B., Pilgrim, C., & Reisert, I. (1992). Sex steroids do not alter sex differences in tyrosine hydroxylase activity of dopaminergic neurons in vitro. *Cell and Tissue Research, 270*(3), 547–552.

Borkhoff, C. M., Hawker, G. A., Kreder, H. J., Glazier, R. H., Mahomed, N. N., & Wright, J. G. (2008). The effect of patients' sex on physicians' recommendations for total knee arthroplasty. *Canadian Medical Association Journal, 178*(6), 681–687.

Buonomano, D. V., & Merzenich, M. M. (1998). Cortical plasticity: From synapses to maps. *Annual Review of Neurosciences, 21,* 149–186.

Bushnell, C. D. (2008). Stroke and the female brain. *Nature Clinical Practice Neurology, 4,* 22–33.

Charchar, F. J., Tomaszewski, M., Strahorn, P., Champagne, B., & Dominiczak, A. F. (2003). Y is there a risk to being male? *Trends in Endocrinology and Metabolism, 14*(4), 163–168.

Clarkson, R. S., Petrovic, M., Einstein, G., & Stewart, D. (2009). Mood and the menstrual cycle: A review of prospective studies. *Psychotherapy and Psychosomatics.* Manuscript submitted for publication.

Craft, R. M., Mogil, J. S., & Aloisi, A. M. (2004). Sex differences in pain and analgesia: The role of gonadal hormones. *European Journal of Pain, 8*(5), 397–411.

de Vries, G. J. (2004). Minireview: Sex differences in adult and developing brains: Compensation, compensation, compensation. *Endocrinology, 145*(3), 1063–1068.

de Vries, G. J., Rissman, E. F., Simerly, R. B., Yang, L. Y., Scordalakes, E. M., Auger, C. J., et al. (2002). A model system for study of sex chromosome effects on sexually dimorphic neural and behavioral traits. *Journal of Neuroscience, 22*(20), 9005–9014.

Diamond, M., & Sigmundson, H. K. (1997). Sex reassignment at birth: Long-term review and clinical implications. *Archives of Pediatrics & Adolescent Medicine, 151*(3), 298–304.

Dulac, C., & Kimchi, T. (2008). Neural mechanisms underlying sex-specific behaviours in vertebrates. *Current Opinion in Neurobiology, 17*(6), 675–683.

Dworkin, R. H., Turk, D. C., Revicki, D. A., Harding, G., Coyne, K. S., Peirce-Sandner, S., et al. (2009). Development and initial validation of an expanded and revised version of the Short-Form McGill Pain Questionnaire (SF-MPQ-2). *Pain, 144*(1–2), 35–42.

Einstein, G. (2007). *Sex and the brain.* Cambridge, MA: MIT Press.

Einstein, G. (2008). From body to brain: Considering the neurobiological effects of female genital cutting. *Perspectives in Biology and Medicine, 51*(1), 84–97.

Einstein, G. (2011). Situated neuroscience: Elucidating a biology of diversity. In R. Bluhm, H. Maibom, and A. J. Jacobson (Eds.), *Neurofeminism: Issues at the intersection of feminist theory and cognitive science.* New York: Palgrave Macmillan.

El-Khayat, H. A., Soliman, N. A., Tomoum, H. Y., Omran, M. A., El-Wakad, A. S., & Shatla, R. H. (2008). Reproductive hormonal changes and catamenial pattern in adolescent females with epilepsy. *Epilepsia, 49*(9), 1619–1626.

Fausto-Sterling, A. (2000). *Sexing the body: Gender politics and the construction of sexuality.* New York: Basic Books.

Fish, E. N. (2008). The X-files in immunity: Sex-based differences predispose immune responses. *Nature Reviews Immunology, 8*(9), 737–744.

Gilbert, F. S. (2006). *Developmental biology.* Sunderland, MA: Sinauer Associates.

Gorman, J. M. (2006). Gender differences in depression and response to psychotropic medication. *Gender Medicine, 3*(2), 93–109.

Grosz, E. (1994). *Volatile bodies: Toward a corporeal feminism.* Bloomington: Indiana University Press.

Harkin, T., Snowe, O. J., Mikulski, B. A., & Waxman, H. A. (2001). *Drug safety: Most drugs withdrawn in recent years had greater health risks for women.* Retrieved December 15, 2010, from http://www.gao.gov/new.items/d01286r.pdf

Harris, G. (1937). The induction of ovulation in the rabbit, by electrical stimulation of the hypothalmo-hypophysial mechanism. *Proceedings of the Royal Society B, 612,* 374–394.

Hayden, E. C. (2010). Sex bias blights drug studies. *Nature, 464,* 332–333.

Herzog, A. G. (2007). Neuroactive properties of reproductive steroids. *Headache, 47*(Suppl. 2), S68–S78.

Humphries, K. H., Pu, A., Gao, M., Carere, R. G., & Pilote, L. (2008). Angina with "normal" coronary arteries: Sex differences in outcomes. *American Heart Journal, 155*(2), 375–381.

Johnson, J., Greaves, L., & Repta, R. (2007). *Better science with sex and gender: A primer for health research.* Vancouver, BC, Canada: Women's Health Research Network.

Kimchi, T., Xu, J., & Dulac, C. (2007). A functional circuit underlying male sexual behaviour in the female mouse brain. *Nature, 448*(7157), 1009–1014.

Kitwood, T., & Bredin, K. (1992). Towards a theory of dementia care: Personhood and well-being. *Ageing & Society, 12,* 269–287.

Krystal, A. D. (2004). Depression and insomnia in women. *Clinical Cornerstone, 6*(Suppl. 1B), S19–S28.

Labad, J., Menchon, J. M., Alonso, P., Segalas, C., Jimenez, S., & Vallejo, J. (2005). Female reproductive cycle and obsessive-compulsive disorder. *Journal of Clinical Psychiatry, 66*(4), 428–435.

Lin, A. E., Neri, G., Hughes-Benzie, R., & Weksberg, R. (1999). Cardiac anomalies in the Simpson-Golabi-Behmel syndrome. *American Journal of Medical Genetics, 83*(5), 378–381.

Liu, P., Death, A., & Handelsman, D. J. (2003). Androgen and cardiovascular disease. *Endocrine Reviews, 24*(3), 313–340.

Lupien, S. J., Maheu, F., Tu, M., Fiocco, A., & Schramek, T. E. (2007). The effects of stress and stress hormones on human cognition: Implications for the field of brain and cognition. *Brain and Cognition, 65*(3), 209–237.

McEwen, B. S., Davis, P. G., Parsons, B., & Pfaff, D. W. (1979). The brain as a target for steroid hormone action. *Annual Review of Neuroscience, 2,* 65–112.

McEwen, B. S., & Goy, R. (1980). Sex differences in behaviour: Rodents, birds, and primates. In B. S. McEwen and R. Goy (Eds.), *Sexual differentiation of* the brain: Based on a work session of the Neurosciences Research Program (pp. 13–58). Cambridge, MA: MIT Press.

Miller, V. M., & Hay, M. (2004). *Principles of sex-based differences in physiology.* Amsterdam: Elsevier.

Modney, B. K., & Hatton, G. I. (1990). Motherhood modifies magnocellular neuronal interrelationships in functionally meaningful ways. In N. A. Krasnegor & R. S. Bridges (Eds.), *Mammalian parenting: Biochemical, neurobiological, and behavioral determinants* (pp. 305–323). New York: Oxford University Press.

Nieminen, M. S., Harjola, V. P., Hochadel, M., Drexler, H., Komajda, M., Brutsaert, D., et al. (2008). Gender related differences in patients presenting with acute heart failure: Results from EuroHeart Failure Survey II. *European Journal of Heart Failure, 10*(2), 140–148.

Nottebohm, F. (1980). Testosterone triggers growth of brain vocal control nuclei in adult female canaries. *Brain Research, 189*(2), 429–436.

Nottebohm, F., & Arnold, A. P. (1976). Sexual dimorphism in vocal control areas of the songbird brain. *Science, 194*(4261), 211–213.

Pardue, M. L., & Wizemann, T. M. (2001). *Exploring the biological contributions to human health: Does sex matter?* [Institute of Medicine report]. Washington, DC: National Academy of Sciences Press.

Payne, J. L., Roy, P. S., Murphy-Eberenz, K., Weismann, M. M., Swartz, K. L., McInnis, M. G., et al. (2007). Reproductive cycle-associated mood symptoms in women with major depression and bipolar disorder. *Journal of Affective Disorders, 99*(1–3), 221–229.

Peterson, L. R., Soto, P. F., Herrero, P., Schechtman, K. B., Dence, C., & Gropler, R. J. (2007). Sex differences in myocardial oxygen and glucose metabolism. *Journal of Nuclear Cardiology, 14*(4), 573–581.

Phoenix, C. H., Goy, R. W., Gerall, A. A., & Young, W. C. (1959). Organizing action of prenatally administered testosterone propionate on the tissues mediating mating behaviour in the female guinea pig. *Endocrinology, 65,* 369–382.

Quiton, R. L., & Greenspan, J. D. (2007). Sex differences in endogenous pain modulation by distracting and painful conditioning stimulation. *Pain, 132*(Suppl. 1), S134–S149.

Raisman, G. (1997). An urge to explain the incomprehensible: Geoffrey Harris and the discovery of the neural control of the pituitary gland. *Annual Review of Neuroscience, 20,* 533–566.

Raisman, G., & Field, P. M. (1973). Sexual dimorphism in the neuropil of the preoptic area of the rat and its dependence on neonatal androgen. *Brain Research, 54,* 1–29.

Rapkin, A. J., Moatakef-Imani, M. B., & Rasgon, N. (2002). The clinical nature and formal diagnosis of premenstrual, postmpartum, and perimenopausal affective disorders. *Current Psychiatry Reports, 4,* 419–428.

Roberts, S. S. (2008). A woman's disease. *Diabetes Forecast, 61*(2), 48–49.

Rubinow, D. R., & Schmidt, P. J. (2006). Gonadal steroid regulation of mood: The lessons of premenstrual syndrome. *Frontiers in Neuroendocrinology, 27,* 210–216.

Sapolsky, R. M. (2004). Mothering style and methylation. *Nature Neuroscience, 7*(8), 791–792.

Seda, O., Tremblay, J., Gaudet, D., Brunelle, P. L., Gurau, A., Merlo, E., et al. (2008). Systematic, genome-wide, sex-specific linkage of cardiovascular traits in French Canadians. *Hypertension, 51*(4), 1156–1162.

Short, R. V., & Balaban, E. (1994). *The difference between the sexes.* Cambridge, UK: Cambridge University Press.

Smith, E. P., Boyd, J., Frank, G. R., Takahashi, H., Cohen, R. M., Specker, B., et al. (1994). Estrogen resistance caused by a mutation in the estrogen-receptor gene in a man. *New England Journal of Medicine, 331*(16), 1056–1061.

Spencer, J. L., Waters, E. M., Romeo, R. D., Wood, G. E., Milner, T. A., & McEwen, B. S. (2008). Uncovering the mechanisms of estrogen effects on hippocampal function. *Frontiers in Neuroendocrinology, 29*(2), 219–237.

Vulink, N. C., Denys, D., Bus, L., & Westenberg, H. G. (2006). Female hormones affect symptom severity in obsessive-compulsive disorder. *International Clinical Psychopharmacology, 21*(3), 171–175.

Weaver, I. C., Cervoni, N., Champagne, F. A., D'Alessio, A. C., Sharma, S., Seckl, J. R., et al. (2004). Epigenetic programming by maternal behaviour. *Nature Neuroscience, 7*(8), 847–854.

Woolsey, R. L., & Singh, S. N. (2000). *Arrhythia treatment and therapy: Evaluation of clinical trial evidence.* New York: Marcel Dekker.

Xerri, C., Stern, J. M., & Merzenich, M. M. (1994). Alterations of the cortical representation of the rat ventrum induced by nursing behaviour. *Journal of Neuroscience, 14*(3, Part 2), 1710–1721.

Xu, J., Taya, S., Kaibuchi, K., & Arnold, A. P. (2005). Spatially and temporally specific expression in mouse hippocampus of Usp9x, a ubiquitin-specific protease involved in synaptic development. *Journal of Neuroscience Research, 80*(1), 47–55.

Xu, J., Watkins, R., & Arnold, A. P. (2006). Sexually dimorphic expression of the X-linked gene *Eif2s3x* mRNA but not protein in mouse brain. *Gene Expression Patterns, 6*(2), 146–155.

Part III

Sex and Gender Research

This section displays an array of research methods where sex and/or gender have been incorporated into research design. The topics range from investigating sexual health among youth, to tobacco use patterns within family systems, to assessing the impact of sex and gender on mortality patterns in urban and rural populations. These examples are not an exhaustive set, but rather serve to illustrate various modes of and issues in operationalizing gender under a range of methods.

The examples range from fieldwork to secondary analysis to discourse analysis. Some of these examples are using more standard methods, such as fieldwork, as described in the contribution by Chabot and Shoveller (see Chapter 6). They describe the impact of gender on fieldwork methods, a well-established approach that includes participation and observation,

among other techniques. Factors such as the gender and social position of the researcher as well as the features of the topic under consideration affect the prospects of discovering new knowledge. They also discuss the conundrum of getting research participants to discuss gender when they may not want to engage with this concept, or perhaps do not understand it or its relevance.

Others are less typical methods, less often used in health research, such as visual methods as illustrated by Haines-Saah, and Oliffe (see Chapter 7). In this example, Haines-Saah and Oliffe describe the investigation of smoking using photographs along with narrative interviews with two separate groups, young women and new fathers. The presentation of self is transmitted through smoking postures of men and women—gendered issues that reflect power, place, identity, and the body. In these two studies, the interviews combined with photographs elicited captions and discussion from two very different groups, surfacing rich data about gender and smoking practices. Again, these researchers comment on the elusive nature of gender in discussion with participants such as these.

Others are secondary analyses, such as the contribution by Ostry and Slaunwhite, looking at a standard data set for a second time, in order to investigate sex- and gender-related issues (see Chapter 8). Ostry and Slaunwhite identify secondary analysis as an opportunity to reconsider extant data, but they also identify the limits placed on secondary analyses by the original design. In this example, the authors reanalyze with a focus on seeking data on age, gender, and place, thereby introducing a set of intersectional variables into a secondary look at a data set. This study presents a series of combinations of variables for analysis, illustrating the impact of geographical location on mortality for both males and females, and reframing the need for prevention and policy initiatives.

Next, Gough and Robertson investigate talk and text surrounding health issues, speculating that these interpretations and reflections of health are also gendered phenomena (see Chapter 9). They illustrate these points through the content analysis of health promotion materials and media reports on topics such as alcohol use, obesity, and hormone replacement therapy. They illustrate how gender and gendered assumptions, as well as gendered identities, mediate messages derived through text. The insights derived from these analyses are directly relevant to knowledge translation.

There are also examples of investigating various aspects of gender itself, such as gender relations. Bottorff and colleagues discuss approaches to investigating gender relations in health research, using examples from a multipart study examining tobacco reduction and use among families expecting babies or with young children (see Chapter 10). Seeing these processes of tobacco reduction as dynamic, gendered phenomena allows for, and requires, gender-sensitive approaches. For example, interviews of the female and male partners in the families were done separately, to limit the influence of gendered power dynamics. A sensitivity to gendered power relations and the potential for escalating tensions in heterosexual couples with respect to tobacco reduction turned out to be critical in carrying out this research.

Finally, Toner and colleagues describe the development of a scale for measuring gender role socialization (see Chapter 11). This scale is designed to investigate the internalization of gender roles as a way of explaining some mental health conditions in women. The scale can also be used to assess the extent of internalization as a way of assessing women as a precursor to psychotherapy. While recognizing that binary and dichotomous conceptualizations of gender are limited, these researchers argue that there is still a lived experience attached to these binaries that can be measured. All of these examples interrogate either the investigation of gender in a health issue or the insertion of gendered considerations in methods, or both. All of these examples contribute to the development of more and better methods in gender, sex, and health research.

Fieldwork 6

Observations and Interviews

Cathy Chabot
Jean Shoveller

Fieldwork involves the collection of data within a particular community, culture, or population using a variety of research techniques. By conducting research in a natural, rather than controlled, setting (e.g., a university laboratory), fieldwork provides researchers with opportunities to observe and record information about everyday life events. During fieldwork, researchers observe community members in the places where they live, work, study, and carry out other day-to-day activities, and they frequently invite community members to provide insights about the social relations and interactions between themselves and their physical, cultural, and social environments (Sobo, 2009). Fieldwork provides opportunities for the researcher to bridge between an entirely etic perspective (i.e., that of an outsider) and a more emic position (i.e., that of an insider) in order to challenge existing presumptions and to develop new insights into a research area. Fieldwork affords researchers glimpses into the ways in which community members understand, define, and classify various aspects of their social and physical worlds (Wolcott, 2005). Fieldwork provides exposure to the community members' perspectives (including the gendered nature of those perspectives) so as to facilitate the development of more nuanced and "grounded" interpretations of the research problem, acknowledging that such interpretations are inextricably linked with their own social position as researchers or outsiders (Thomas, 1993; Wolf, 1996).

The effect of gender on the dynamics of insider–outsider relations in fieldwork is complex. For example, in communities where women are regarded as having primary or sole responsibility for contraception, researchers can use fieldwork to observe community members' behavior that is rooted in their perceptions about the ways in which biological sex, gender roles, and other sociocultural forces affect contraceptive practices. Clearly, it would be naive to assume that researchers who are women are necessarily more adept at bridging the etic–emic perspectives in such fieldwork settings. Rather, what fieldwork can offer is the opportunity to be exposed to situations where one can observe and problematize the roles of gender as well as other crucial aspects of social relations within such settings that may simultaneously affect the insider–outsider interface (e.g., ethnicity, socioeconomic status).

First developed by anthropologists and sociologists in the 19th and 20th centuries, traditional definitions of fieldwork emphasized researchers spending long periods of time (typically a year or more) living with a community as well as observing and participating in community members' daily lives (Delamont, 2004; Fetterman, 1998; Mason, 1996). While fieldwork techniques are often associated with ethnography, it is important to note that researchers from other disciplines, such as health sciences, have adapted these techniques for use in a variety of methodologies (e.g., grounded theory, phenomenology, interpretive description, ethnoscience) (Bernard, 2006; Wolcott, 2005).

This chapter focuses on the use of qualitative fieldwork methods in gender and health research. We introduce a variety of fieldwork strategies and discuss their benefits and challenges. Drawing on examples from our own research related to youth sexual health, we compare naturalistic and participant observational techniques, and describe particular observational and interview approaches. Key questions are posed to guide the use of fieldwork in gender and health research. We also describe how "entry," standpoint, and power relations can affect fieldwork. In closing, we discuss innovations in fieldwork and address some strengths and limitations associated with the use of fieldwork in gender and health research, again drawing on examples from our program of research on sexual health.

Fieldwork Techniques in Sex, Gender, and Health Research

OBSERVATIONAL STRATEGIES AND TECHNIQUES

The use of *naturalistic observation* during fieldwork (Sobo, 2009) provides opportunities to develop nuanced, contextualized understandings of the research topic, although such observations do not give a *complete* picture of people's beliefs, experiences, and social relations. *Direct observation*, in which researchers observe people without actively participating or interacting with them (Yin, 1998), can be conducted in two ways: *reactive observations*, where those who are being observed are aware of what the researcher is doing, and *nonreactive observations*, conducted without the knowledge of those who are being observed (Bernard, 2006). The use of nonreactive observations raises questions about deception and the observed individuals' rights to privacy and informed consent (Bernard, 2006; Wolcott, 2005). We exclude nonreactive observation from all of our youth sexual health research because we believe it is important to inform potential participants and offer them the choice of whether to participate.

In a study examining youth's experiences with sexually transmitted infection (STI) testing services, we conducted 23 direct observations in 10 youth sexual health clinics in British Columbia, Canada (Goldenberg, Shoveller, Koehoorn, & Ostry, 2008; Shoveller et al., 2009). Our observations were directed by detailed guidelines (Cresswell, 1994) developed at the outset of the study and subsequently revised based on feedback from research team members to provide greater clarity and detail where necessary (see Table 6.1). The observation guidelines covered a range of topics, from providing physical descriptions of the clinic and the surrounding neighborhood to observations about who the researcher saw in the clinic as well as people's behaviors and interactions in the waiting area. The guidelines also reminded researchers to think reflexively about how perceptions and interpretations of what was observed are influenced by sociocultural factors of gender, age, ethnicity, and sexuality, as well as personal experiences. Researchers were encouraged to reflect on how the interactions between their behaviors and feelings and those being observed might influence what observations were recorded and represented in field notes as well as their subsequent interpretations (Thomas, 1993).

Successfully gaining *entry* (e.g., building rapport in order to be permitted to observe a community's social interactions and/or to participate in those interactions) is one of the most important steps in conducting fieldwork. One common approach is to work with community members who agree to act as intermediaries between the community and the research team (Adler & Adler, 2001; Oliffe, 2010). In studies related to youth sexual health, we have been able to establish good working relationships with many agencies and groups including youth health care workers and social services providers. However, we have encountered difficulties recruiting young men, a challenge cited by other researchers (Butera, 2006; Oliffe & Mróz, 2005). Some young men have said that they are uncomfortable engaging in our studies on sexual health because of gender (and age) differences between them and our female research team members, while others said that our recruitment materials were not appealing. They were also reluctant to volunteer for a study about sexual health. Using community members or gatekeepers who work with young men (e.g., teachers, youth center workers) can facilitate recruitment. The gender of the gatekeeper may have an impact on recruitment. For example, in our studies related to youth sexual health, we have found that it is easier to recruit women than men.

Table 6.1   Guidelines for Site Visit Observation

Description	Neighborhood	*Surrounding businesses* *"Type" of area* *Cleanliness* *Traffic (e.g., buses? cars? people?)*
	Clinic site	*Size* *Décor (e.g., paint, flooring, wall hangings, plants, extras)* *Reading materials (e.g., types of magazines, books, pamphlets, ads) and appearance (e.g., new, well-used)* *Cleanliness* *Lighting* *Overall impressions (e.g., comfortable, shabby, clinical, nice energy)* *Operation (e.g., hours of operation, number of staff, types of clients)*
	Staff	*Verbal and nonverbal communication (e.g., with other staff and clients, with researcher)* *Appearance (e.g., age, gender, ethnicity, dress)* *Overall impressions (e.g., do they create a friendly atmosphere?)* *Roles/procedures (e.g., what does the receptionist/doctor/nurse do?)* *Power dynamics (among staff and/or with clients)*
	Clients	*Verbal and nonverbal communication (e.g., with staff and other clients, with researcher)* *Appearance (e.g., age, gender, ethnicity, dress)* *Overall impressions (e.g., do they seem comfortable? nervous?)* *Did any clients take any pamphlets/info sheets that were in the waiting area? Were they given any pamphlets/info sheets by staff?*

What the observer did during the site visit	Did you take in the surrounding area?
	How long were you there?
	What were your interactions with others (i.e., staff, clients)?
	How do you think you were perceived?
Reflexivity: your interpretations of how you perceived those you observed and interviewed. How did you interpret observable cues that might give you insight into their perceptions? How might your behavior and feelings affect your interpretations of what you observed?	Body language—self and others
	Specific factors that might have affected (positively or negatively) your interpretations of what you observed. How do you think others perceived you?
Take home	Were you given anything to take home?
	Did you take any pamphlets or other information that were not given to you by someone?
Follow-up	What to do next time
	People to contact
	Ideas for interview questions, coding
Photos/sketches	Provide a short written description with each photo. Indicate where each photo was taken and what it is, why you took the photo, and its potential importance to the study.
	Draw a "map" of the clinic space (e.g., layout of clinic, relative size of rooms, doorways and windows).

Source: Adapted from guidelines used for our study "Sex, Gender and Place: An Analysis of Youth's Experiences With STI Testing," funded by the Canadian Institutes of Health Research. See Shoveller, Johnson, et al., 2007.

We have used respondent-driven sampling techniques (e.g., asking women to refer their male partners) as an effective way to recruit men (Heckathorn, 1997; Oliffe & Mróz, 2005; Salganik & Heckathorn, 2004).

In preparing to launch our study on young women's and men's experiences with STI testing, we considered how we (being a team of four female researchers and one male researcher) would negotiate the etic–emic continuum during fieldwork. Having previously reviewed statistics that elucidated the fact that most staff, clients, and volunteers at the clinics included in our study were female, we surmised that the women on our research team would "fit" relatively seamlessly into the fieldwork setting, and that the experience of our one male researcher might be different. We also designed the staffing for our study team so that interview participants could be offered the choice to be interviewed by either a woman or a man.

What our fieldwork experience revealed in actuality was that our genders, although important considerations, were only one of many features that were influential in producing the set of social relations that we cocreated and observed at the clinics. Our primarily female research team experienced a fairly smooth "entry" into most clinic settings, although we felt more connected and welcomed in some than others (e.g., it was especially challenging to integrate into the very small and rural clinics, where the presence of any "stranger"—woman or man—was easy to note). Moreover, because we were required by our university ethics board to clarify to all of the people we encountered during our observational work that we were researchers (not staff, volunteers, or clients), our entire team was firmly established as outsiders—albeit outsiders who were by and large welcomed to see and do tasks that were normally performed only by insiders (e.g., filing, booking follow-up appointments).

During clinic observations, we introduced ourselves to clients after they sat down in the waiting area, explained what we were doing, and invited them to contact us if they wished to participate in an individual interview at a later date. In clinic waiting rooms and reception areas, we recorded the ratio of women to men using clinic services and whether they were alone or accompanied by a partner, friend, or family member, and we observed the dynamics between service providers and youth according to their gender and other social positions. Outside of clinic operating hours, we spoke informally with health care providers about their experiences providing STI testing, and the policies and practice guidelines regarding their work. Service providers gave us tours of their clinics (after closing to avoid disrupting client services) and permitted us to photograph clinic spaces.

The tours and photographs provided opportunities to observe the degree to which clinic décor and design might be gendered. Most clinics featured stereotypical feminine décor (see Image 6.1), and pink and rose tones of paint and fabric were the norm; nearly all the posters and brochures in the waiting areas featured pregnancy or breast cancer (usually characterized as women's health issues). Service providers told us that they would like to see increases in the number of young male clients. However, few efforts were made to adapt décor in ways that might encourage more men to seek STI testing or other sexual health services. For example, some clinic receptionists, nurses, and physicians suggested that it would be useful to have health care providers of different genders on staff, men-only clinic hours, and clinic spaces decorated in ways that appeal to youth of different genders and sexualities—but few such changes had been implemented.

As we were curious to see how youth might react to the décor and design of clinic spaces, we shared photographs of clinic spaces with study participants in follow-up individual interviews. Many of them, particularly young men, told us that they would not feel comfortable seeking testing at clinics that they perceived to be overtly feminized spaces. This finding was shared with STI testing service providers at the end of our study (Shoveller, Johnson, et al., 2007; Shoveller et al., 2009).

Participant observation can be naturalistic whereby researchers participate in the activities of those they are observing (Wolcott, 2005). Researchers record detailed field notes about the environment and the content of informal conversations, along with notes about their interpretations. Researchers can obtain a more nuanced understanding of the perspectives and opinions of study participants by spending time in the field speaking with key informants (including community members identified by participants as experts in a particular area), observing the social structure and relations of the communities, and compiling comprehensive field notes and materials.

Image 6.1 STI Clinic Décor

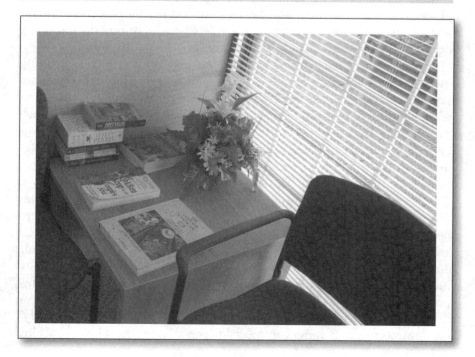

Recruitment for in-depth interviews can also be facilitated through fieldwork, and gender features in this process. For example, in our fieldwork, we have used purposive approaches to recruit samples that fit the purpose of our research questions. Because we are often interested in researching the ways in which our questions about youth sexual health intersect with gender, we spend a significant amount of time at the outset of our fieldwork to develop an appropriate sampling frame and recruitment strategy—one that attempts to reflect, where appropriate, the experiences of men and women—as well as diversity within those two broad (and potentially essentializing) characterizations of "gender." In our studies, we have found that it takes more time (in general) to recruit sufficient numbers of men/boys than women/girls (similar to a well-established pattern in studies that rely on surveys) (Fenton, Johnson, McManus, & Erens, 2001), but we also are interested in "moving beyond the binary" to recruit diverse samples that have the capacity to provide insights into an issue (e.g., STI testing) from various standpoints along the gender continuum. Our recruitment and other fieldwork strategies are developed in concert with the sampling framework and are tailored to each of those populations (e.g., working with community groups whose membership reflects the populations of interest, designing posters that are eye-catching to particular age-groups, ensuring our study brochures are available in both female and male washroom stalls). We also have found it helpful to be familiar with critiques of conventional research approaches (e.g., randomized clinical trials) and the ways in which they have failed to fully address gender (e.g., in terms of sampling bias as well as other forms of bias) (Iyer, Sen, & Ostlin, 2010; Ruiz-Cantero et al., 2007), which emphasize the importance of addressing gendered assumptions during study design and execution, including fieldwork.

In our youth sexual health studies, we were successful in recruiting interview participants after people had spoken with us informally and a rapport had been developed. This is particularly important when working with members of vulnerable groups, because many (although not all) such people may feel coerced to participate in light of power differentials between themselves and the researcher. As well, some people may be unfamiliar with their rights as study participants and therefore may not be likely to enact their right to refuse to participate (Leadbeater & Glass, 2006). Researchers need to take the necessary time to establish rapport, review study participants' rights, and wait for participants to consent before launching interviews during fieldwork. For example, during our Youth STI Testing Study (Shoveller, Johnson, et al., 2007; Shoveller et al., 2009), we conducted fieldwork at several youth sexual health clinics, including observations that we conducted at one particular clinic on many occasions. The clinic's nurse manager invited us to assist with administrative tasks while we conducted our observations. This included inventorying contraceptives, helping volunteers dispense birth control pills, packing up STI samples for shipment to the lab for testing, and assisting with filing. These activities provided us with opportunities to develop insights into what it could be like to work as a volunteer within the clinic and helped us to describe in more depth our interpretations of what we did and observed. Performing some workplace duties facilitated the development of more nuanced understandings of the clinic's policies and practices. From the observations and subsequent interviews, it became clear that the gendered use of clinical sexual health services reflects, in part, our society's dominant social mores (e.g., women are often expected to be the caretakers of sexual health), as well as prevailing norms within clinical practice that make women's bodies more likely to be examined via systematic, organized efforts (i.e., STI screening, annual gynecological exams).

In another study, we examined how the lives of young mothers (aged 15–25 years) are shaped by sociocultural conditions and policy structures in a northern British Columbian community (Chabot, Shoveller, Johnson, & Prkachin, 2010; Shoveller, Chabot, Johnson, & Prkachin, 2010). During this "Young Mums Study," we conducted seven 1-week fieldwork sessions over an 8-month period that included participant observation, in-depth semistructured and unstructured interviews, and focus groups with young mothers and their health and social service providers. This iterative design provided us with opportunities to analyze the data between each fieldwork session and guided subsequent data collection.

At the beginning of our fieldwork, we (a female professor and two female research staff) spent time "hanging out" at two alternative school programs and an at-risk parenting program for young mothers. We observed students', teachers', and other service providers' interactions in and around classes (e.g., mathematics, English, science). We also participated in program activities, such as parenting skills and cooking classes. We had frequent informal conversations with young mothers, family members, and staff at each site regarding our study, specific services offered, and personal parenting experiences. From these conversations we learned about the social relations within each site and how gender norms are enacted and challenged. Although we do not pretend to adopt completely emic perspectives (we are female researchers, not teen mothers or service providers), our fieldwork provided sufficient exposure to the study participants' perspectives so as to help us "ground" our interpretation of the data in what we understood to be participants' everyday realities.

Early in our fieldwork, most young mothers were hesitant to participate in interviews. As privileged, White, female adult researchers, we occupied a different social position than the young mothers. We were sometimes mistaken for service providers (a misperception we always corrected). These young women needed time to get to know us before they could begin to trust us and consider participating in the study. By "hanging out" at each site, the young mothers had many opportunities to get to know us and saw that we were genuinely interested in understanding their experiences.

Informal conversations helped us (and study participants) to negotiate the potential communication challenges that might have arisen from differences in our current life situations (e.g., our ages, academic achievements, perceived privileges and disadvantages). For example, participants often talked among themselves and with us about a party that they had attended or a new boyfriend one of them was seeing—common conversation topics for many teenagers. Perhaps the rapport that we developed with the young mothers was influenced by the fact that we (the researchers and study participants) were women—albeit women representing a range of femininities, cultural/ethnic identities, and socioeconomic status. We acknowledge that these important differences between the researchers and the participants affected the data collection and analysis during fieldwork (Ramzan, Pini, & Bryant, 2009; Reinharz, 1992). We suggest that the researcher–participant dynamics would have been different for a team of male researchers working in this setting, in part because our observations of the everyday experiences in these settings found that these settings do not generally feature men (e.g., fathers or other men were rarely observed at any of the sites). As well, during our fieldwork we noted that the mothers and service providers frequently (although not exclusively) characterized men, especially young fathers, in a negative light (e.g., failure to provide child support, being abusive). As well, issues of gendered power imbalances also were discussed openly (e.g., patriarchy within families, the job market), something that might have taken on a different dynamic in the presence of male researchers.

In the Young Mums Study, we also photographed and sketched characteristic features of the community's physical environment to help us understand how the spatial relations (e.g., distances between homes and services, availability of public transit) might affect young women and their families. We collected and analyzed a wide variety of media (e.g., photographs; newspaper articles; social service pamphlets and resources; videos about parenting, sex education, and drug use). This analysis provided background on the community's history, economy, services, and social relations, and further informed our understanding of the local culture. For example, our analysis of local social services identified a dearth of services specifically designed for young fathers. This finding was echoed by mothers and a few service providers, who commented that stereotypes of young fathers as "uninvolved or irresponsible" are in fact reinforced by a lack of services to help young men become more engaged with their children.

Interview Strategies and Techniques

Health researchers examining gender can employ a variety of interview approaches, including unstructured interviews, semistructured interviews, and focus groups. *Unstructured interviews* are often conducted during participant observation activities. In some circumstances, researchers may elect to use deception when conducting their research (e.g., "secret-shopper" studies of pharmacists' knowledge of and attitudes toward emergency contraception; Bennett, Petraitis, D'Anella, & Marcella, 2003). In situations where researchers wish to avoid deception, participants must understand that they are being interviewed, and what they say will be recorded and/or written down (Bernard, 2006). Although unstructured, "conversational" interviews afford more flexibility for participants to talk about an issue at length, researchers should have a clear plan of what they want to ask participants (Fontana & Frey, 2000). Based on our previous experience, it can be challenging to ask youth (or adults) to speak directly about "gender"—due to the somewhat esoteric nature of this concept. To address this issue during fieldwork (and particularly during in-depth interviews), we ask questions about the potentially gendered aspects of some very "concrete" experiences (e.g., seeking/using STI testing, locating a clinic and getting there; discussing results with partners, peers; seeking information online related to STI/HIV testing). During our interviews, we also prompt participants to describe how the activities in their daily lives might be influenced by factors within their social contexts that are linked with their gender (e.g., inequitable distribution of power and other resources). For example, we ask participants to address issues related to their previous use of STI testing services and invite them to begin to unpack how gender (e.g., gender stereotypes about who should bear most responsibility for contraception) may be incorporated and/or communicated during clinical interactions (e.g., differential expectations of their interactions when they are served by a female doctor vs. a male doctor).

The flexibility and informality of unstructured interviews can facilitate rich, ongoing, and sometimes far-ranging dialogue—rather than abbreviated responses to questions—when conducting sex and gender health research. Feminist sociologist Ann Oakley (2005) has argued that conventional interviewing techniques emphasizing impartiality reflect masculine values such as "objectivity, detachment, hierarchy and 'science' as an important cultural activity which take priority over people's more individualized concerns" (p. 221). By opening up interviews to reflect conversations, emphasizing that there are no right or wrong answers, and acknowledging the role of gender relations in interviews, the dynamics between Oakley and her participants may have enhanced the richness of her interview data. Such conversational approaches have likewise been found to work well in interviews with men in health research (Oliffe & Mróz, 2005; Shoveller, Knight, Johnson, Oliffe, & Goldenberg, 2010).

In our work, we have conducted unstructured individual interviews, most notably during the Young Mums Study while driving around the city accompanied by young mothers. During these "drive-around" interviews, we invited each young woman to give us a tour of and provide commentary about her city. Through this approach we learned about young mothers' interpretations of the physical, social, and cultural structures that feature in their lives. These interviews were audio-recorded and accompanied by field notes that included the tour route plotted on a city map. This enabled our research team to see the distance between the places they showed us while reading the young women's narratives about their city. The tours also afforded women opportunities to share their perspectives about the city including places such as schools they attended, where they lived or hung out, and the businesses and services they used. These tours reflect the interactions that the young women have with their communities. Perhaps some of the same places (and some different places) would have been highlighted during a tour with young fathers.

USING SEMISTRUCTURED INTERVIEWS DURING FIELDWORK

In researching youth sexual health, we regularly conduct in-depth *semistructured interviews* during fieldwork. This method (not exclusive to fieldwork) relies on an interview guide and framework, while affording some flexibility for both the researcher and the participant. The order or phrasing of questions may vary according to conversational flow, while still yielding data that can be compared across interviews (Kvale, 1996; Sobo, 2009).

Investigating gender through semistructured interviews can be challenging, particularly when participants do not understand or relate to these theoretical constructs. In research with adolescents regarding gender and marijuana use, for example, Haines, Johnson, Carter, and Arora (2009) found that most participants were unable or unwilling to talk about how patterns of marijuana use might be influenced by gender performance and social norms. In our interviews for the Youth STI Testing Study (Shoveller, Johnson, et al., 2007; Shoveller et al., 2009), we developed questions in non-academic language that helped us integrate gendered explanations about sex differences between young men's and women's testing experiences. These questions included how young women and men describe the physical aspects of their STI experiences (e.g., symptom expression, physical sensations associated with testing techniques) and what it means to undergo STI testing. We also wanted to understand how young women's and men's productions and practices around femininities and masculinities affected their STI testing experiences. Because gender is influenced by other social positions (Women's Health Bureau, Health Canada, 2003; Risman, 2004; Wolf, 1996), we asked each participant how his or her STI testing experience was affected by, or changed, his or her self-perception with regard to sexual orientation, gender identity, and ethnicity.

Listening to what participants say during interviews and observations is important, but paying close attention to *how* people talk about a particular issue also provides insight into the meaning and significance of their com-ments (Hill, 2005; Hutchinson, Marsaglio, & Cohan, 2002; Sobo, 2009). These narratives "are important not only because they offer an unmatched window into subjective experience, but also because they are part of the image people have of themselves" (Ochberg, in Hydén, 1997, p. 50). We can observe how people perform gender, as well as how structural forces rein-force or challenge gender norms, without asking specifically about gender (Datta, 2008; Emslie, Ridge, Ziebland, & Hunt, 2006). For example, during interviews, women are often more willing to share intimate feelings and details of their lives, while many men prefer to speak in an impersonal tone or portray themselves as experts on a topic (Coates, 2002, 2004). Also, par-ticipants often use gender-specific language to express gender. For example, a female clinician who participated in our Youth STI Testing Study explained that young women were less likely than men to arrive alone for testing. She said that girls "drag their friend in with them and [the friend then] says, 'Oh I think I'll get tested too.' . . . Girls come in gaggles [laughs]." While this clinician understood that young women preferred to visit the clinic in pairs or groups to provide moral support, her choice of language—"girls come in gaggles"—connotes a noisy group, and her laughter suggests dissatisfaction with this feminine parody and practice. This became clear later in the interview when she said that it takes up to an hour to counsel and test women (three times longer than it does for male clients), challeng-ing nurses' ability to see everyone within limited clinic hours.

The data that researchers are able to obtain can be influenced by their gender (Bye, 2009; Finch, 1984; Pini, 2005), perceived sexual orientation (Fields, 2007), and racial or ethnic identity (Archer, 2002; Lichtenstein, 2004). In some cases, it is helpful that researchers and study participants are of the same gender. For example, in our Young Mums Study, most participants told us they would not have been comfortable being inter-viewed by a man. In other instances, the inverse may be true. In our Youth STI Testing Study, many young men (but not all) told us that they pre-ferred to be interviewed by women because they perceived women as empathetic and less intimidating. Although they did not explicitly cite homophobia, many men hinted at their discomfort in talking with another man about sexual issues, suggesting that men (in general) would prefer to adopt an aura of bravado or to remain silent and stoic during their inter-actions with other men regarding sexual health issues.

Sex and gender differences between researchers and participants also can yield important insights into a research topic (Williams & Heikes, 1993). Pini (2005) experienced this while interviewing male farmers in Australia about the lack of female representation in farming associations. Her gender, young age, and research topic led participants to feel threatened and con-tributed to a heightened enactment of hegemonic masculinity by farmers during interviews. To better understand how participants perform gender, Pini notes that researchers "need to extend their proposed question for analysing gender and interviewing to 'Who is asking who about what and where?'" (p. 212). We suggest that, whenever possible, it is important to offer study participants the option to be interviewed by a female or male interviewer. Interviewers should also emphasize that there are no right or wrong answers to research questions and ensure that their body language is open and nonthreatening (Oliffe & Mróz, 2005). When writing field notes, researchers need to include reflections on how gender relations may affect the dynamics of the interview or observations and use these insights to inform future data collection and analysis (Hutchinson et al., 2002).

USING FOCUS GROUPS IN FIELDWORK

Focus group interviews are used in many types of studies, including those that employ fieldwork techniques. Focus groups are facilitated group discussions about a specific topic that can yield a range of responses about an issue when time or resources are limited (Bernard, 2006). Focus groups also offer opportunities to examine features of group interaction, as well as their verbal content/data. These social interactions help bring to our attention shared cultural norms, in addition to the ways in which people in focus groups may reify or contest gender norms and stereotypes (Hyde, Howlett, Brady, & Drennan, 2005; Sobo, 2009). In these ways, focus groups can produce data that would be less accessible without the interactions among group members.

Generally speaking, homogeneity among focus group participants (e.g., shared gender, ethnicity, occupation, or age) can foster relational dynamics (Hyde, Drennan, Howlett, & Brady, 2009; Krueger & Casey, 2000). For example, some researchers suggest women participants may feel uncomfortable or silenced when there are male focus group participants present (Burgess, 1996; Krueger & Casey, 2000), or that men may challenge women's comments more than those of other men (Kim & Motsei, 2002). However, mixed focus group interviews can produce a range of responses and provide researchers with opportunities to observe how gender norms compare, inform, and influence participants (Burgess, Harrison, & Maiteny, 1991; Sobo, 2009).

Focus group interviews can be both beneficial and challenging when doing health research. We have found them to have limited effectiveness because of the sensitive nature of much of our youth sexual health research. For example, in a study exploring young women's knowledge, attitudes, and experiences related to emergency contraception (EC) (Shoveller, Chabot, Soon, & Levine, 2007), we initially aimed to conduct 12 focus groups with approximately 60 participants. We limited our sample to women only because EC is rarely, if ever, sought by or dispensed to men. After weeks of recruiting, no women had volunteered; a number of service providers suggested that many young women, especially those from conservative social and cultural backgrounds, would be reluctant to discuss such sensitive issues in a focus group. We modified our data collection strategy so that women could choose to be interviewed individually or in a focus group, resulting in 40 individual semistructured interviews and three focus groups. To allow for comparisons between the data sets, interview schedules for both methods were as similar as possible.

When conducting qualitative interviews it is important to make detailed notes about the interview, its context, and any preliminary observations about the data. In some instances, it may not be possible to take notes during an interview because it is logistically impossible. Whether note taking is perceived as disruptive or as a cue to the study participants that the researcher values their statements is open to debate. A number of qualitative researchers have written at length about how to take notes during interviews and how to write field notes (see, for example, Bernard, 2006; Emerson, Fretz, & Shaw, 1995; Sobo, 2009). For a detailed list of what we recommend to include in your interview notes, see Table 6.2.

Table 6.2 Guidelines for Interview Notes

Description of where the interview took place	*Neighborhood or "type" of area (e.g., industrial, residential, poor, rich)*
	Cleanliness, size, décor of interview space (e.g., paint, flooring, wall hangings, plants, extras), lighting
	Overall impressions of the space
Summary of discussion with participant before, during, and after recording	*Discussions you had*
	General description of participant's appearance (e.g., age, ethnicity, dress)
	Overall impressions (e.g., does the participant seem comfortable? nervous?)
	Did the participant say anything in particular that stood out to you as very important and/or memorable?
	Did the participant give you any feedback on the interview process and/or materials that you gave her or him?
	How long were you there?
	Did you have any interactions with others while at the interview location?
	How do you think you were perceived by the participant and/or any others you encountered at the interview location?

(Continued)

Table 6.2 (Continued)

Reflexivity: your interpretations of how you perceived those you interviewed. How did you interpret observable cues that might give you insight into their perceptions? How might your behavior and feelings affect your interpretations of the data?	*Body language—self and others*
	Specific factors that might have affected (positively or negatively) your interpretations of what you observed and discussed in the interview. How do you think the participant perceived you?
Follow-up	*Are there any interview questions that might need revision, any interview questions that worked particularly well, or any new questions that should also be asked?*
	If you interviewed a youth, is she or he interested in doing a follow-up interview?
	Other people to contact for an interview (e.g., a particular service provider that a participant mentioned in the interview who might be worth interviewing as well)
	Preliminary ideas for coding the data

Source: Adapted from guidelines used for our study "Sex, Gender and Place: An Analysis of Youth's Experiences With STI Testing," funded by the Canadian Institutes of Health Research. See Shoveller, Johnson, et al., 2007.

Additional Considerations When Conducting Fieldwork

Before embarking on a fieldwork-based study, there are a number of questions that researchers should consider. First is feasibility. How much time and money do you have available for this study? If you have limited or no funding for your project, fieldwork may not be a viable method. Fieldwork requires an investment of time, which in many cases also entails financial resources (e.g., salary, travel expenses). Second, are you prepared to negotiate entry and explore potentially provocative experiences and situations? For example, conducting observations in youth clinics can provide opportunities to see discordance between what youth say they want and what service providers are prepared to deliver—which means that the researcher must carefully and openly negotiate these kinds of situations. Third, how will you acknowledge and honestly negotiate with study participants the complexities of power relations—which are highly gendered—that may arise during fieldwork (Canadian Institutes of Health Research, Natural Sciences & Engineering Research Council of Canada, & Social Sciences and Humanities Research Council of Canada, 1998 [see 2005 update]; Chabot et al., 2010; Leadbeater & Glass, 2006)? Last, what may seem like mundane, practical issues also need to be considered and planned for prior to launching fieldwork. What are the most feasible modes of transportation to reach the fieldwork location? Where will you be able to conduct interviews? Will you have adequate privacy and a quiet space to conduct interviews? Can you realistically balance the commitments of fieldwork (e.g., immersion and substantial periods of time spent in the field) with competing demands for your time and attention (e.g., other work commitments)?

Conclusion

Some unique innovations are being used in fieldwork to investigate complex issues within a variety of health research contexts. For example, Cohen and colleagues (2000) developed a "broken window index" to measure health inequalities. Using census data and observations of neighborhood conditions (e.g., graffiti, quality of housing, abandoned cars) to examine the linkages between those conditions; i.e., "broken windows" and gonorrhea rates in New Orleans, Louisiana, the researchers found that the most physically deteriorated neighborhoods had higher rates of gonorrhea. This novel technique provided a more accurate indicator than poverty indexes that measured income, employment, and education level. Within the health services realm, Sobo (2009), an applied medical anthropologist, notes that "ethnographically informed" studies can yield valuable, reliable results within relatively short time frames (p. 74). Applying sex and gender analyses in health research can also advance health promotion efforts. For example, recent research by Bottorff and colleagues (2010) with heterosexual couples who recently became parents examined how the men's smoking habits and attempts to quit are influenced by gender relations. These findings can inform new health promotion programs that take into consideration how gender dynamics impact smoking cessation efforts (Bottorff et al., 2010).

Fieldwork offers researchers opportunities to immerse themselves in the social context of communities, while simultaneously engaging in reflexive practices that challenge or dislodge assumptions about the ways in which health status reflects experiences in the social world. Fieldwork techniques (and, in the case of participant observation, techniques that involve participatory interactions between researchers and communities to generate data) provide insights into the ways in which the physical world and the social world "get under the skin" to affect health. Although fieldwork is not intended to fully bridge the emic–etic divide, it can provide opportunities to see (and sometimes feel) the impacts of various social and structural forces that may differentially affect women and men.

One of the greatest strengths of fieldwork may also be viewed as a limitation by some: Fieldwork occurs in natural settings, not in controlled laboratory-like environments, rendering many positivist assumptions extraneous. What fieldwork offers is a "window" into the particular local context, with efforts to understand the links between localized observations and broader macro-level structures. In attempting to understand the particular, researchers also need to be cautious that they do not blindly apply their preconceived understandings of sex and gender (and their hypothesized impacts on health) without also considering how sex and gender themselves may be embedded in local context and enacted in particular ways in that locale.

References

Adler, P. A., & Adler, P. (2001). The reluctant respondent. In J. F. Gubrium & J. A. Holstein (Eds.), *Handbook of interview research: Context and method* (pp. 515–536). Thousand Oaks, CA: SAGE.

Archer, L. (2002). "It's easier that you're a girl and that you're Asian": Interactions of "race" and gender between researchers and participants. *Feminist Review, 72*(1), 108–132.

Bennett, W., Petraitis, C., D'Anella, A., & Marcella, S. (2003). Pharmacists' knowledge and the difficulty of obtaining emergency contraception. *Contraception, 68*(4), 261–267.

Bernard, H. R. (2006). *Research methods in anthropology: Qualitative and quantitative approaches* (4th ed.). Lanham, MD: AltaMira.

Bottorff, J. L., Oliffe, J. L., Kelly, M. T., Greaves, L., Johnson, J. L., Ponic, P., et al. (2010). Men's business, women's work: Gender influences and fathers' smoking. *Sociology of Health and Illness, 32*(4), 583–596. doi:10.1111/j.1467-9566.2009.01234.x

Burgess, J. (1996). Focusing on fear: The use of focus groups in a project for the Community Forest Unit, Countryside Commission. *Area, 28*(2), 130–135.

Burgess, J., Harrison, C. M., & Maiteny, P. (1991). Contested meanings: The consumption of news about nature conservation. *Media, Culture and Society, 13*(4), 499–519.

Butera, K. J. (2006). Manhunt: The challenge of enticing men to participate in a study on friendship. *Qualitative Inquiry, 12*(6), 1262–1282.

Bye, L. M. (2009). "How to be a rural man": Young men's performances and negotiations of rural masculinities. *Journal of Rural Studies, 25*(3), 278–288.

Canadian Institutes of Health Research, Natural Sciences & Engineering Research Council of Canada, & Social Sciences and Humanities Research Council of Canada. (1998). *Tri-council policy statement: Ethical conduct for research involving humans* [With 2000, 2002, and 2005 amendments]. Retrieved December 20, 2010, from http://www.pre.ethics.gc.ca/eng/archives/tcps-eptc/Default/

Chabot, C., Shoveller, J. A., Johnson, J. L., & Prkachin, K. (2010). Morally problematic: Young mothers' lives as parables about the dangers of sex. *Sex
Education: Sexuality, Society and Learning, 10*(2), 201–215.

Coates, J. (2002). *Men talk: Stories in the making of masculinities.* Oxford, UK: Basil
Blackwell.

Coates, J. (2004). *Women, men and language.* London: Pearson/Longman.

Cohen, D., Spear, S., Scribner, R., Kissinger, P., Mason, K., & Wildgen, J. (2000).
"Broken windows" and the risk of gonorrhea. *American Journal of Public
Health, 90*(2), 230–236.

Cresswell, J. W. (1994). *Research design: Qualitative and quantitative approaches.*
Thousand Oaks, CA: SAGE.

Datta, A. (2008). Spatialising performance: Masculinities and femininities in a
"fragmented" field. *Gender, Place and Culture, 15*(2), 189–204.

Delamont, S. (2004). Ethnography and participant observation. In C. Seale,
G. Gobo, J. F. Gubrium, & D. Silverman (Eds.), *Qualitative research practice*
(pp. 217–229). London: SAGE.

Emerson, R. M., Fretz, R. I., & Shaw, L. L. (1995). *Writing ethnographic fieldnotes.*
Chicago: University of Chicago Press.

Emslie, C., Ridge, D., Ziebland, S., & Hunt, K. (2006). Men's accounts of depression: Reconstructing or resisting hegemonic masculinity? *Social Science and
Medicine, 62*(9), 2246–2257.

Fenton, K. A., Johnson, A. M., McManus, S., & Erens, B. (2001). Measuring sexual
behaviour: Methodological challenges in survey research. *Sex Transmitting
Infections, 77,* 84–92.

Fetterman, D. M. (1998). *Ethnography step by step* (2nd ed.). Thousand Oaks, CA:
SAGE.

Fields, J. (2007). Knowing girls: Gender and learning in school-based sexuality
education. In N. Teunis & G. Herdt (Eds.), *Sexual inequalities and social justice* (pp. 67–85). Berkeley: University of California Press.

Finch, J. (1984). "It's great to have someone to talk to": The ethics and politics of
interviewing women. In C. Bell & H. Roberts (Eds.), *Social researching:
Politics, problems, practice* (pp. 70–87). London: Routledge.

Fontana, A., & Frey, J. H. (2000). The interview: From structured questions to
negotiated text. In N. K. Denzin & Y. S. Lincoln (Eds.), *Handbook of qualitative research* (2nd ed., pp. 645–672). Thousand Oaks, CA: SAGE.

Goldenberg, S., Shoveller, J. A., Koehoorn, M., & Ostry, A. (2008). Barriers to STI
testing among youth in a Canadian oil/gas community. *Health and Place,
14*(4), 718–729.

Haines, R. J., Johnson, J. L., Carter, C. I., & Arora, K. (2009). "I couldn't say, I'm
not a girl": Adolescents talk about gender and marijuana use. *Social Science
and Medicine, 68*(11), 2029–2036.

Heckathorn, D. D. (1997). Respondent-driven sampling: A new approach to the
study of hidden populations. *Social Problems, 44*(2), 174–199.

Hill, J. H. (2005). Finding culture in narrative. In N. Quinn (Ed.), *Finding culture
in talk: A collection of methods* (pp. 157–202). New York: Palgrave Macmillan.

Hutchinson, S., Marsaglio, W., & Cohan, M. (2002). Interviewing young men about sex
and procreation: Methodological issues. *Qualitative Health Research, 12*(1), 42–60.

Hyde, A., Drennan, J., Howlett, E., & Brady, D. (2009). Young men's vulnerability
in constituting hegemonic masculinity in sexual relations. *American Journal
of Men's Health, 3*(3), 238–251.

Hyde, A., Howlett, E., Brady, D., & Drennan, J. (2005). The focus group method: Insights from focus group interviews on sexual health with adolescents. *Social Science and Medicine, 61*(12), 2588–2599.

Hydén, L.-C. (1997). Illness and narrative. *Sociology of Health and Illness, 19*(1), 48–69.

Iyer, A., Sen, G., & Ostlin, P. (2010). Inequalities and intersections in health: A review of the evidence. In G. Sen & P. Ostlin (Eds.), *Gender equity in health: The shifting frontiers of evidence and action* (pp. 70–95). New York: Routledge.

Kim, J., & Motsei, M. (2002). "Women enjoy punishment": Attitudes and experiences of gender-based violence among PHC nurses in rural South Africa. *Social Science and Medicine, 54*(8), 1243–1254.

Krueger, R. A., & Casey, M. A. (2000). *Focus groups: A practical guide for applied research* (3rd ed.). Thousand Oaks, CA: SAGE.

Kvale, S. (1996). *An introduction to qualitative research interviewing.* Thousand Oaks, CA: SAGE.

Leadbeater, B., & Glass, K. (2006). Including vulnerable populations in community-based research: New directions for ethical guidelines and ethics research. In B. Leadbeater, E. Banister, C. Benoit, M. Jansson, A. Marshall, & T. Riecken (Eds.), *Ethical issues in community-based research with children and youth* (pp. 248–266). Toronto, ON, Canada: University of Toronto Press.

Lichtenstein, B. (2004). Caught at the clinic: African American men, stigma, and STI treatment in the Deep South. *Gender and Society, 18*(3), 369–388.

Mason, J. (1996). *Qualitative researching.* London: SAGE.

Oakley, A. (2005). Interviewing women: A contradiction in terms? In A. Oakley (Ed.), *The Ann Oakley reader* (pp. 217–231). London: Policy Press.

Oliffe, J. L. (2010). Bugging the cone of silence with men's health interviews. In S. Robertson & B. Gough (Eds.), *Men, masculinities and health: Critical perspectives* (pp. 67–91). London: Palgrave.

Oliffe, J., & Mróz, L. (2005). Men interviewing men about health and illness: Ten lessons learned. *Journal of Men's Health and Gender, 2*(2), 257–260.

Pini, B. (2005). Interviewing men: Gender and the collection and interpretation of qualitative data. *Journal of Sociology, 41*(2), 201–216.

Ramzan, B., Pini, B., & Bryant, L. (2009). Experiencing and writing indigeneity, rurality and gender: Australian reflections. *Journal of Rural Studies, 25*(4), 435–443.

Reinharz, S. (1992). *Feminist methods in social research.* Oxford, UK: Oxford University Press.

Risman, B. J. (2004). Gender as a social structure: Theory wrestling with activism. *Gender and Society, 18*(4), 429–450.

Ruiz-Cantero, M. T., Vives-Cases, C., Artazcoz, L., Delgado, A., del Mar García Calvente, M., Miqueo, C., et al. (2007). A framework to analyse gender bias in epidemiological research. *Journal of Epidemiology & Community Health, 61*(Suppl. II), ii46–ii53.

Salganik, M. J., & Heckathorn, D. D. (2004). Sampling and estimation in hidden populations using respondent-driven sampling. *Sociological Methodology, 34*(1), 193–239.

Shoveller, J., Chabot, C., Johnson, J. L., & Prkachin, K. (2010). "Ageing out": When policy and social orders intrude on the "disordered" realities of young mothers. *Youth & Society.* doi:10.1177/0044118X10386079

Shoveller, J., Chabot, C., Soon, J. A., & Levine, M. (2007). Identifying barriers to emergency contraception use among young women from various sociocultural groups in British Columbia, Canada. *Perspectives on Sexual and Reproductive Health, 39*(1), 13–20.

Shoveller, J., Johnson, J., Rosenberg, M., Greaves, L., Patrick, D., Oliffe, J. L., et al. (2007). *Seeking a better deal. Community report. Sex, gender & place: An analysis of youth's experiences with STI testing.* Vancouver, BC, Canada: Authors.

Shoveller, J. A., Johnson, J., Rosenberg, M., Greaves, L., Patrick, D., Oliffe J., et al. (2009). Youth's experiences with STI testing in four communities in British Columbia, Canada. *Sexually Transmitted Infections, 85*(5), 397–401.

Shoveller, J. A., Knight, R., Johnson, J., Oliffe, J., & Goldenberg, S. (2010). Not the swab! Young men's experiences with STI testing. *Sociology of Health & Illness, 32*(10), 57–73.

Sobo, E. J. (2009). *Culture and meaning in health services research: A practical field guide.* Walnut Creek, CA: Left Coast Press.

Thomas, J. (1993). *Doing critical ethnography.* Qualitative research methods series, 26. Newbury Park, CA: SAGE.

Williams, C. L., & Heikes, E. J. (1993). The importance of researcher's gender in the in-depth interview: Evidence from two case studies of male nurses. *Gender and Society, 7*(3), 280–291.

Wolcott, H. F. (2005). *The art of fieldwork* (2nd ed.). Walnut Creek, CA: AltaMira.

Wolf, D. L. (1996). Situating feminist dilemmas in fieldwork. In D. L. Wolf (Ed.), *Feminist dilemmas in fieldwork* (pp. 1–55). Boulder, CO: Westview Press.

Women's Health Bureau, Health Canada. (2003, June). *Exploring concepts of gender and health.* Ottawa, ON, Canada: Author. Retrieved December 20, 2010, from http://www.hc-sc.gc.ca/hl-vs/alt_formats/hpb-dgps/pdf/exploring_concepts.pdf

Yin, R. K. (1998). The abridged version of case study research: Design and method. In L. Bickman & D. J. Rog (Eds.), *Handbook of applied social research methods* (pp. 229–259). Thousand Oaks, CA: SAGE.

Visual Methods in Gender and Health Research

7

Rebecca J. Haines-Saah

John L. Oliffe

This chapter provides an introduction to using visual methodologies in contemporary research on gender and health. Drawing from photographic research projects with men and women who smoke, we demonstrate the unique possibilities of visual methods for unpacking and theorizing the gendered aspects of health practices. We show that, more than just a novel or creative methodology, engaging research participants with the visual has the potential to demonstrate complex theoretical ideas and provide material that illustrates seemingly elusive concepts in social research (Sweetman, 2009). We argue that while gender has an important visual dimension, it is important that the collection and interpretation of images take place within the context of a theoretical framework that accounts for the socially situated nature of gender and health practices. In addition to taking up current methodological debates within the arena of visual research and analysis in this chapter, we position our photographic work in tobacco control as an ethical intervention within a research context where the "smoker's view" has been frequently marginalized or absent, and as a way to engage broader theoretical questions regarding the social (re)production of identities, bodies, gender, and health.

Introduction to Visual Methods

Visual methods have long been used in the social sciences, often to complement or augment ethnographic methods such as naturalistic observation, or through historical analyses of photographic archives and other visual materials. In early modernist approaches photographs were taken exclusively by the ethnographer, a practice that privileged the researcher's point of view. Postcolonial approaches to anthropology and the interdisciplinary field of visual studies have problematized the relationship between photographer and subject, drawing attention to power relations and the need to be reflexive about constructions of the Other within photographs and visual media. Poststructuralist theorizing has also privileged a semiotic and discursive approach to seeing, with an emphasis on representation and symbolism rather than literal interpretations of the visual. Parallel to these theoretical and epistemological shifts in visual research, methodological developments have brought photography, video, and other visual methods into the arena of feminist, community-based, and participatory action research (PAR) strategies, placing cameras in the hands of "the researched" as a way to prioritize participants' experiences and ways of seeing. In addition to the goal of empowering research participants, visual findings are also seen as providing creative opportunities for knowledge translation and for communicating research results to policymakers and other stakeholders outside the academy (Rhodes & Fitzgerald, 2006; Wang, Burris, & Xiang, 1996).

Although visual methods can utilize drawings, photography, or video/film, the use of participant-driven photography has been prominent in health and illness research during the last two decades. This is largely owing to use of a method known as Photovoice, which was developed by Caroline Wang and colleagues at the University of Michigan School of Public Health as a participatory research method in working with women from marginalized communities (Wang & Burris, 1997). Photovoice is intended as a method to empower participants as public health advocates by providing cameras and photographic training that enables people to document a shared health and social issue, frequently at the community or neighborhood level. Photographers write explanatory, text-based captions for their images, and the resulting photographs are presented in a group discussion format where participants jointly select several images to publicly display and bring forward as part of an advocacy platform or community event. To this end, participant-generated photography is often used to address gender in relation to broader, social determinants of health such as women and communities experiencing homelessness (Killion & Wang, 2000; Klitzing, 2004; Wang, Cash, & Powers, 2000), poverty

(Duffy, 2008; Wang, Yi, Tao, & Carovano, 1998), and violence (Frohman, 2005; McIntyre, 2003).[1]

Outside of the goals of PAR, photographic methods are also used to engage participants in critical reflection about images at an individual level. Stemming from psychology, this use of photography in health research is informed by arts-based approaches to counseling and psychotherapy. In methods such as autodriving or photo-elicitation interviewing (PEI) (Harper, 1986; Heisley & Levy, 1991), the researcher engages with individual participants in a narrative interview about their photographs, as opposed to the photo discussion group that is a central feature of Photovoice. In gender and health research PEI is typically framed as a means for people to document intimate aspects of the illness experience not routinely shared with others, in particular their health care providers. For example, photography has been used to explore men's experience of living with prostate cancer (Oliffe, 2003, 2009; Oliffe & Bottorff, 2007), women's accounts of appearance change while undergoing chemotherapy (Frith & Harcourt, 2007), and transgendered men's access to health services (Hussey, 2006). Photographic methods are also used to access the experiences of persons that might be more engaged by visual as opposed to verbal forms of expression in research, such as children (Epstein, Stevens, McKeever, & Baruchel, 2006; Tinkler, 2008), youth (Allen, 2008; Strack, Magill, & McDonagh, 2004), and adults with intellectual disabilities (Booth & Booth, 2003; Jurkowski & Paul-Ward, 2007).

Visual methods such as Photovoice and other PAR using images are typically seen as more empowering alternatives to traditional health research as they seek to engage participants in the research process, thereby privileging their interpretations and experiences. However, the notion of empowerment through method alone—what Sweetman (2009) refers to as the "fetishization" of method—can be a problematic assumption, as photographs and the process of taking pictures for research can be decontextualized, without a theoretical framework for interpreting images. More often than not, photographs and other visual data are taken at face value, or interpreted by researchers post hoc. In PAR methods such as Photovoice, images are not typically coded or analyzed using any preexisting theoretical framework, other than the group process of participants selecting those images and issues that they think are the most critical to bring forward to a public audience (Killion & Wang, 2000). Scholars of the visual have been careful to problematize the issue of truth in photographs and to emphasize that how images are produced, viewed, and interpreted is very much context dependent and subjectively experienced (Becker, 1978; Clark-Ibanez, 2004;

---

[1]Photo-interviewing methods in social research are also known as photo-elicitation (Harper, 2002), reflexive photography (Berman, 2001), and photo novella (Wang & Burris, 1994).

Rhodes & Fitzgerald, 2006). While rich in detail, visual data, like interview texts, represent a temporal reality or one version of truth or "reality" (Becker, 1998; Harrison, 2002). Indeed, the content of photographs is not static; cultural interpretations of imagery are transient, and subject to shifts in meaning over time. Therefore, whether the primary research method employed is narrative, visual, or a combination of the two, the researcher must be reflexive about the epistemological assumptions that guide these forms of data collection (Moran-Ellis et al., 2006). Finally, the collection and dissemination of photographs also raises ongoing ethical and privacy concerns, as researchers must ensure that images are produced and shared in a manner that protects the rights of participants at all times.[2]

Visual Research on Gender and Smoking

While previous visual research has focused on women's and men's health experiences, there is little work that uses participant photography to explore how health and illness practices are gendered, or that adopts a critical approach to theorizing masculinity and femininity in relation to health. In our visual work with persons who smoke, gender is the primary analytical concern, in an effort to theorize the social production of gender and to show how masculinities and femininities are present in people's photographs about smoking. This is a relatively new area of focus for tobacco research, which has more often prioritized sex differences but typically paid less attention to the social significance of gender. Since the mid- to late 1990s there has been an increased presence of social scientists in the tobacco field, along with recognition that theoretical work addressing the social context of smoking practices is essential to the future of tobacco control (Poland et al., 2006).[3] Prioritizing a sociological view of both men's and women's tobacco use as a gendered cultural practice linked to social context, identity, and place, our research projects employed participant-driven photography to access participants' views of gender and gender relations.

---

[2]See Wang and Redwood-Jones (2001) for best practice guidelines and Photovoice ethics.

[3]For research that focuses on how health inequalities shape tobacco use and a gender-based analysis of smoking among vulnerable women and girls, see Amos, Sanchez, Skar, and White (2008); Graham (1993); Greaves (2007); and Greaves and Jategaonkar (2006). For feminist accounts of the cultural symbolism of women's smoking, see Amos and Haglund (2000); Greaves (1996); and Tinkler (2006). With exceptions (e.g., Dewhirst & Sparks, 2003; Nichter et al., 2006; Pavis & Cunningham-Burley, 1999), critical gender research on men's smoking is less prominent.

In both research studies narrative interviews were combined with a form of participant-driven photography. Study A (Haines) was carried out with young women ages 16 to 19 and was concerned with how gender, youth cultures, and social context shape young women's smoking status. Study B (Oliffe) was carried out with men who were new fathers, and focused on how gender and couple dynamics influence smoking in pregnancy and the postpartum period.[4] In both studies a theoretical framework based on the sociology of Pierre Bourdieu (1930–2002) was used to position smoking as more than just an individual-level "habit," but a social practice intimately tied to identity, the body, power relations, and place (Poland et al., 2006). While Study A focused on how gender domination and symbolic violence (Bourdieu, 2001) inform the habitus of young women's tobacco use, Study B was concerned with how habitus (Bourdieu, 1984) and hegemonic masculinities (Connell & Messerschmidt, 2005) intersect with fathering to shape men's smoking practices following the birth of a child. Subsequent to a brief overview of the Bourdieusian perspectives guiding our research, we draw from a small selection of participant photographs generated from these two projects to show how visual methods are useful in unpacking gender and the social reproduction of health practices.

The Gendering of Smoking Bodies, Identities, and Practices

To understand how Bourdieu positions the gendering of bodies through practice, it is important to first comprehend his theorization of the habitus, the idea that is central to his analysis of social identity (Lawler, 2004). Habitus shapes our preferences, tastes, and practices in a gentle or unconscious manner, so people reproduce certain dispositions and lifestyles as normal or "natural" (Bourdieu, 1984). Bourdieu used the metaphor of a sport or playing field to illustrate the interdependency of habitus and social fields, as social relations are reproduced through acts of willing participation or "playing along." Fields have taken-for-granted or transparent "rules of play" that structure the practices therein, amid field-specific forms of capital (Bourdieu, 1990; Bourdieu & Wacquant, 1992). In addition to economic or material capital, Bourdieu delineated social, cultural, and symbolic capitals that establish the power and status of groups and their hierarchical organization within fields (Bourdieu, 1986). In this view, a practice—whether healthy or "harmful," as in the case of smoking—has

---

[4]For extensive descriptions of the studies, their methodological procedures, and ethical considerations, see Haines (2008) and Oliffe, Bottorff, Kelly, and Halpin (2008). In another joint publication we explore the implications of visual research for tobacco control policy and practice (Haines, Oliffe, Bottorff, & Poland, 2010).

an inherent logic (i.e., it "makes sense" to people) when considered within the context of a field. Practices are acts of consumption that are at once material and symbolic, as taste preferences and ability to consume are shaped by the social conditioning of the habitus.[5]

Not only is habitus socially embedded and unknowingly reproduced; for Bourdieu it is also the embodiment of the social. Habitus and cultural capital are seen as having a tangible component that is visibly manifested in physical actions and as something that is "socially inscribed" upon people's bodies (Williams, 1995). It is through certain ways of being or presenting the body, through "acts of labour" *done with* the body, that people reproduce social identities and structures (Garrett, 2004). Following the work of Mauss (1930/1979), Bourdieu's notion of bodily hexis illustrates how social position is discernible through variations in bodily stance and gestures, how physical actions are performed, and how people carry and hold their bodies (comportment) (Bourdieu, 1984, 1990). Gender is fundamental to the social reproduction of habitus and bodily hexis, observable in everyday physical practices and ways of being in the world (Bourdieu, 2001). For Bourdieu, habitus is both "gendered and gendering" (Bourdieu & Wacquant, 1992, p. 172), an imperceptible force that enables unequal social relations where men dominate over women.[6] As with other dispositions of the habitus, gender is an embodied social difference that not only shapes subjective systems of meaning, but also structures the types of practice possible for men and women within social fields.

EMBODIED PRACTICE

Reviews of the photographs from our two studies revealed support for locating tobacco use as unconsciously reproduced and embodied practice. In participants' images showing themselves and other people smoking, the bodily hexis of smoking was shown through images that repeated a certain stance, posture, or pose (i.e., how one "does" smoking with the body). In Study A, an image that appeared within several sets of photographs was

---

[5]Researchers have also made prominent use of Bourdieu's theory of practice to understand the social production of disease and illness including the embodied experience of Alzheimer's disease (Kontos, 2004); the habitus of long-term home care recipients (Angus, Kontos, Dyck, McKeever, & Poland, 2005); mothers' work at securing symbolic capital for children with physical disabilities (McKeever & Miller, 2004); the habitus of men with muscular dystrophy (Gibson, Young, Upshur, & McKeever, 2007); and the socially embedded nature of smoking (Poland, 2000).

[6]Bourdieu was largely dismissive of contemporary feminist thought, which he characterized as essentialist "grand theory." In turn, Bourdieu has been criticized for promoting a determinist and androcentric view of gender. For an overview of feminist critiques and responses to Bourdieu, see, for example, Adkins and Skeggs (2005); Dillabough (2004); and McLeod (2005).

the close-up of a hand curled around a cigarette, held between the middle and index fingers. As one young woman explained in her written caption, this picture represents the "typical image that just about every smoker loves. It's great having a fresh cigarette ready to be lit, especially after a long day of fiending," meaning craving a cigarette. When these hand-focused images were put forward to the participants in a final research discussion group, the young women said the significance of this imagery was that it represents the smoker's point of view (i.e., what people see each time they smoke a cigarette). The images could also be read as signifying how the cigarette becomes a part of the smoker's identity, with smoking practices embodied through daily repetition.

Similarly, in Study B the participant's rationale for taking Image 7.1 was that he wanted to show researchers what he sees each time he lights up: "Mostly I was trying to capture the smoke, to get it the same as like where you get the lines going up . . . so it was like the blowout." For this new father, the image captured a particular "cigarette hold," or bodily hexis, whereby the cigarette was carefully nestled between the thumb and fingers and was being smoked outside on his balcony—the long sleeve suggesting cold weather—to ensure that his newborn was not exposed to secondhand smoke. While the smoking ritual was central to his identity and daily

Image 7.1

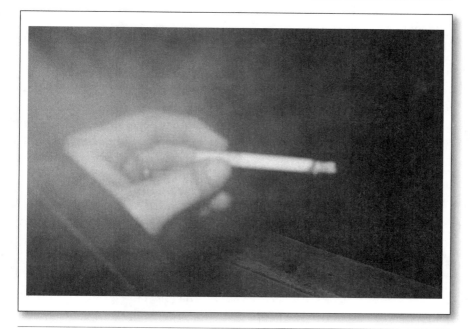

Source: Joan Bottorff and John Oliffe Research Image: Families Controlling and Eliminating Tobacco (FACET): A Gender Analysis of Tobacco Use in Families During Pregnancy, Postpartum and Early Childhood

routine, it was also clear from his narration that relations within the domestic field had undergone a shift to accommodate his newborn. To this end, "taking it outside" was a means for him to reconcile his smoking with fathering ideals around protector roles.

Gendered Bodily Hexis

In terms of images of smokers in Study A, a prevalent image of both female and male photo subjects was that of a smoker holding his or her hand up to his or her mouth and inhaling, or holding the cigarette near the face between puffs. Although this type of image is a simple way of showing what smoking looks like, when asked about the significance of this pose the young women explained that this represented a so-called "classic" image of smoking. From a Bourdieusian perspective, the articulation of a classic smoking image suggests these young women have come to internalize and reproduce the bodily hexis associated with smoking, along with the taken-for-granted stances, gestures, and physical displays associated with tobacco use that would not typically be articulated in everyday contexts, outside of the context of photographic research. Looking specifically at women smokers, Image 7.2

Image 7.2

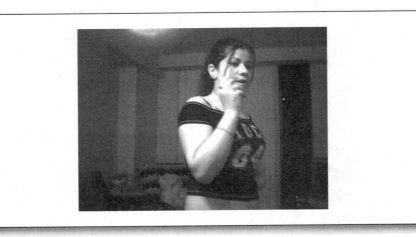

Source: Rebecca Haines Research Image: "Smoke, In My Eyes"—a qualitative project with young women that smoke

"Showing smoking with the hand up—closer to the face. It depends on what I'm doing—sometimes I keep it up, other times down" (Study A, Participant 08).

shows another frequent stance, holding the cigarette up and away from the face while exhaling.

Akin to the previous example of reflecting on the symbolism of holding a cigarette in one's hand, this participant shows an awareness of smoking as a bodily practice. However, this was only one of a few occasions where a participant wrote a caption directly addressing the bodily hexis of smoking. This apparent lack of conscious reflection about "how" one smokes is consistent with Bourdieu's conceptualization of habitus and bodily hexis as operating at an unconscious or prereflexive level, typically taken for granted by the body in practice. As a result, even within the context of a photographic activity, it might not occur to persons to reflect directly on how they smoke, or to explain this type of normative bodily practice to others. While perhaps not discernible to participants in their individual collections of photographs, looking across the visual findings the gendered bodily hexis of smoking is immediately visible in the images of young men and young women. Compiled from the findings of Study A, Image 7.3

Image 7.3

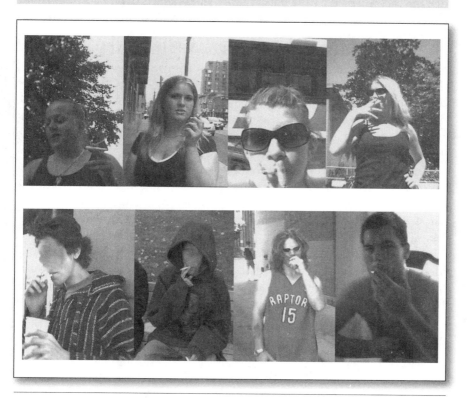

Source: Rebecca Haines Research Image: "Smoke, In My Eyes"—a qualitative project with young women that smoke

is a collage illustrating possible gender distinctions in the bodily hexis of smoking.[7]

Based on initial readings of these images there appear to be differences in the stances adopted by young men and women smokers when posing for the camera. For example, men were more likely to be seen smoking with palm down or with the hand held cupping the cigarette in a manner suggesting concealment, much like the stance employed when smoking marijuana. By comparison, female smokers were more likely to have the palm of the hand facing toward them, with their fingers held loose and spread out.

Study B included many participant-produced photographs depicting men's vehicles and workplaces as familiar fields in which to smoke. In terms of habitus, vehicles were social spaces delinked from home and/or direct fathering, in which men's imagery located smoking as a distinctly masculine practice and often solitary pursuit. For example, Image 7.4 reveals the smoker's view while driving, affording a glimpse of how the hand that strategically holds the cigarette near the open window also effortlessly steers the vehicle. The connectivity between tobacco use and driving is confirmed by the participant's statement "I drive a lot so I smoke a lot," and he located smoking as providing respite from his commute: "It's so boring, just check lines and stop signs, so you smoke."

Surveying the various smoking poses and stances within the photographs also presents a possible difficulty in terms of how to interpret and theorize imagery showing gendered bodily hexis. Unlike the visual trope of the hand up and away from the face that appeared to be the exclusive domain of feminine smoking style, what might be seen as a typically masculine pose—the cigarette dangle—appeared in photographs of both women and men in Study A.

The collage of pictures included in Image 7.5 shows three people photographed at their workplace by the same participant. The images in the middle and to the right of the collage were accompanied by captions about the stresses of the workplace, while the image to the left appeared captionless alongside another photograph of the subject lighting her cigarette. The immediate impression is that the male smoker clearly embodies an identifiably "masculine" style, letting his cigarette dangle from his mouth, lips closed around it without a hand to hold it up to or away from the face. Like the pictures of the hand with a cigarette, these mouth-dangle images

---

[7]As per the researcher's photo consent guidelines, faces have been blurred where the participant photographers did not obtain consent from their subjects. The young women seen in the photographs were research participants and gave their consent to share these images. The young men pictured in Image 7.3 were friends and romantic partners of the female research participants, with the exception of one subject who was a stranger, randomly approached on the street by a participant.

Image 7.4

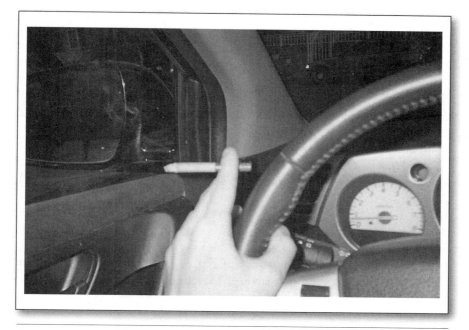

Source: Joan Bottorff and John Oliffe Research Image: Families Controlling and Eliminating Tobacco (FACET): A Gender Analysis of Tobacco Use in Families During Pregnancy, Postpartum and Early Childhood

Image 7.5

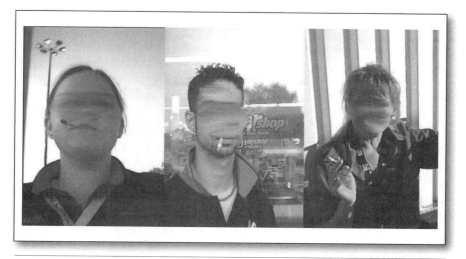

Source: Rebecca Haines Research Image: "Smoke, In My Eyes"—a qualitative project with young women that smoke

also symbolize the idea of the cigarette as an extension of the body, where it is attached to the mouth and seemingly effortlessly held in place. However, in the image to the left, the younger female smoker also projects a tough "attitude" through her stance. Therefore, it might be argued that her cigarette dangle shows a type of gender-based coolness, seen in the way this subject holds her cigarette in her mouth, pointed outward while she stares directly into the camera. Turning to the pose of the older woman to the right of the collage, the bodily stance perhaps suggests an age-based dimension of bodily hexis, as this woman poses for the camera holding the cigarette in a manner that denotes a more mature and composed style compared with the younger woman's stance.

Similarly, in the context of Study B a new dad spoke about the diverse smoking and nonsmoking practices he and his (male) buddies embodied. In building the narrative around his solo portrait in Image 7.6, masculine ideals are adhered to, but also interrogated in typically homosocial ways. The scene is set as the participant's patio where smoking occurs to punctuate the beers and conversation shared among the larger group of friends inside the home. While the participant expresses some concerns about the (health) effects of smoking, hedonism ultimately prevails to reify his smoking as a masculine marker.

In this example, smoking occurs outside, again, as a means to protect a newborn from secondhand smoke. It is clear that dominant masculine ideals can both potentiate smoking (i.e., by linking it with mateship and related pursuits including alcohol consumption) and restrict such practices by questioning the acceptability of smoking. Gender diversity or masculinities emerge here, albeit briefly, before the men privilege autonomy and freedom in accepting some men's choice to smoke. Image 7.6 reveals comfort and satisfaction, with the hanging cigarette a signifier of the man's self-assured, relaxed bodily hexis.

The photographic findings from our study support the Bourdieusian notion of how habitus shapes bodily hexis, and the socially distinct nature of bodily practices. As well, the gendering of smoking was of particular note in repetition of certain poses and stances and the physical ways of smoking seen in the participant-produced photographs. The images we collected from participants pointed to the presence of a gendered "smoker's habitus" that establishes capital related to tobacco use and the "correct" way to smoke (Haines, Poland, & Johnson, 2009). Smokers quickly adopt these bodily competencies, and through repetition these become habitual and observable in a gendered bodily hexis of smoking. Bourdieu's theory is valuable in this sense, as it posits that these stances are the unconscious, gendered embodiment of practice *and* a bodily representation of smoker's capital. In other words, these stances are not consciously adopted or artificially "put on," but are socially reproduced and inculcated within the body. Offering much more information than could narrative findings alone, these participant-produced images provide a preliminary means of

Image 7.6

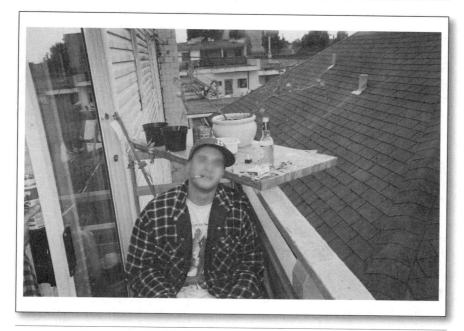

Source: Joan Bottorff and John Oliffe Research Image: Families Controlling and Eliminating Tobacco (FACET): A Gender Analysis of Tobacco Use in Families During Pregnancy, Postpartum and Early Childhood

Researcher [R]: So the nonsmoker [buddy] would come to the door?

Participant [P]: Just to say something stupid.

R: You guys would be outside?

P: Make fun of us or something.

R: He'd make fun of you about smoking?

P: No, no really, oh yeah, he'd say, "Oh, you guys stink." Like we come inside from outside, and then he would say, "Oh, you guys stink." When I worked with him I'd have a cigarette outside while working, and again, he'd say, "Why don't you get out? You stink." But he doesn't mean it.

R: He's just sort of playing around?

P: Yeah, he wants to see me quit, but yeah.

R: And what about the other guys? Do they want to see you quit?

P: Yeah, he [pointing to a picture of his friend] probably, he'd be like "That's cool," you know, to quit.

R: But he smokes?

P: He smokes.

R: Does he want to quit?

P: He's quit enough stuff in his life I don't know if he really wants to quit cigarettes right now.

seeing that representations of smoking are gendered, and that there are masculine and feminine ways of smoking and of establishing one's bodily competency as a genuine, experienced smoker competent in various smoking practices.

Having pointed to some of the typically "feminine" and "masculine" examples of the bodily hexis of smoking, it should be noted that these images represent only a small portion of our findings. When analyzing images it should be remembered that photographs are socially constructed and subject to socially reproduced interpretations (Rhodes & Fitzgerald, 2006; Rose, 2001). This includes photo subjects (who might have consciously posed for the camera in a certain way), photographers (who decided on the types of images they wanted to portray), and finally the viewer or researcher, who brings to bear his or her own analytical framework for interpreting the gendered aspects of the photographs.

Conclusion

This chapter has used the example of visual methods to illustrate the importance of theory-driven methodological practice in gender and health research. Bourdieu's theorization of the habitus and bodily hexis illustrates how gender is a prereflexive category, reproduced, embodied, and displayed in unconscious, naturalized ways. Yet it is because gender identities and practices operate at an unconscious level that these are often elusive concepts, ideas that research participants find awkward to speak about. Likewise, it can be challenging for researchers to apprehend perceived gendered meanings from the text of narrative transcripts alone. Health researchers can be faced with a dilemma when accessing gender through interview and focus group methodologies, as their theoretically sophisticated frameworks for understanding masculinities and femininities might not easily translate to tangible questions that can be understood by participants (Haines, Johnson, Carter, & Arora, 2009). Photography can provide another, creative way of "getting at gender" in research. As the photographs from persons that smoke illustrate, visual methods can reveal social phenomena as embodied experience in ways that narrative techniques alone cannot (Pink, 2001).

Using participant-driven photography in Study A allowed young women to represent gendered practices of smoking in a tangible and direct manner, something that was much more difficult for them to do within the context of a one-to-one interview (Haines, 2008). Although the long interview has become the gold standard in qualitative health research as a technique for privileging the experiences and views of those whose voices are not typically heard, there is also much to be gained by seeing the perspectives of those persons or groups who are often invisible. This is a particularly important issue to consider in research that is concerned with the relational production of gender. For instance, in the case of Study B, although there are other ethnographic tools at our disposal, it is generally unfeasible to observe people's gendered interactions within the context of intimate relationships (i.e., couple dynamics), as they can be constrained when a third party is watching. This is not to suggest that visual methods are a panacea, but they do allow participants to show us ways of doing gender, as opposed to only telling it, through speaking.

References

Adkins, L., & Skeggs, B. (2005). *Feminism after Bourdieu.* Oxford, UK: Blackwell/ The Sociological Review.

Allen, L. (2008). Young people's "agency" in sexuality research using visual methods. *Journal of Youth Studies, 11*(6), 565–577.

Amos, A., & Haglund, M. (2000). From social taboo to "torch of freedom": The marketing of cigarettes to women. *Tobacco Control, 9*(1), 3–8.

Amos, A., Sanchez, S., Skar, M., & White, P. (2008). *Exposing the evidence: Women and secondhand smoke in Europe.* Brussels, Belgium: INWAT-Europe & ENSP.

Angus, J., Kontos, P., Dyck, I., McKeever, P., & Poland, B. (2005). The personal significance of home: Habitus and the experience of receiving long-term home care. *Sociology of Health and Illness, 27*(2), 161–187.

Becker, H. S. (1978). Do photographs tell the truth? *Afterimage, 5*(February), 9–13.

Becker, H. S. (1998). Visual sociology, documentary photography, and photojournalism. In J. Prosser (Ed.), *Image-based research: A sourcebook for qualitative researchers* (pp. 84–96). London: Routledge Falmer.

Berman, H. (2001). Portraits of pain and promise: A photographic study of Bosnian youth. *Canadian Journal of Nursing Research, 32*(4), 21–41.

Booth, T., & Booth, W. (2003). In the frame: Photovoice and mothers with learning difficulties. *Disability & Society, 18*(4), 431–442.

Bourdieu, P. (1984). *Distinction: A social critique of the judgment of taste.* Cambridge, MA: Harvard University Press.

Bourdieu, P. (1986). The forms of capital. In J. Richardson (Ed.), *Handbook of theory and research for the sociology of education* (pp. 241–258). New York: Greenwood Press.

Bourdieu, P. (1990). *The logic of practice.* Stanford, CA: Stanford University Press.

Bourdieu, P. (2001). *Masculine domination.* Oxford, UK: Polity Press.

Bourdieu, P., & Wacquant, L. J. D. (1992). *An invitation to reflexive sociology.* Chicago: University of Chicago Press.

Clark-Ibanez, M. (2004). Framing the social world with photo-elicitation interviews. *American Behavioral Scientist, 47*(12), 1507–1527.

Connell, R., & Messerschmidt, J. (2005). Hegemonic masculinity: Rethinking the concept. *Gender & Society, 19*(6), 829–859.

Dewhirst, T., & Sparks, R. (2003). Intertextuality, tobacco sponsorship of sports, and male smoking culture: A selective review of tobacco industry documents. *Journal of Sport & Social Issues, 27*(4), 372–398.

Dillabough, J. (2004). Class, culture and the "predicaments of masculine domination": Encountering Pierre Bourdieu. *British Journal of Sociology of Education, 25*(4), 489–506.

Duffy, L. R. (2008). Hidden heroines: Lone mothers assessing community health using Photovoice. *Health Promotion Practice.* doi:1524839908324779v1

Epstein, I., Stevens, B., McKeever, P., & Baruchel, S. (2006). Photo elicitation interview (PEI): Using photos to elicit children's perspectives. *International Journal of Qualitative Methods, 5*(3), Article 1. Retrieved January 10, 2010, from http://www.ualberta.ca/~iiqm/backissues/5_3/pdf/epstein.pdf

Frith, H., & Harcourt, D. (2007). Using photographs to capture women's experiences of chemotherapy: Reflecting on the method. *Qualitative Health Research, 17*(10), 1340–1350.

Frohman, L. (2005). The Framing Safety Project: Photographs and narratives by battered women. *Violence Against Women, 11*(11), 1396–1419.

Garrett, R. (2004). Negotiating a physical identity: Girls, bodies and physical education. *Sport, Education and Society, 9*(2), 223–237.

Gibson, B. E., Young, N. L., Upshur, R. E. G., & McKeever, P. (2007). Men on the margin: A Bourdieusian examination of living into adulthood with muscular dystrophy. *Social Science & Medicine, 65*(3), 505–517.

Graham, H. (1993). *When life's a drag: Women smoking and disadvantage.* London: HMSO.

Greaves, L. (1996). *Smoke screen: Women's smoking and social control.* London: Scarlet University Press.

Greaves, L. (2007). Gender, equity and tobacco control. *Health Sociology Review, 16*(2), 115–129.

Greaves, L., & Jategaonkar, N. (2006). Tobacco policies and vulnerable girls and women: Toward a framework for gender sensitive policy development. *Journal of Epidemiology and Community Health, 60*(Suppl. 2), ii57–ii65.

Haines, R. (2008). *Smoke in my eyes: A Bourdieusian account of young women's tobacco use.* PhD dissertation, University of Toronto, Canada.

Haines, R. J., Johnson, J. L., Carter, C. I., & Arora, K. (2009). "I couldn't say, I'm not a girl": Adolescents talk about gender and marijuana use. *Social Science & Medicine, 68*(11), 2029–2036.

Haines, R. J., Oliffe, J. L., Bottorff, J. L., & Poland, B. D. (2010). "The missing picture": Tobacco use through the eyes of smokers. *Tobacco Control, 19*(3), 206–212.

Haines, R. J., Poland, B. D., & Johnson, J. L. (2009). Becoming a "real" smoker: Cultural capital in young women's accounts of substance use. *Sociology of Health & Illness, 31*(1), 66–80.

Harper, D. (1986). Meaning and work: A study in photo-elicitation. *Current Sociology, 34*(3), 24–36.

Harper, D. (2002). Talking about pictures: A case for photo elicitation. *Visual Studies, 17*(1), 13–26.

Harrison, B. (2002). Seeing health and illness worlds—Using visual methodologies in a sociology of health and illness: A methodological review. *Sociology of Health and Illness, 24*(6), 856–872.

Heisley, D. D., & Levy, S. J. (1991). Autodriving: A photoelicitation technique. *Journal of Consumer Research, 18*(3), 257–272.

Hussey, W. (2006). Slivers of the journey: The use of Photovoice and storytelling to examine female to male transsexuals' experience of health care access. *Journal of Homosexuality, 51*(1), 129–158.

Jurkowski, J. M., & Paul-Ward, A. (2007). Photovoice with vulnerable populations: Addressing disparities in health promotion among people with intellectual disabilities. *Health Promotion Practice, 8*(4), 358–365.

Killion, C. M., & Wang, C. C. (2000). Linking African American mothers across life stage and station through Photovoice. *Journal of Health Care for the Poor and Underserved, 11*(3), 310–325.

Klitzing, S. W. (2004). Women living in a homeless shelter: Stress, coping and leisure. *Journal of Leisure Research, 36*(4), 483–512.

Kontos, P. (2004). Ethnographic reflections on selfhood, embodiment and Alzheimer's disease. *Aging & Society, 24*(6), 829–849.

Lawler, S. (2004). Rules of engagement: Habitus, power and resistance. In L. Adkins & B. Skeggs (Eds.), *Feminism after Bourdieu* (pp. 110–128). Oxford, UK: Blackwell /The Sociological Review.

Mauss, M. (1979). *Sociology and psychology: Essays.* London: Routledge & Kegan Paul. (Original work published 1930)

McIntyre, A. (2003). Through the eyes of women: Photovoice and participatory research as tools for reimagining place. *Gender, Place and Culture, 10*(1), 47–66.

McKeever, P., & Miller, K. (2004). Mothering children who have disabilities: A Bourdieusian interpretation of maternal practices. *Social Science & Medicine, 59*(6), 1177–1191.

McLeod, J. (2005). Feminists re-reading Bourdieu: Old debates and new questions about gender habitus and gender change. *Theory and Research in Education, 3*(1), 11–30.

Moran-Ellis, J., Alexander, V. D., Cronin, A., Dickinson, M., Fielding, J., Sleney, J., et al. (2006). Triangulation and integration: Processes, claims and implications. *Qualitative Research, 6*(1), 45–59.

Nichter, M., Nichter, M., Lloyd-Richardson, E. E., Flaherty, B., Carkoglu, A., & Taylor, N. (2006). Gendered dimensions of smoking among college students. *Journal of Adolescent Research, 21*(3), 215–243.

Oliffe, J. (2003). *Prostate cancer: Anglo-Australian perspectives.* PhD dissertation, Deakin University, Melbourne, Australia.

Oliffe, J. L. (2009). Positioning prostate cancer as the problematic third testicle. In A. Broom & P. Tovey (Eds.), *Men's health: Body, identity and social context* (pp. 33–62). London: John Wiley & Sons.

Oliffe, J. L., & Bottorff, J. L. (2007). Further than the eye can see? Photo-elicitation and research with men. *Qualitative Health Research, 17*(6), 850–858.

Oliffe, J. L., Bottorff, J. L., Kelly, M., & Halpin, M. (2008). Analyzing participant produced photographs from an ethnographic study of fatherhood and smoking. *Research in Nursing & Health, 31*(5), 529–539.

Pavis, S., & Cunningham-Burley, S. (1999). Male youth street culture: Understanding the context of health-related behaviours. *Health Education Research, 14*(5), 583–596.

Pink, S. (2001). More visualizing, more methodologies: On video, reflexivity and qualitative research. *The Sociological Review, 49*(4), 586–599.

Poland, B. (2000). The "considerate" smoker in public space: The micro-politics and political economy of "doing the right thing." *Health & Place, 6*(1), 1–14.

Poland, B., Frohlich, K., Haines, R. J., Mykhalovskiy, E., Rock, M., & Sparks, R. (2006). The social context of smoking: The next frontier in tobacco control? *Tobacco Control, 15*(1), 59–63.

Rhodes, T., & Fitzgerald, J. (2006). Visual data in addictions research: Seeing comes before words? *Addiction Research and Theory, 14*(4), 349–363.

Rose, G. (2001). *Visual methodologies.* Thousand Oaks, CA: SAGE.

Strack, R. W., Magill, C., & McDonagh, K. (2004). Engaging youth through Photovoice. *Health Promotion Practice, 5*(1), 49–58.

Sweetman, P. (2009). Revealing habitus, illuminating practice: Bourdieu, photography and visual methods. *The Sociological Review, 57*(3), 491–511.

Tinkler, P. (2006). *Smoke signals: Women, smoking and visual culture in Britain.* Oxford, UK: Berg.

Tinkler, P. (2008). A fragmented picture: Reflections on the photographic practices of young people. *Visual Studies, 23*(3), 255–266.

Wang, C., & Burris, M. (1994). Empowerment through photo novella: Portraits of participation. *Health Education Quarterly, 21*(2), 171–186.

Wang, C., & Burris, M. (1997). Photovoice: Concept, methodology, and use for participatory needs assessment. *Health Education and Behaviour, 24*(3), 369–387.

Wang, C., Burris, M., & Xiang, Y. (1996). Chinese village women as visual anthropologists: A participatory approach to reaching policymakers. *Social Science and Medicine, 42*(10), 1391–1400.

Wang, C. C., Cash, J., & Powers, L. S. (2000). Who knows the streets as well as the homeless? Promoting personal and community action through Photovoice. *Health Promotion Practice, 1*(1), 81–89.

Wang, C. C., & Redwood-Jones, Y. A. (2001). Photovoice ethics: Perspectives from Flint Photovoice. *Health Education and Behaviour, 28*(5), 560–572.

Wang, C. C., Yi, W. K., Tao, Z. W., & Carovano, K. (1998). Photovoice as a participatory health promotion strategy. *Health Promotion International, 13*(1), 75–86.

Williams, S. J. (1995). Theorising class, health and lifestyles: Can Bourdieu help us? *Sociology of Health and Illness, 17*(5), 577–604.

Secondary Analysis—Gender, Age, and Place 8

Gender, Place, and the Mortality Gap Between Urban and Rural Canadians

Aleck Ostry

Amanda Slaunwhite

Several studies in recent years have demonstrated a consistent deficit in health status among rural compared with urban Canadians (Boland, Staines, Fitzpatrick, & Scallan, 2005; Canadian Institute for Health Information, 2006; Lagacé, Mesmeules, Pong, & Heng, 2007; McNiven, Puderer, & Janes, 2000; Mitura & Bollman, 2003; Ostry et al., 2009; Pohar, Majumdar, & Johnson, 2007). The most comprehensive of these recent Canadian studies was conducted by the Canadian Institute for Health Information (CIHI; 2006). This original CIHI analysis demonstrated consistent gradients in health outcomes, including mortality, across the urban–rural continuum in Canada. In this chapter we conduct an age-, gender-, and place-based reanalysis of this secondary data set produced in CIHI's original study in order to more clearly demonstrate the role played by age, gender, and place in rural–urban differences in mortality, ultimately, in order to better develop policy to reduce the mortality gap in rural compared with urban places.

Secondary analysis of population health data is commonly used in Canadian and international research to explore differences in the prevalence of disease, behavioral risk factors, and health care utilization in particular demographic groups and in different regions (Andrew, McNeil, Merry, & Rockwood, 2004; Cooper, Smaje, & Arber, 1998; Cronk & Sarvela, 1997; Haworth-Brockmann, Donner, & Isfeld, 2007; Reijneveld, 2002). One strength of conducting secondary analysis is that the data are already available. However, analysis of secondary data also has limitations as researchers are confined within the variables, topic area, and geographic scale of the original investigation, which limits the ability of these studies to be extended and expanded (Bibb, 2007).

Notwithstanding this latter limitation, the database utilized in the CIHI study of rural health in Canada is suitable for a more in-depth analysis to better understand mortality differences between men and women. Secondary data analysis is perhaps most appropriate where there has been little research completed on a topic, and exploratory studies are needed to form the foundation for more in-depth future research. Given the lack of research on gender differences in mortality across the rural–urban continuum in Canada, this CIHI data set lends itself well to secondary analysis. This data set is particularly useful as it is based on a large population, and the investment in time and dollars has already been made to gather these data.

This chapter is organized as follows. The methodology section begins by outlining how *urban* and *rural* are defined and with a review of the methods used to gather and analyze data in the original CIHI study. Then, the approach used to develop our secondary analysis is outlined. We also revisit the original study results and resynthesize and present them in such a way that age, gender, and place are more integral to the analysis of the gap in mortality between residents of urban compared with rural Canada. The results of this reanalysis are presented. This is followed by a discussion about and suggestions for how to use the results from this secondary analysis to develop targeted policy to reduce the current gap in mortality between urban and rural communities in Canada.

Methods

RESEARCH DESIGN

In the original investigation, CIHI researchers aggregated records from the Canadian Mortality Database (CMD) to the census subdivision (CSD) level for each of the years beginning in 1986 and ending in 1996. Because some census district boundaries changed over this time period, mortality data from each of these years were fitted to 1996 CSD boundaries.

Next, each CSD was categorized into one of seven possible metropolitan influenced zones (MIZs) (see Table 8.1) (McNiven et al., 2000). These MIZs characterize rural areas in terms both of population size and proximity and of the influence exerted by nearby urban areas. By using the MIZ classification scheme, communities are differentiated from one another based on population size, which has been shown to have an influence on social, economic, and health care service structures that impact population health (Rosenberg & Wilson, 2000).

Once mortality data were made available for all CSDs in Canada for each of these years and each CSD was categorized into one of the seven MIZ categories, statistical comparisons of mortality outcomes for major causes of death were made across five MIZ categories for different age-groups and genders. Causes of death were extracted from the ICD-9 codes found in the CMD.

Table 8.1 Standard Area Classification (SAC) Codes (MIZ System)

	SAC Code	Zone Label	Definition
Urban CSDs	1	Census metropolitan area (CMA)	Population > 100,000
	2	Tracted census agglomeration (CA)	Population > 10,000
	3	Nontracted CA	Population > 10,000
Rural CSDs	4	Strongly influenced MIZ	More than 30% of residents commute
	5	Moderately influenced MIZ	5%–30% of residents commute
	6	Weakly influenced MIZ	0%–5% of residents commute
	7	Not influenced (remote)	Fewer than 40 residents commute

Note: *In the original CIHI study, SAC codes 1, 2, and 3 were amalgamated into one "urban" category, and SAC codes 4, 5, 6, and 7 were left intact so that all analyses were with five place categories as follows: urban, strong MIZ, moderate MIZ, weak MIZ, and remote.

The results section of the original CIHI report and the appendix contained a number of tables with data on mortality rates for major causes of death by MIZ classification, age-group, and gender. The original report presented general results with discussion based on each major cause of death. Results were tabulated for each cause of death by gender and age-groups (usually 0–4, 5–19, 20–44, 45–64, and 65+).

Calculations were performed to determine the proportion of excess deaths occurring in each of the four different types of rural places, relative to deaths in urban places. These calculations were performed for each gender and age-group. In this way, the age, gender, and rural place-specific characteristics of mortality gradients for major causes of death were highlighted. This reanalysis provides new insights into the gender and place dimension of the mortality gap between urban and rural Canadians and can be utilized to more effectively develop health prevention policy in rural Canada.

RESULTS

1. *All-cause mortality by gender and across the urban/rural continuum.* Table 8.2 shows that, for all causes of death (except cancer), age-standardized mortality

Table 8.2   Annual Mortality Rates (per 100,000) in Canada by Residence and Gender

		Urban	Strong MIZ	Moderate MIZ	Weak MIZ	Remote
All cause	Men	908	838.9	946.3	940.7	1010.4
	Women	542.4	515.2	563.5	557.7	585.1
Circulatory disease	Men	354.5	339.8	368.6	366.9	377.7
	Women	214.1	215.1	226.5	221.9	229.2
Respiratory disease	Men	88.8	79.8	93.2	92.1	91.8
	Women	42.1	37.8	42.6	44.8	43.2
All cancer mortality	Men	247	221.3	245.4	238.7	250.1
	Women	155.1	140.8	152.2	149.9	150.1
Diabetes	Men	18.8	15.4	18.1	18	19.2
	Women	13.6	13.3	15.9	15.8	18.5
Injury or poisoning	Men	61.9	79.2	97.3	101.2	142.5
	Women	25.6	29	33.3	34	48.5
Suicide	Men	19.3	21.4	27.3	27.1	38.4
	Women	5.7	4	5.1	4.9	7.9

Source: Canadian Institute for Health Information (2006).

rates are higher in rural areas compared with strong MIZs and that male mortality for all causes of death and within each place category is always greater than female mortality.

Figure 8.1 illustrates the presence of a rough gradient in all-cause mortality for both genders moving from strong MIZs to remote regions. All-cause mortality rates for both men and women are approximately 20% greater in remote compared with strong MIZ regions.

In order to better understand the drivers of this gradient in mortality across the urban–rural continuum, it is necessary to look more closely at its age and gender structure.

2. *Variation in all-cause mortality between residents of urban regions and residents of rural regions in Canada by age and gender.* Subanalyses were conducted separately for males and females with age-groups 0–4, 5–19, 20–44, 45–64, and over 65. As shown in Figure 8.2a, there is only a slight gradient in age-standardized all-cause mortality across the rural–urban continuum for men and women over age 45. In contrast, a strong gradient exists for all-cause mortality among girls and women and boys and young men (see Figure 8.2b).

These data demonstrate that the seemingly small gradient in all-cause mortality across the urban/rural continuum observed for the

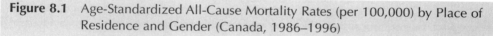

Figure 8.1   Age-Standardized All-Cause Mortality Rates (per 100,000) by Place of Residence and Gender (Canada, 1986–1996)

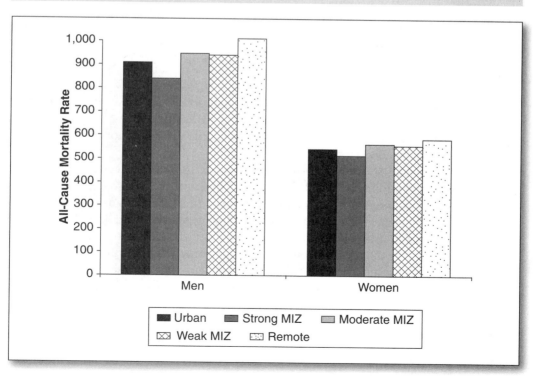

Figure 8.2a   Age-Standardized All-Cause Mortality Rates (per 100,000) Among Women and Men (Over Age 44) by Place of Residence (Canada, 1986–1996)

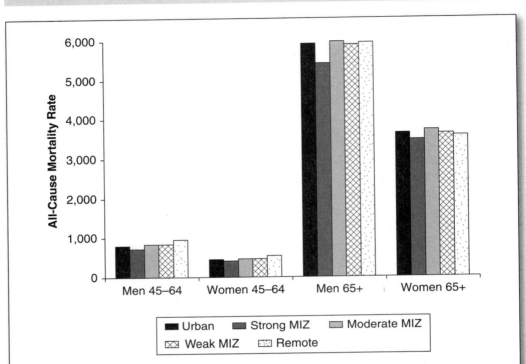

entire population (see Figure 8.1) is driven by steep gradients in mortality among people younger than age 45. As well, the highest all-cause mortality rates for males and females under age 45 are found in age-group 0 to 4.

3. *The effect of place on the gradient from urban to increasingly rural places.* Figure 8.3 compares all-cause mortality in urban places for those under age 45 with mortality in strong MIZs, moderate MIZs, weak MIZs, and remote places to illustrate the excess all-cause mortality in each of these rural places.

Excess mortality in rural compared with urban places was highest for boys and girls ages 5–19 and lowest for boys and girls ages 0–4. For boys and girls ages 5–19 living in remote communities, all-cause mortality rates were, respectively, 164% and 157% higher for boys and girls the same age living in urban places.

Given that deaths from injury or poisoning, suicides, and motor vehicle accidents make up the bulk of deaths occurring in those under age 45, the gradients across place, in mortality for these causes of death, are next explored.

Figure 8.2b Age-Standardized All-Cause Mortality Rates (per 100,000) Among Boys, Men, Girls, and Women (Under Age 45) by Place of Residence (Canada, 1986–1996)

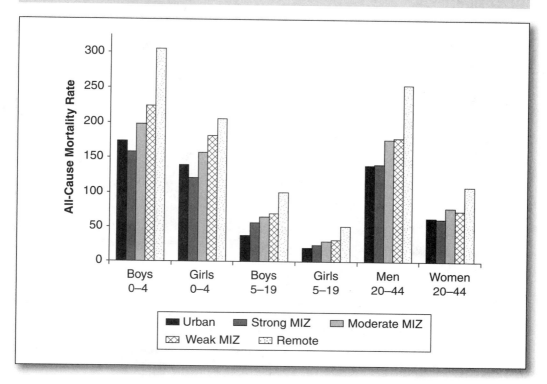

4. *The effect of gender and age on mortality gradient from urban to increasingly rural places for suicide, injury or poisoning, and motor vehicle accidents.* Excess suicide mortality for girls and boys ages 5–19 living in remote places is, respectively, 533% and 329% greater than that for girls and boys of the same age residing in urban places. In weak MIZs, excess suicide mortality for 5- to 19-year-olds is similar for girls and boys and is "only" 50% greater than that for those of the same age living in urban places (see Figure 8.4).

As in the case of suicide mortality, excess rural compared with urban injury or poisoning deaths tend to increase with decreasing age. In remote places, injury or poisoning deaths among boys ages 0–4 are 374% greater than they are for boys of the same age residing in urban places. Compared with the same age-groups in urban places, excess deaths due to injury or poisoning for girls ages 0–4, girls ages 5–19, and boys ages 5–19 in remote places were approximately 250% greater than in urban places (see Figure 8.5).

Figure 8.3   Excess All-Cause Rural Relative to Urban Mortality by Age and Gender

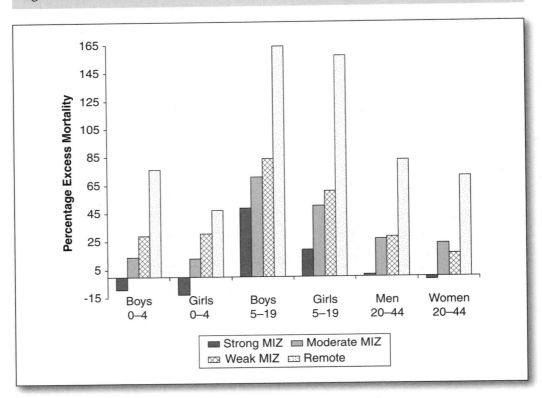

Mortality from motor vehicle accidents (MVAs) is higher in all rural compared with urban places. Unlike in the case of suicide and injury or poisoning mortality, there is relatively little difference in the observed patterns of excess rural mortality across age-groups. Excess MVA mortality in remote places is in the 175%–225% range for all age-groups. In weak MIZs, excess MVA mortality for girls ages 0–4 is 275% compared with a figure in the 125% range for boys and girls and men and women in other age-groups (see Figure 8.6).

Discussion

Recent work has supported the utility of a geographic lens in understanding health inequalities across the urban–rural continuum by documenting variations in the experience (Crooks & Chouinard, 2006) and treatment of illness (Bierman, 2007; Fowler et al., 2007) by gender and geographic location in relation to health care services (Dyck, 2003; Parr, 2002;

Figure 8.4   Excess Rural Suicide Relative to Urban Mortality by Age and Gender

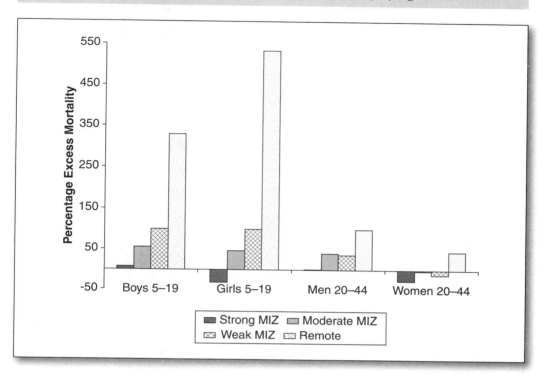

Ross, Rosenberg, Pross, & Bass, 1994; Williams & Garvin, 2004). Gender differences have been found in the type and use of preventative measures (Bird et al., 2007), diagnostic screening (Ross et al., 1994), treatment regimes (Curtis et al., 2007; Hernandez et al., 2007; Young, 2007), and health care utilization (Cloutier-Fisher & Kobayashi, 2009; Drapeau, Richard, & Alain, 2009; Kazanjian, Morettin, & Cho, 2003), influencing the likelihood of appropriate and timely diagnosis and treatment for some life-threatening diseases and conditions.

Using a geographic lens, several studies in recent years have demonstrated a consistent deficit in health status among rural compared with urban Canadians (CIHI, 2006; Mitura & Bollman, 2003, 2004). In this chapter we have reanalyzed a CIHI data set with a geographic as well as a gender lens in order to more fully understand the gender dynamics of the mortality gap between rural and urban places in Canada.

There are five main conclusions drawn from this chapter. First, mortality rates move in a similar gradient across place for most causes (i.e., they tend to be worse moving from urban to remote regions) except in the case of strong MIZs, where rates tend to be lower than they are in urban places and other rural areas. Second, these differences in mortality across the

Figure 8.5   Excess Rural Injury/Poisoning Relative to Urban Mortality by Age and Gender

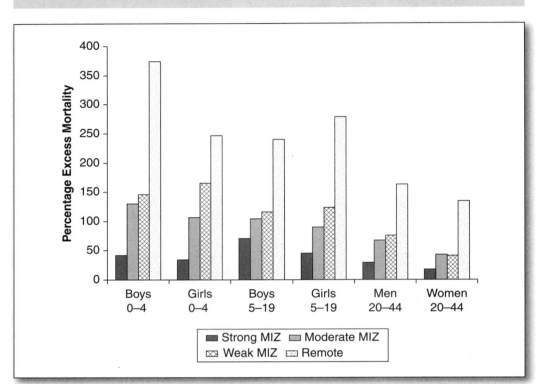

urban–rural continuum are mainly driven by people under age 45 and particularly due to deaths caused by injury or poisoning, motor vehicle accident, and suicide. Third, the proportion of excess deaths relative to urban places for those under age 45 increases with decreasing age. Fourth, remote places have the highest excess in mortality for suicide, MVA, and injury or poisoning relative to urban places.

Fifth, although absolute mortality for all age-groups and in all regions is higher for males than it is for females, the relative impact of place (in terms of the proportion of excess deaths) in rural versus urban Canada is remarkably consistent across gender for the three major causes of death for those under age 45. In other words, for those under age 45, the relative impact, in terms of excess mortality, of living increasingly farther away from Canadian cities is, in general, equally adverse for males and females.

This reanalysis shows that life outside Canadian cities is much more dangerous, in relative terms, for *both* boys and girls than it is for their counterparts in urban places. Many studies have shown that higher absolute risk of injury for young males compared with young females is mainly due to male tendencies to take more risks while engaging in dangerous behavior. While this is likely true for absolute risks faced by young males,

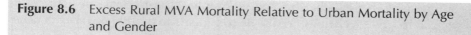

Figure 8.6   Excess Rural MVA Mortality Relative to Urban Mortality by Age and Gender

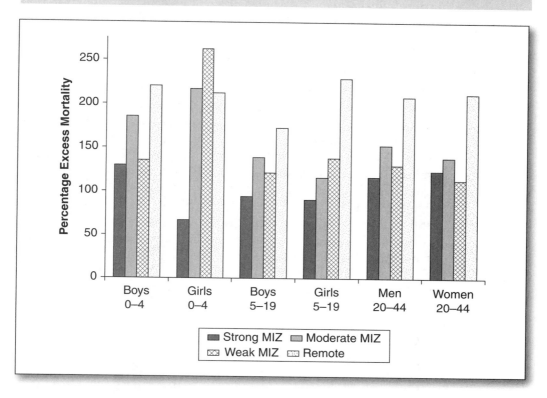

our results indicate that risks for excess mortality faced by both and girls and boys (including social and physical environment) at young ages are much higher in remote and rural places than they are in urban places. This observation has implications for policy. In particular, there is a need for prevention policies and awareness programs targeted at both boys and girls that work to prevent suicide, injury or poisoning, and MVAs. Given commonly held beliefs about riskier young male behavior, it is likely that, to the extent that these programs are available, they may be oriented toward the needs of young males more than young females. These programs need to be a particular priority in remote places where excess deaths, relative to urban places, are astoundingly high. In designing these programs, the importance of place to the social structure and the delivery of prevention, diagnosis, and treatment programs ought to be considered in relation to gender roles within urban, rural, and remote communities that heavily influence health status (Little, 1987). While this study was unable to dissect the complex relationship of gender to health status due to limitations associated with using mortality data, future work examining the complex dynamics between geography, gender, and health ought to consider the importance of gender roles and their associated behaviors to engaging in risk behaviors and seeking health care. Social structures and gender power relations need to be considered to capture how health determinants influence men and women differently (Hankivsky, 2007; Johnson, Greaves, & Repta, 2009).

Similarly, differences in health status by age structure need to be emphasized in the formulation of public policy responses to reducing the mortality gap between urban, rural, and remote areas. The original CIHI analysis showed that the differences in health status across the rural–urban continuum are small for those over age 45 so that the rural health disadvantage is largely a problem for children, youth, and young adults. The results for suicide are alarming particularly for boys and girls ages 15–19. Research from Australia, Norway, and the United Kingdom has found the largest increases in suicide rates for young adults since the 1970s occurred among residents in rural regions (Dudley et al., 1998; Kelly, Charlton, & Jenkins, 1995; Mehlum, Hytten, & Gjertsen, 1999). The high rates in rural Canada seen in this study may also reflect recent increases. Access to mental health services in rural areas is generally more limited than in urban areas, and awareness of symptomatology and treatment may also be restricted among physicians and parents, drawing attention to the need for study into the prevalence of mental illness in rural and remote communities and treatment utilization to design appropriate place-specific initiatives to reduce suicide risk (Boydell et al., 2006; Offord et al., 1987; Philo, Parr, & Burns, 2003).

This chapter has documented the use of secondary analysis to examine the mortality gap between urban, rural, and remote areas of Canada by gender using data collected from the CIHI. To build on this research, more in-depth study of the gender-specific factors that influence risk behaviors associated with increased injury, motor vehicle accidents, and suicide in these demographic groups is needed. As well, a gender focus to research must be designed into original investigations, especially those that are expensive, difficult, and likely to produce important results, so that research outcomes and policy recommendations that follow have a gender lens that is essential to and embedded in the initial study design.

References

Andrew, M. K., McNeil, S., Merry, H., & Rockwood, K. (2004). Rates of influenza vaccination in older adults and factors associated with vaccine use: A secondary analysis of the Canadian Study of Health and Aging. *BMC Public Health, 4*(36), 24–37.

Bibb, G. S. (2007). Issues associated with secondary analysis of population health data. *Applied Nursing Research, 20*(2), 94–99.

Bierman, A. S. (2007). Sex matters: Gender disparities in quality and outcomes of care. *Canadian Medical Association Journal, 17*(12), 1520–1521.

Bird, C. A., Fremont, A., Bierman, S., Wickstrom, M., Shah, T., Rector, T., et al. (2007). Does quality of care for cardiovascular disease and diabetes differ by gender for enrollees in managed care plans? *Women's Health Issues, 17*(3), 131–138.

Boland, M. A., Staines, P., Fitzpatrick, P., & Scallan, E. (2005). Urban-rural variation in mortality and hospital admission rates for unintentional injury in Ireland. *Injury Prevention, 11,* 38–42.

Boydell, K. M., Pong, R., Volpe, T., Tilleczek, K., Wilson, E., & Lemieux, S. (2006). Family perspectives on pathways to mental health care for children and youth in rural communities. *The Journal of Rural Health, 22*(2), 182–188.

Canadian Institute for Health Information. (2006). *How healthy are rural Canadians? An assessment of their health status and health determinants.* Ottawa, ON, Canada: Author.

Cloutier-Fisher, D., & Kobayashi, K. (2009). Examining social isolation by gender and geography: Conceptual and operational challenges using population health data in Canada. *Gender, Place & Culture: A Journal of Feminist Geography, 16*(2), 181–199.

Cooper, H., Smaje, C., & Arber, S. (1998). Use of health services by children and young people according to ethnicity and social class: Secondary analysis of a national survey. *British Medical Journal, 317,* 1047–1051.

Cronk, C. E., & Sarvela, P. D. (1997). Alcohol, tobacco, and other drug use among rural/small town and urban youth: A secondary analysis of the Monitoring the Future data set. *American Journal of Public Health, 87*(5), 760–764.

Crooks, V. A., & Chouinard, V. (2006). An embodied geography of disablement: Chronically ill women's struggles for enabling places in spaces of health care and daily life. *Health & Place, 12*(3), 345–352.

Curtis, L. H., Al-Khatib, S. M., Shea, A. M., Hammill, B. J., Hernandez, A. F., & Schulman, K. A. (2007). Sex differences in the use of implantable cardioverter-defibrillators for primary and secondary prevention of sudden cardiac death. *Journal of the American Medical Association, 298,* 1517–1524.

Drapeau, A., Richard, B., & Alain, L. (2009). The influence of social anchorage on the gender difference in the use of mental health services. *Journal of Behavioral Health Services & Research, 36*(3), 372–384.

Dudley, M., Kelk, N., Florio, T., Waters, B., Howard, J., & Taylor, D. (1998). Coroners' records of rural and non-rural cases of youth suicide in New South Wales. *Australian and New Zealand Journal of Psychiatry, 32*(2), 242–251.

Dyck, I. (2003). Feminism and health geography: Twin tracks or divergent agendas. *Gender, Place & Culture, 10*(4), 361–368.

Fowler, R. A., Sabur, N., Li, P., Juurlink, D. N., Pinto, R., Hladunewich, M. A., et al. (2007). Sex- and age-based differences in the delivery and outcomes of critical care. *Canadian Medical Association Journal, 177,* 1513–1519.

Hankivsky, O. (2007). Gender-based analysis and health policy: The need to rethink outdated strategies. In M. Morrow, O. Hankivsky, & C. Varcoe (Eds.), *Women's health in Canada: Critical perspectives on theory and policy* (pp. 143–168). Toronto, ON, Canada: University of Toronto Press.

Haworth-Brockmann, M., Donner, L., & Isfeld, H. (2007). A field test of the gender-sensitive core set of leading health indicators in Manitoba, Canada. *International Journal of Public Health, 52*(1), S49–S57.

Hernandez, A. F., Fonarow, G. C., Liang, L., Al-Khatib, S. M., Curtis, L. H., LaBresh, K. A., et al. (2007). Sex and racial differences in the use of implantable cardioverter-defibrillators among patients hospitalized with heart failure. *Journal of the American Medical Association, 298*, 1525–1532.

Johnson, J. L., Greaves, L., & Repta, R. (2009). Better science with sex and gender: Facilitating the use of a sex and gender-based analysis in health research. *International Journal for Equity in Health, 8*(14), 94–102.

Kazanjian, A., Morettin, D., & Cho, R. (2003). Health care utilization by Canadian women. *Women's Health Surveillance Report.* Ottawa, ON, Canada: Canadian Institute for Health Information.

Kelly, S., Charlton, J., & Jenkins, R. (1995). Suicide deaths in England and Wales, 1982–1992: The contribution of occupation and geography. *Population Trends, 80*, 16–25.

Lagacé, C., Mesmeules, M., Pong, R., & Heng, D. (2007). Non-communicable disease and injury-related mortality in rural and urban places of residence. *Canadian Journal of Public Health, 98*(Suppl. 1), 562–569.

Little, J. (1987). Gender relations in rural areas: The importance of women's domestic role. *Journal of Rural Studies, 3*(4), 335–342.

McNiven, C., Puderer, H., & Janes, D. (2000). *Census metropolitan area and census agglomeration influenced zones (MIZ), a description of the methodology* [Catalogue No. 92F0138MIE2000002]. Ottawa, ON: Statistics Canada.

Mehlum, L., Hytten, K., & Gjertsen, F. (1999). Epidemiological trends of youth suicide in Norway. *Archives of Suicide Research, 5*, 193–205.

Mitura, V., & Bollman, R. D. (2003). The health of rural Canadians: A rural urban comparison of health indicators. *Rural and Small Town Canada Analysis Bulletin, 4*(6), 23.

Mitura, V., & Bollman, R. D. (2004). Health status and behaviours of Canada's youth: A rural-urban comparison. *Rural and Small Town Canada Analysis Bulletin, 5*(3), 22.

Offord, D. R., Boyle, M. H., Szatmari, P., Rae-Grant, N. I., Links, P. S., Cadman, D. T., et al. (1987). Ontario Child Health Study: II. Six-month prevalence of disorder and rates of service utilization. *Archives of General Psychiatry, 44*(9), 832–836.

Ostry, A., Maggi, S., Hershler, R., Louise, A., Chen, L., & Hertzman, C. (2009). A case control study of differences in non-work injury and accidents among sawmill workers in rural compared to urban British Columbia, Canada. *BMC Public Health, 9*, 432.

Parr, H. (2002). Medical geography: Diagnosing the body in medical and health geography, 1999–2000. *Progress in Human Geography, 26*(2), 240–251.

Philo, C., Parr, H., & Burns, N. (2003). Rural madness: A geographical reading and critique of the rural mental health literature. *Journal of Rural Studies, 19*(3), 259–281.

Pohar, S., Majumdar, S., & Johnson, J. (2007). Health care costs and mortality for Canadian urban and rural patients with diabetes: Population-based trends from 1993–2001. *Clinical Therapeutics, 29*, 1316–1324.

Reijneveld, S. A. (2002). Neighbourhood socioeconomic context and self reported health and smoking: A secondary analysis of data on seven cities. *Journal of Epidemiology & Community Health, 56*, 935–942.

Rosenberg, M. W., & Wilson, K. (2000). Gender, poverty and location: How much difference do they make in the geography of health inequalities? *Social Science & Medicine, 51,* 275–287.

Ross, N., Rosenberg, M., Pross, D. C., & Bass, B. (1994). Contradictions in women's health care provision: A case study of attendance for breast cancer screening. *Social Science & Medicine, 39*(8), 1015–1025.

Williams, A., & Garvin, T. (2004). Taking stock: Geographical perspectives on women and health in Canada. *The Canadian Geographer, 48*(1), 29–34.

Young, L. E. (2007). Women's health and cardiovascular care: A persistent divide. In M. Morrow, O. Hankivsky, & C. Varcoe (Eds.), *Women's health in Canada: Critical perspectives on theory and policy* (pp. 456–476). Toronto, ON, Canada: University of Toronto Press.

Content and Discourse Analysis 9

Brendan Gough

Steve Robertson

There has been a long-standing theoretical and empirical interest in "differences" between "men's talk" and "women's talk" (e.g., Coates, 2004; Tannen, 2001).[1] Such differences relate not only to the content of such talk but also to the meanings associated with words and phrases, and the consideration of meaning when words are not forthcoming—that is, consideration of the meaning of silences and silenced voices. Yet it is not just differences in the nature and meaning of direct talk by men and women that are of interest and significance. Specific "texts," such as media texts, literary texts, and policy texts (to name a few), frequently carry explicit or implicit content and meaning in relation to gender and health. Talk and texts are therefore a significant area for study in relation to (a) considering how men and women might (and, as important, might not) talk differently about health and health-related matters and (b) considering the role that health talk and texts have in constructing and/or replicating particular "norms" or gendered expectations. In short, talk and texts can be considered both as representative of held views and as (re)constructive of normative forms of gendered health practices.

This chapter considers two approaches that can be adopted to examine the content and meaning of health talk and text. It first describes how content analysis may be used to make sense of health publications such as

---

[1]It is by no means accepted, though, that any differences exist to the extent that some claim (e.g., Aries, 1997).

government-produced health promotion materials, health-related magazine features, and television advertisements. It then makes a case for moving beyond content analysis to take a discursive approach to analyzing these and other health-related data. Specifically, we suggest that an analysis of discursive resources (i.e., culturally dominant ideals) and discursive practices (i.e., rhetorical strategies used in talk) can help illuminate the social construction of gender, health, and illness in defined contexts.

Content analysis (CA) often constitutes the first wave of analysis before moving to a more "branded" methodology such as grounded theory or discourse analysis. Indeed, this two-stage analytic approach has been used by various researchers working in the areas of health and/or gender (see Gough, 2006; Willott & Griffin, 1997). Discourse analysis emerged as an approach to qualitative research in the last 20 years within social psychology (and beyond), but with intellectual influences traced to continental philosophy (particularly the work of Foucault, 1980) and ethnomethodology (e.g., Garfinkel, 1967; Goffman, 1961). There is now a plethora of particular methodologies that can be placed under the discourse analysis (DA) umbrella, ranging from critical discourse analysis (e.g., Fairclough, 1995) to discursive psychology (Edwards & Potter, 1992) to conversation analysis (Hutchby & Wooffitt, 2008) and membership categorization analysis (e.g., Eglin & Hester, 2003) (see Wetherell, Taylor, & Yates, 2001, for a good overview).

Content Analysis (CA)

Content analysis can be used in a predominantly quantitative or qualitative fashion. In the former sense, we start with preconceived categories derived from a theory and simply look for evidence of these categories in the data set. For example, we might be interested in the attributions people make concerning the perceived cause of their illness, and have three significant conceptual dimensions to consider: external-internal (e.g., environmental vs. individual contribution); stable-unstable (e.g., cause remains consistent vs. changes over time); global-specific (cause concerns all body problems vs. this illness only). We would then go through the available data, say accounts provided by patients during brief research interviews, and identify instances of each dimension before producing a frequency count. The fact that 80% of attributions turn out to be external (i.e., due to chance, circumstances), or that 60% of women use global attributions (i.e., not just the specific illness but generalized to all bodily problems) compared with 40% of men, might reveal something about how people think about and manage their illnesses, and the role of gender in accounting for sex differences in this context. So, this type of research is theoretically informed and quantitative, and can produce useful information concerning trends and patterns in the data. However, quantitative CA need not be theory driven, and can be deployed as part of a wider, qualitative project that is more inductive or open-ended. Qualitative CA does not generally employ theory in advance; instead, the data are analyzed in-depth and bottom-up, with the goal being to generate new categories rather than test for the presence and salience of already chosen categories. As mentioned, quantitative and qualitative CA can be used in tandem within a broader qualitatively oriented project. For example, a CA of *Cosmopolitan* magazine might yield results concerning the prevalence of specific sex-related terms within the editions covered (e.g., 235 mentions of *sexual problems*; 127 mentions of *sex therapy*; 58 mentions of *sex toys*) while also presenting more interpretative or conceptual categories, say *sex as pleasure* and/or *sex as conflict*. The data associated with these categories could then be analyzed for constructions of gender; for example, to what extent are men constructed as sex objects (by the editors) to be gazed upon and fantasized about by women readers? Who is designated as primarily responsible for contraceptive decisions and practices, men or women? Such analyses of contemporary mediated sexualities could also tell us something about modern-day gendered ideals and practices.

There is no one "correct" way of doing CA, although useful guidelines have been published (e.g., Weber, 1990). As with other (particularly qualitative) methods, one's approach to analyzing data in practice tends to draw from an array of options. Once you have decided on your research topic and focus, the first important step is to delineate the data set to be analyzed. Let's say the topic is media representations of gender and alcohol consumption; you need to decide which type of media you will focus on—print media such as newspapers and magazines, television programs such as soap operas and detective shows, or Internet data such as news websites and discussion forums? Moreover, within each genre there are further decisions to be made. For example, in studying national newspaper coverage of gender and drinking, decisions are necessary about which particular publications to include—just tabloids, tabloids and broadsheets, or tabloids, broadsheets, and "middle-brow" newspapers? Also, do we confine the focus to one country, or should we consider newspapers from other countries to give the project an international dimension? And then there is the question of time period—are we interested in very recent articles—say in the last month or over the past year? Or might we consider a comparison between a previous period—say 20 years ago—and the present? These and other choices will be influenced by researcher resources, scope of the project, existing literature, and data availability, among other things.

If, for example, you have decided to focus on UK newspaper representations of gender and alcohol consumption over the past year and, initially at least, you will not exclude any particular national publication, the next step is to locate an online database that allows searches by key words.

A good one for UK national newspapers is Nexis UK—http://www
.lexisnexis.co.uk/—and you might try a range of key words in different
combinations: *gender* and *drinking; men* and *drinking; women* and *drinking; gender* and *alcohol; men* and *alcohol; women* and *alcohol;* and so on.
This topic will generate many hits given the current intense media coverage of binge drinking in the United Kingdom (and other Western nations),
especially in relation to particular subgroups such as young women and
men (e.g., college students), mothers, and working-class men (e.g., manual
laborers) (see Measham & Brain, 2005). You may have a target number of
features in mind that will be influenced by resource constraints, so if your
search generates hundreds of hits, then further selection is required. For
example, search by type of newspaper (e.g., tabloids only) or time period
(e.g., last 6 months only).

Once the data set has been retrieved (e.g., producing 100 articles), then
each unit (article) will need to be read a number of times. Reading through
the material in this way will likely stimulate ideas about significant themes,
so it is best to note your ideas in a folder as you go along—these notes can
then guide your analysis at a later stage. Following this reading stage, each
article should be read closely and themes generated in a line-by-line fashion for each paragraph or section—this process will generate lots of
low-level themes to begin with for each article. These descriptive themes
simply restate in a succinct way what is presented in each line or two.
Periodically, it is worth pausing to consider themes so far developed with
a view to forming clusters of themes that link together in some way; for
example, several themes might relate to women, drinking, and pregnancy,
while others might relate to men, drinking, and violence. Such clusters
develop, mutate, and reform over time within and between articles: The
goal is to move from descriptive to conceptual clusters/categories, and to
work toward settling on relatively few higher-order (conceptual) themes.
For example, a core theme from a newspaper data set on gender and alcohol consumption might revolve around "gendered moral judgements,"
subsuming themes concerning tolerance of men's drinking and condem-
nation of women's drinking. An in-depth qualitative CA aims to produce
theoretical insights into the phenomenon in question and, when applied
to contemporary media reports, helps to signal something of the cultural
common sense around gender and health issues (see Day, Gough, &
McFadden, 2004; Gannon, Glover, & Abel, 2004).

Discourse Analysis (DA)

In recent years, discourse analysis has been increasingly applied to
health-related topics, and following Wetherell (1998), we can usefully distinguish between discursive resources and discursive practices. Discursive

resources refer to those ideals and ideologies that inform our understanding of objects, events, and people. For example, conventional ideals of masculinity that specify strength, emotional suppression, and endurance of pain can influence how men experience and report (or do not report) health-related complaints. Discursive practices refer to the actual strategies people use in talk (or in texts such as magazine articles) to perform certain functions such as defending oneself from accusations, giving compliments, or presenting oneself in a positive light. For example, a speaker may cite scientific evidence or the opinions of noted experts to validate what he is saying and reinforce his own practices and gender identities (consuming beer might be linked to media reports of research invoking positive health benefits for men, thus reinforcing valued masculinized drinking practices) (see Potter, 1996, for a comprehensive review of such discursive practices).

These days there are various sets of guidelines available for doing DA—most qualitative methods textbooks feature at least one chapter on DA, while there are many books also devoted to explaining a particular version of DA (e.g., Edwards & Potter, 1992). DA studies can focus on a range of data, including printed media, focus group discussions, and natural conversations. A few brief examples give a flavor of the breadth and focus of DA work in gender and health. Sue Wilkinson (2003) used DA to understand how women with breast cancer cope with the disease and manage their identities and relationships. Sally Wiggins (2004) studied video recordings of family interactions during mealtimes and looked at how members orient to and use health promotion advice in their talk. Ken Gannon and colleagues (2004) explored the social construction of male infertility and masculinity through newspaper accounts of a declining sperm count, and Dariusz Galasiński (2008) contrasted men's gendered experiences of depression with diagnostic and screening tools using a DA approach. In what follows, we share three extended examples to show how a discursive approach can contribute insights into gender and health issues.

Gough (2009) used aspects of DA to critically examine a men's health "manual" designed to encourage overweight and obese male readers to lose weight and lead a healthier lifestyle. This "HGV Man" text, as with other texts in the "Man" series, is sponsored by Haynes (UK) car manuals and deliberately adopts the recognized style and format of these manuals (for details about the book see Banks, 2005). The focus of this DA is on how masculinity is constructed within the text, and the implications of such constructions for men's health promotion. A key theme of the article is the mechanization of the male body, which is perhaps an unsurprising finding in a car-themed format, but which certainly seems odd within a text supposedly focusing on the flabby male body. Here is a sample extract:

Do you spend as much time looking after yourself, thinking about what fuel you need to perform well and how best to recharge your batteries as you do your vehicle?

Do you service and MoT[2] your body and mind and consider what will keep you mentally and physically in peak condition? (Manual, Section 2.5)

The emphasis on the male body as a solid, performance-oriented vehicle sensitive to physical inputs is perhaps rather peculiar in the context of male obesity—but this makes sense in terms of preserving men's sense of "masculinity" in a potentially threatening situation such as being an overweight reader receiving health advice. So, the discursive resources employed revolve around traditional notions of masculinity as hard bodied and performance orientated. In terms of discursive practices, note the use of a three-part list (Jefferson, 1990)—"looking after yourself . . . thinking about what fuel . . . how best to recharge . . ."—a known strategy commonly used to reinforce a point, in this case the necessity of caring for your body-machine. The use of *you* is also prominent (rather than, say, *men* or *they*), a footing device (Goffman, 1961) that in this case facilitates a direct appeal to the reader.

Gough (2009) goes on to argue that the actual obese male body is absented within the text, with a major focus being on the male mind:

Make your decisions based on logical discussion with yourself rather than allowing them to be a fait accompli. (Manual, Section 2.5)

Knowing how powerful your thoughts are will give you another tool for your kitbag. (Manual, Section 2.6)

Weight management is just a matter of choosing the right foods. (Manual, Section 4.11)

Here the male mind is depicted as rational, capable of making logical decisions and controlling key activities. This foregrounding of mental reasoning links to historically dominant notions of men as logical thinkers (and women as tied to nature and therefore more emotional and less rational) (Seidler, 1994, 1997). Discursive practices underline such gendered constructions; for example, the effort required to lose weight is minimized (see Pomerantz, 1986)—"*just* a matter of choosing the right foods"—as if men's naturally rational approach can easily be applied to the task at hand.

In line with the hard bodies and rational minds advertised, specific health-promoting activities are remasculinized in order to appeal to male readers:

When you're walking, do your pelvic floor exercises. This will not only help relieve boredom, but also boosts circulation to the prostate

---

[2]*MoT* stands for Ministry of Transport. It is used as shorthand in the United Kingdom for the compulsory, annual check that every vehicle must pass to be legally allowed to drive on the roads.

(important to help prevent cancer), and because it increases blood-flow to that area, can significantly improve erectile function! (Manual, Section 8.10)

There is a concern, then, that men's needs should be fulfilled while engaged in healthy activities, in this case more/better sex. Perhaps because pelvic floor exercises are conventionally construed as feminine, an extra "manly" ingredient is required to make things more interesting and acceptable to men. It is also interesting to note that male sexuality is treated in a rather medicalized and functional way ("circulation to the prostate"; "increases blood-flow"; "improve erectile function"), an account that prioritizes the stimulation of phallocentric performance (and omits notions of agency, relationship, and emotion). In conclusion, Gough (2009) suggests that the preoccupation with preserving and protecting traditional masculinities could actually undermine health promotion efforts since aspects of conventional masculinities have been associated with men's poor health (see Courtenay, 2000; Gough, 2006). With regard to the HGV manual, the subordination of soft, loose, and flabby bodies in favor of idealistic hard bodies and a focus on the rational mind means that the embodied reality of being overweight or obese, and by extension the emotional consequences of such "deviant" embodiment within a health- and weight-conscious culture, is neglected.

As noted above, DA can also be used—indeed is more commonly used—to study social interaction. Our second extended example is taken from the work of Seymour-Smith (2009) on the negotiation of masculinity relating to participation in a support group for men with testicular cancer (TC). In the following extract, Paul and Cal, who belong to a TC support group, talk about the challenge of encouraging men to attend (Sarah is the researcher).

1. Paul   I think they expect to come along and find a load of ill people=

2. Cal   =yeah yeah (laughs)

3. Paul   [and you know (inaudible due to over talking)

4. Sarah   [yeah

5. Cal   [yeah it's er I think it's erm a bit of a I always use this one

6. but a bit of an alcoholics anonymous thing (2)

7. Sarah   yeah

8. Cal   stand up you know my names Cal Jackson I've had testicular

9. cancer and then burst into tears and all that sort of thing and

10. blokes don't like that sort of [thing

11. Sarah   [they just think I'm not going to do that

12. Cal   I don't want anybody to cry in front of me or anything like

13. that=

14. Sarah   =no

15. Cal   so they don't want to come along (p. 100)

First, you will note the transcription symbols that pepper this extract—discourse analysts (especially those using discursive psychology and/or conversation analysis) transcribe interactions in detail to include immediate responses (=), timed pauses (2), and overtalking ([) (for more information on transcription conventions, see Potter, 1996). At the start of the extract, Paul suggests that men might expect to find "a load of ill people" at the group (line 1). Cal then sets up a familiar image of self-help groups with reference to Alcoholics Anonymous (lines 6–9). Cal dramatizes the activities of this type of group by saying, "Stand up you know my name's Cal Jackson I've had testicular cancer and then burst into tears and that sort of thing" (lines 8–9). The upshot of this portrayal is then provided: "Blokes don't like that sort of thing" (line 10), a gendered explanation for why more men do not come forward for group meetings. The potential for emotional displays, rendered excessive here ("burst into tears," etc.), is presented as inappropriate for men in general while Cal and Paul's participation is legitimated because they know the reality rather than the stereotype. Elsewhere in the data, the feminized, emotion-driven nature of such groups is explicitly presented:

1. Matt   you know (.) but they seemed to be more erm she said er the woman

2. that run it she had breast cancer and she belonged to the breast

3. cancer er group and she said it was like a mothers' meeting you

4. know it was

5. Sarah   right

6. Matt   erm (1) you know th there was coffee mornings and stuff like that =

7. Sarah   =yeah (laughs)

8. Matt   guys don't er don't want that sort of thing anyway=

9. Sarah   =no

10. Matt   and that was how I perceived a self help group to be that it

11. was this sort of=

12. Sarah   =yeah

13. Matt   you know touchy-feely

14. Sarah   yeah

15. Matt   yeah you know [(laughter) they get hold of you and once they

16. Sarah [(laughter)

17. Matt   have you can't escape

18. Sarah   (laughs) they hug you to death (laughs)

19. Matt   yeah yeah (pp. 99–100)

Here, Matt discusses another local self-help group and in doing so builds up a comical portrayal of such groups as being "like a mothers' meeting" (line 3), where there are "*coffee mornings* and *stuff like that*" (line 6). In lines 10 through 19 Matt concludes his narrative of the group by positioning himself as somebody who perceives self-help groups in this way. *Touchy-feely* (line 13) is the term he draws upon, and he adds that such a group would "get hold of you and once they have you can't *escape*" (lines 15–17). With the "you know" (lines 13 and 15), Matt frames the interviewer as aware that self-help groups are parodied in such ways. Furthermore, the interviewer's laughter (lines 16 and 18) and co-construction (line 18) orient to this consensus. The point underlined here is that ordinarily men will be deterred from joining such caricatured women-centered group sessions. Seymour-Smith (2009) goes on to argue that the presentation of identity had a material consequence for the members of the self-help group interviewed—they changed the name of their group from "testicular cancer self-help group" to a new title, which omitted the troubling "self-help" concept. This has implications for health promotion. First, the name of self-help groups should be carefully considered, especially if men are to be attracted. Second, perhaps health education campaigns need to consider targeting men in ways that appeal or even conform to what we could describe as hegemonic masculine ideals (such as bravado, humor, or discretion)—although, as highlighted elsewhere, care perhaps needs to be taken not to replicate potentially damaging aspects of hegemonic masculinity by appealing to aspects of it when "marketing" health to men in this way (Robinson & Robertson, 2010).

In our final example, we draw from the work of Christine Stephens, Jenny Carryer, and Clair Budge (2004) that considered the identity and subject positions women negotiated in relation to hormone replacement therapy (HRT).[3] In the following two extracts, the women participants

---

[3]While we present only two discursive repertoires here, the full paper provided many more and a far more detailed discussion of the negotiations between these repertoires as subject positions are constructed and contested.

draw on what the authors termed a "biomedical" repertoire to explain the use of HRT:

1. I was just going to say that when I was younger I thought that menopause was females and sometimes males, who were aged around 45 to 50 who were grumpy. But I thought, you know, it wasn't really related to menstruation and that just stopped along the way. Causes them to be grumpy, bad tempered . . .

2. As I understand it having read as much as I have, that the body as you get older, the body stops producing these specific hormones and the benefit of the HRT tablet is to replace, um, hormones. (p. 337)

The use of HRT "tablets" is supported here by the use of a "biomedical" repertoire that includes descriptors of menopausal experience in terms of "symptoms" ("grumpy, bad tempered"; stopping "menstruation") brought on by an aging body ("as you get older") that ceases to function adequately ("stops producing these specific hormones"). As the authors highlight, the subject position taken up by women using this repertoire was one of a "rational decision maker who desired control over a potentially problematic body" (Stephens et al., 2004, p. 336). In contrast to this, other women drew on a "natural" repertoire to resist notions of the menopause as a "threatening change," and to oppose the use of HRT:

He [doctor] knows I prefer not to take drugs. So I went to a homeopath and, um, had some treatment there. I also have to say that I'm very much into I suppose trying to know my own body. I'm very physical and for the last probably 15 years have been a regular gym attender and to me it was always, "How can I get to know my body better?" Not that so I can beat it but so I can live with it and really appreciate the process without it being a burden. (p. 338)

Here the menopause is constructed as a bodily process requiring understanding ("trying to know my own body"; "know my body better") in order to reduce any impact on everyday life ("appreciate the process without it being a burden"). HRT is no longer a "tablet" to assist with maintaining a biological balance but now labeled a "drug" ("I prefer not to take drugs"), with the associated negative, addictive connotations, and therefore is to be (morally) avoided. The subject position taken up here is one of a woman who is "closer to the body's real needs, and who takes a more gentle and understanding approach to its control" (Stephens et al., 2004, p. 338).

Discussion and Conclusion

Within these three examples, we see how exploring discursive resources and practices can provide valuable insights to the relationships between gender and health. As we have suggested, the historical linking of men to the mind and rationality and women to the body and emotionality sets some parameters for the discursive resources drawn upon here. The men in Example 2 make it clear that the potential of self-help groups to be places of emotional expression is problematic for men when control, rationality, and stoicism form the dominant (hegemonic) discursive resource for understanding masculinity. Yet, for some women in Example 3, discursive resources formed in the linking of women with the body and emotionality provide an important opportunity to support a "natural" understanding of menopause (and concomitant rejection of HRT use)— an understanding established on an intimate knowing and understanding of the body based less in biology and more on listening, feeling, and expe-riencing. However, it is important also to note that exploring discourses shows similarities (as well as differences) in health discourses reproduced (and resisted) between men and women. In both Example 1 and Example 3 the discursive practice of "rational decision making" is employed to implore men to take care of their bodies and to sustain a biomedical view of menopause (and using HRT), respectively. This is because gendered discourses do not stand alone but interact (compete) with other dis-courses. One likely competing discursive resource here is that of "medical-ization," the precedence within that discourse given to professional (biomedical) knowledge and how adherence to suggested medical advice therefore represents the logical (rational *and* morally correct) decision.

Within this chapter we have summarized key features of content analy-sis and discourse analysis and provided some gender and health examples. The value of discursive analyses in particular has been emphasized; we have suggested that DA can bring forth fascinating insights into the social construction of health and gender through a focus on how cultural and contextual meanings are negotiated in practice. Such analyses are also well placed to critically inform ongoing health promotion campaigns—for example, making suggestions concerning the recruitment of men to health promotion (self-help) groups, calling for more diverse and embodied rep-resentations of the overweight male in self-help texts, and understanding the different subject positions and therefore decision-making processes of women in relation to HRT. The growing literature on DA as well as pub-lished papers in health and gender journals (e.g., *Journal of Health Psychology, Social Science & Medicine*) that employ DA to explore how men and women co-construct health in diverse contexts and how various texts play a role in (re)creating gendered "norms" in relation to health practices should further guide researcher efforts.

References

Aries, E. (1997). Women and men talking: Are they worlds apart? In M. R. Walsh (Ed.), *Women, men and gender: Ongoing debates* (pp. 91–100). New Haven, CT: Yale University Press.

Banks, I. (2005). *The HGV man manual.* Somerset, UK: Haynes.

Coates, J. (2004). *Women, men and language: A sociolinguistic account of gender differences in language.* London: Longman.

Courtenay, W. H. (2000). Constructions of masculinity and their influence on men's well being: A theory of gender and health. *Social Science and Medicine, 50,* 1385–1401.

Day, K., Gough, B., & McFadden, M. (2004). "Warning! Alcohol can seriously damage feminine health": A discourse analysis of recent British newspaper coverage of women and drinking. *Feminist Media Studies, 4*(2), 165–185.

Edwards, D., & Potter, J. (1992). *Discursive psychology.* London: SAGE.

Eglin, P., & Hester, S. (2003). *The Montreal massacre: A story of membership categorization analysis.* Waterloo, ON, Canada: Wilfrid Laurier University Press.

Fairclough, N. L. (1995). *Critical discourse analysis: The critical study of language.* Harlow, UK: Longman.

Foucault, M. (1980). *Power/knowledge: Selected interviews and other writings 1972–1977.* Brighton, UK: Harvester Press.

Galasiński, D. (2008). *Men's discourses of depression.* Basingstoke, Hampshire, UK: Palgrave Macmillan.

Gannon, K., Glover, L., & Abel, P. (2004). Masculinity, infertility, stigma and media reports. *Social Science and Medicine, 59*(6), 1169–1175.

Garfinkel, H. (1967). *Studies in ethnomethodology.* Englewood Cliffs, NJ: Prentice Hall.

Goffman, E. (1961). *Encounters: Two studies in the sociology of interaction.* Oxford, UK: Bobbs-Merrill.

Gough, B. (2006). Try to be healthy, but don't forgo your masculinity: Deconstructing men's health discourse in the media. *Social Science & Medicine, 63,* 2476–2488.

Gough, B. (2009). Promoting "masculinity" over health: A critical analysis of men's health promotion with particular reference to an obesity reduction "manual." In B. Gough & S. Robertson (Eds.), *Men, masculinities and health: Critical perspectives* (pp. 125–142). Basingstoke, Hampshire, UK: Palgrave Macmillan.

Hutchby, I., & Wooffitt, R. (2008). *Conversation analysis.* Cambridge, UK: Polity.

Jefferson, G. (1990). List construction as a task and resource. In G. Psathas (Ed.), *Interaction competence* (pp. 63–92). Washington, DC: University Press of America.

Measham, F., & Brain, K. (2005). "Binge" drinking, British alcohol policy and the new culture of intoxication. *Crime, Media, Culture, 1*(3), 262–283.

Pomerantz, A. (1986). Extreme case formulations. *Human Studies, 9,* 219–230.

Potter, J. (1996). *Representing reality: Discourse, rhetoric and social construction.* London: SAGE.

Robinson, M., & Robertson, S. (2010). The application of social marketing to promoting men's health: A brief critique. *International Journal of Men's Health, 9*(1), 50–61.

Seidler, V. (1994). *Unreasonable men: Masculinity and social theory*. London: Routledge.

Seidler, V. (1997). *Man enough: Embodying masculinities*. London: SAGE.

Seymour-Smith, S. (2009). Men's negotiations of a "legitimate" self-help group identity. In B. Gough & S. Robertson (Eds.), *Men, masculinities and health: Critical perspectives* (pp. 93–108). Basingstoke, Hampshire, UK: Palgrave Macmillan.

Stephens, C., Carryer, J., & Budge, C. (2004). To have or to take: Discourse, positioning, and narrative identity in women's accounts of HRT. *Health: An Interdisciplinary Journal for the Social Study of Health, Illness and Medicine, 8*(3), 329–350.

Tannen, D. (2001). *You just don't understand: Women and men in conversation*. London: Harper.

Weber, R. P. (1990). *Basic content analysis*. London: SAGE.

Wetherell, M. (1998). Positioning and interpretative repertoires: Conversation analysis and post-structuralism in dialogue. *Discourse & Society, 9*, 387–412.

Wetherell, M., Taylor, S., & Yates, S. J. (Eds.). (2001). *Discourse theory and practice: A reader*. London: SAGE.

Wiggins, S. (2004). Good for "you": Generic and individual healthy eating advice in family mealtimes. *Journal of Health Psychology, 9*(4), 535–548.

Wilkinson, S. (2003). Focus groups. In J. A. Smith (Ed.), *Qualitative psychology: A practical guide to research methods* (pp. 184–204). London: SAGE.

Willott, S., & Griffin, C. (1997). Wham bam, am I a man? Unemployed men talk about masculinities. *Feminism and Psychology, 7*, 107–128.

Approaches to Examining Gender Relations in Health Research

Joan L. Bottorff

John L. Oliffe

Mary T. Kelly

Natalie A. Chambers

U nderstanding the influence of gender (i.e., masculinities and femininities) on health experiences and practices, and addition-ally how interplay *within and between genders,* vis-à-vis gender relations, mediates those practices, has begun to receive research attention (Krieger, 2003; Lyons, 2009; Schofield, Connell, Walker, Wood, & Butland, 2000). However, one of the challenges facing researchers is the lack of well-developed methods to study gender relations. Accordingly there is an urgent need for developing and applying gender relations methods in health research (Johnson, Greaves, & Repta, 2009). In this chapter we describe some conceptualizations of gender relations and follow by detailing methods that we have used to examine the connec-tions between gender, couple interactions, and tobacco reduction efforts. The chapter concludes with recommendations for future devel-opment of gender relations research methods.

Gender Relations and Health

Theories of masculinity and femininity contend that gender is socially constructed and reenacted in the daily activities of our lives including health and illness practices (Connell, 2005; Lyons, 2009). The ways in which we relate to the health of our body and the practices we engage in to be healthy are infused with culturally constructed masculine and feminine ideals to such an extent that it is akin to performing gender (Saltonstall, 1993). For example, research that has explored the relationships between gender and health behaviors demonstrates that masculine ideals are reproduced by men's practice of risky health behaviors, such as using alcohol or drugs to self-medicate depression (Oliffe & Phillips, 2008; Oliffe, Robertson, Kelly, Roy, & Ogrodniczuk, 2010), and that idealized versions of femininity tend to embody health-seeking and self-help practices (Lyons, 2009).

In the field of gender relations, these distinctly different idealized masculine and feminine health practices are deconstructed, with particular emphasis on unraveling the ways that culturally dominant forms of practicing gender are negotiated, coproduced, and performed within interpersonal relationships. In addition, examinations of gender relations focus on describing activities and transactions that give meaning to interactions within specific cultural, historic, and social contexts. For example, household relations such as spousal relationships play a critical role in shaping health practices. In these domestic interactions, men and women in heterosexual households tend to be influenced by prevailing gendered expectations that reflect dominant cultural values (Smiler & Epstein, 2010).

In some cultures, women are known to positively influence health behaviors among the men in their lives (Bottorff et al., 2010; Robertson, 2007; Westmass, Wild, & Ferrence, 2002) in part because of alignments to feminine ideals around nurturing, caring, and concern for others' well-being and, perhaps, as compensatory measures for masculine identities that typically embody disregard for self-health. As such, research that explores the influence of gender relations on health behavior has the potential to inform health interventions in ways that are responsive to these relationships. Although there are diverse gender relations, contextualized by culture and social location, the examples in this chapter are drawn from our research, which focuses on heterosexual relationships in Canada.

Current Conceptualizations of Gender Relations

Conceptualizations of gender relations have begun to emerge amid growing interest in gender influences in everyday life. In Connell's (2005) influential work, masculinities are constructed in relation to idealized characteristics and practices to influence men's identities and behaviors, and as an active "place" of connection within gender relations. Some forms of masculinity are hegemonic, and function in ways that subordinate other masculinities as well as femininities. This is reflected in Connell's classification of masculinities comprising *complicit* masculinities that reflect sustained hegemony by enacting traditional Western social practices that position men as family providers, stoic and autonomous; *subordinate* forms of masculinity that typically embody practices traditionally associated with femininities, including domesticity, weakness, and lack of authority; and *marginalized* masculinities that are often linked to race, class, and ethnic demographics that are de-privileged because they do not resemble and/or conform to Western, White, middle-class masculine ideals (Connell, 2005).

Although theorizing femininities has received less attention (Lyons, 2009), some attention has been focused on developing concepts of femininity as a way to explore male-dominant gender relations. For example, Howson (2006) further developed Connell's work on hegemonic masculinity by identifying and describing the tripartite relationships of femininity to hegemonic masculinity as *emphasized, ambivalent,* or *protest*. *Emphasized* femininity is complicit with, and accommodates, hegemonic masculinity; *ambivalent* femininities strategically resist and/or cooperate with hegemonic masculinity; and *protest* femininities challenge the foundation of the gender order, contesting assumptions of the hierarchies governing intrarelational constructs configuring masculinities and femininities. Efforts to theorize femininity as a gendered phenomenon without reference to male dominance are also needed.

In revising Connell's theory of gender hegemony, Schippers (2007) argues that in addition to social *practices,* the symbolic and discursive meaning and value of femininity and masculinity must be included. She adjusted Connell's definition of hegemonic masculinity, proposing to make the relationship between masculinity and femininity central to the theory, and developed an alternative means of conceptualizing femininities that allows for the concept of *hegemonic femininity*. Rather than conceiving masculinity and femininity as separate from each other, Schippers insisted that an understanding of how gender hegemony is produced requires focusing on the relationships between masculinity and femininity. As a result, her theory highlights the idealized relationships between masculinity and femininity that comprise configurations of gender dominance, as opposed to separate configurations of gender that exist as relating exclusively to hegemonic masculinity. In this schema, *hegemonic femininity* is superior to subordinate or "pariah" femininities precisely because it embodies the *relationship* between masculinity and femininity characteristic of gender hegemony (e.g., women desire men who are strong and authoritative, thus making those qualities unavailable to women, who then must be weak and require protection). Schippers argued that a focus on gender relations will help researchers avoid confining masculinity and femininity to men and women respectively. By opening up space for conceptualizing male femininities and female masculinities, it becomes possible to reflect the fluidity of gender and locate the practices of men and women on a gender continuum, thereby extending the study of gender relations in the broad context of social life.

Social constructionist health researchers have increasingly lobbied for a more nuanced relational theory of masculinities and femininities, and a few approaches are theoretically and empirically emergent (Lyons, 2009; Schippers, 2007). However, it is clear that there are some specific areas requiring further theoretical and methodological attention, including (1) understanding the relational aspects of gender and paying attention to the intersectional aspects of masculinities and femininities (Howson, 2006); (2) identifying the ways in which masculinities and femininities are embodied (Lyons, 2009); (3) questioning which characteristics are manly or womanly, and of these practices which position femininity as complementary and/or inferior to masculinity (Schippers, 2007); (4) interrogating and describing hegemonic masculinities that are characterized by power dynamics that subordinate women and some men (Connell, 2005); and (5) examining the micro-, meso-, and macro-level social processes that produce gender inequalities (Ferree & Hall, 2000).

Gender Relations in Health Research

Health researchers interested in gender relations have primarily focused on social processes and interactions influencing health as they occur between men and women, and among men and among women. Schofield and associates (2000) argue, for example, that men's and women's experiences of health occur in the context of interactive gender relations within specific social contexts and settings. They contend that by using a gender relations approach it is possible to examine men's and women's interactions, and the means by which these interactions influence health opportunities and constraints. Such an approach to gender relations provides the opportunity to investigate and include relational constructs connecting masculinities and femininities, the relational positioning of intramasculinities and intrafemininities, and the relationship of these gender dynamics to the social environment.

Although few researchers have examined gender relations in the context of health-related experiences, some important directions have been identified. Smith and Robertson (2008), for example, recommend that gender and health researchers investigate the everyday lived experiences of women and men with the aim of developing an understanding about how power is negotiated in gender relations. In this way, they echo the work of

Schippers (2007), Connell (2005), Howson (2006), and critical feminists who insist research approaches to gender relations need to account for the reproduction of gender hegemony and acknowledge and interrogate cultural norms around power and inequality in society.

We located a few empirical studies where researchers examined the influence of gender relations on men's and women's health using qualitative methods. For example, Mumtaz and Salway (2009) conducted four phases of fieldwork to collect data in their ethnographic study of how gender influences contraceptive practices and pregnancy. They started with broad informal house-to-house surveys in a Punjabi village in Pakistan to understand general kinship, class, and economic structures. This was followed by many informal observations and interviews, as well as more formal semistructured interviews with women, their husbands, and their mothers-in-law focusing on gender relations in the context of reproductive and contraceptive health practices. Finally, the researchers chose five case studies to follow more closely by conducting a series of interviews and observation to examine power and gender relations. The findings, drawn from constant comparative methods, demonstrated how attention to men and masculinities and woman-to-woman bonds in addition to husband-wife relationships in the village, was central to understanding gender relations and women's reproductive health. Their approach mustered important understandings about the complex nature of and the influence of locale-specific gender orders.

In a related example, researchers in Ghana (Tolhurst, Amekudzi, Nyonator, Squire, & Theobald, 2008) drew on two consecutive studies to explore the gendered dynamics of intrahousehold bargaining related to children's treatment for malaria in rural communities. The first study employed a large situational approach involving government workers in a cross section of health districts who were trained by the researchers to conduct focus group discussions and lead community meetings and mapping exercises, role plays, and critical incidence interviews. This participatory approach to examine gender relations was an intervention in and of itself. In the second study, the researchers conducted in-depth interviews with 14 women in various marital situations, as well as participatory learning discussions in community-based formats. These data collection methods allowed the researchers to explore the complex dynamics between men and women in household bargaining that influenced children's health. Using this approach, the authors learned that while women were responsible for detecting illness in the family, the decision about whether a child received formal treatment for malaria was linked to payment, something that fell to men, who often preferred to use the money for other expenses such as plowing fields, drinking, or having multiple wives. The findings illustrated the ways in which the women attempted to persuade men to contribute or borrow money for treatment. As a result of their micro-level research methods, these researchers were able to recommend how different approaches to gender mainstreaming at the broader political and social level might produce different results at the individual and familial level. These studies reveal the potential for qualitative approaches to uncover important connections between gender relations and family health practices and provide direction for future methodological considerations as well as program and policy development.

In summary, data collection and analytical tools to guide researchers seeking to investigate gender relations are still very much under development. In the following section, we describe approaches to qualitative data collection and analysis that were developed in a research program investigating tobacco reduction and have demonstrated potential to support research on gender relations.

Developing Methods for Gender Relations in Health Research: The FACET Example

The Families Controlling and Eliminating Tobacco (FACET) project provided an opportunity to develop gender relations approaches in health research. This program of research focused on examining women's tobacco reduction efforts during pregnancy and the postpartum period in the context of couple interactions (Bottorff, Kalaw, Johnson, Chambers, et al., 2005; Bottorff, Kalaw, Johnson, Stewart, & Greaves, 2005; Greaves et al., 2003). We were interested in situating our research program in the micro-social context of the home in order to examine the influence of household dynamics on women's smoking. The home represents an ideal context to study gender relations because it is a location where gender is most intimately practiced and negotiated. The importance of gender relations is reflected in descriptions of spousal relationships as behavioral systems encompassing divisions of labor, expressions of affection, and hostility. In the following sections we highlight the research strategies used to support our efforts to study the influence of gender relations. In keeping with the exploratory and descriptive aims of the FACET project, qualitative research methods were used.

PARTICIPANT RECRUITMENT AND DATA COLLECTION FOR GENDER RELATIONS RESEARCH

Recruitment and data collection methods in studies focusing on gender relations are important considerations, particularly when the research involves couples and socially stigmatized health behaviors such as smoking and other substance use. Although qualitative interviews have been noted for the benefits that participants receive by telling their stories, expressing unspoken feelings and unresolved issues in an atmosphere of sympathetic understanding (Ortiz, 2001), they can also create negative situations. For example, we have observed how interviews that invite participants to consider changes to their own substance use (e.g., requests to comply with smoking restrictions) can lead to interaction styles that have the potential to contribute to conflict and tension between couple participants (Bottorff, Kalaw, Johnson, Stewart, et al., 2005; Greaves, Kalaw, & Bottorff, 2007). In our FACET research, efforts to protect potentially vulnerable participants guided our approaches to recruitment and data collection, the specificities of which are described below.

In the FACET study we recruited women who had reduced or stopped smoking during pregnancy along with their partners. Because smoking during pregnancy is highly stigmatized in Canada, women are often pressured by their partners and others to quit smoking during pregnancy. This pressure to remain smoke free can continue into the postpartum period. Hypothesizing that the pregnant and postpartum woman is the most vulnerable member of the couple-dyad, we decided that women should be approached first for the study. When they expressed an interest in participating in the study, we asked them to obtain agreement from their partners to participate before we set up the first interview. The absence of their partner at initial contact made it possible for women to refuse to participate without involving their partner, thereby minimizing possible conflicts for women who may have otherwise been vulnerable to manipulation or coercion to participate or not (Bottorff, Kalaw, Johnson, Chambers, et al., 2005).

No guidelines exist regarding qualitative data collection for health research with a gender relations focus. The challenge of safely gathering data on gender relations within the context of tobacco use during pregnancy was contingent on ensuring confidentiality for individual partners, so that they were comfortable sharing their views and experiences regarding sensitive or socially stigmatized issues. Although some researchers have recommended the use of conjoint couple interviews to elicit rich information and observe interactions, individual interviews may be more appropriate when exploring sensitive topics because participants often refuse to disclose certain kinds of information in the presence of a partner (Racher, Kaufert, & Havens, 2000). In our research related to tobacco reduction and pregnancy, protecting women's vulnerability to increased pressure and conflict with partners about smoking (e.g., as might be the case if women had slipped or relapsed to smoking during pregnancy without their partner's knowledge and this information was revealed in a joint interview) was a key consideration (Bottorff, Kalaw, Johnson, Stewart, et al., 2005). For this reason we utilized separate, sequential individual interviews with dyad partners. In the context of an individual interview, participants could be more comfortable discussing behaviors about which their partners might be sensitive (e.g., nagging or coercive behavior) or of which they might be critical (e.g., sneaking cigarettes).

We recognized that within the context of open-ended individual interviews, the researcher and each partner co-constructed an account of the couple experience. Using a semistructured interview guide to collect data about gendered interactions and tobacco, we posed similar open-ended questions to both women and their partners to help us understand common events and experiences from both partners' experiences. To obtain interactional data, we asked participants what we would hear if we were present when discussions with their partner about smoking took place. We also asked participants to share specific examples of their discussions related to tobacco issues and encouraged them to provide as much detail as possible about what each person said. These questions provided important clues about the nature of tobacco-related interactions for some participants. After analyzing the initial interviews, we realized that most tobacco issues were not addressed or negotiated in focused discussions. Rather, interactions about tobacco use were often threaded across other spousal interactions about domestic duties, stress and coping, child care and parenting, finances, and recreational time. With additional interview questions, we obtained rich descriptions of specific contexts in which tobacco issues are raised either directly or indirectly in gendered ways.

ANALYTICAL TOOLS FOR GENDER RELATIONS ANALYSIS

In the FACET research we also developed several analytical strategies to investigate gender relations within and across couple-dyads. The first involves the use of dyad summaries for analyzing individual interviews conducted with couples. The second involves the use of the Minnesota-based Domestic Abuse Intervention Project's Power and Control Wheel as an analytical framework, and in the third approach we engaged Howson's (2006) conceptualization of masculinities and femininities as a theoretical lens to guide gender relations data analysis.

The Dyad Summary

Because the interview is a "site of meaning making" (Warren, 2002, p. 86), the account each partner shared with the interviewer was considered an actively produced version of the couple's reality (Valentine, 1999). In the analytic process, it was important to interpret the two accounts (the mother's account and the father's account) to produce a "joint" description of each couple's experiences. In developing summations of each couple's everyday gender relations involving tobacco we needed to capture the complexity of individual stories, perceptual differences between partners, discrepant accounts within dyads, changes in couple interactions from pre-pregnancy to postpartum, and the range of different experiences among couples. In developing an analytic tool for constructing the couple's experience from the individual interviews, we drew on Knafl and Ayres's (1996) approach of family case summaries, an analytic strategy to manage large amounts of data and preserve the integrity of the family unit.

We developed a framework for dyad summaries with "at-a-glance" background information (e.g., whether pregnancy was planned, number of children, smoking status) (Bottorff, Kalaw, Johnson, Stewart, et al., 2005) and categories of interactions that would help to bring together and organize data in such a way as to reflect couple experiences. To complete the dyad summaries, we thoroughly reviewed individual interviews and field notes for each couple, compared and synthesized the transcribed data from the participants in each dyad, and referenced transcript line numbers to link summaries to supporting data. In addition, we structured the dyad summaries to include memos about the couples' experiences gained in the process of conducting the interviews and analyzing data. The summaries typically reduced the two interview transcripts for each dyad (representing 40 to 50 pages) to 5- to 10-page single-spaced summaries. The dyad summaries provided the research team with a detailed and systematic interpretation of each couple's experiences of tobacco reduction and facilitated constant comparison of data within and across dyads over time. If structured appropriately, dyad summaries provide a useful starting point for examining gender relations.

The Power and Control Wheel

A second analytical tool that we used to examine gender relations in the FACET study is the Power and Control Wheel. The Minnesota-based Domestic Abuse Intervention Project's Power and Control Wheel identifies eight aspects of abuse in intimate heterosexual relationships, including economic abuse, coercion, intimidation, emotional abuse, isolation, blaming, using children, and using male privilege to exert control (Domestic Abuse Intervention Programs, 2008). Using a case study approach combined with elements of the Power and Control Wheel helped us understand gender relations as they played out among heterosexual couples when women were engaged in tobacco reduction during pregnancy. The Power and Control Wheel also provided a useful analytic framework for the examination of couple dynamics within the context of substance use (Smith, 2000) and was particularly suitable for our research purposes, because it identified specific, coercive dynamics of abuse within relationships and related these dynamics to external social forces, thus providing an ideal approach to examining gender relations (Greaves et al., 2007).

Using a maximum variation sampling approach, we carefully chose three dyad cases that represented distinctly different interaction types from our earlier FACET findings (Bottorff et al., 2006). We began by constructing narrative summaries of each dyad from the point of view of the women. However, we also drew on data from men partners to validate and extend our interpretation of the effect of interaction patterns on women. Representative examples in these data illustrating relationships between the elements of power and control and the use of tobacco were used to make comparisons among the three cases. For example, gendered interaction patterns such as limiting the women's access to money to purchase cigarettes (economic control), threatening to expose their smoking to family members (using isolation), and the use of verbal tactics or argumentativeness to pressure them to stop smoking (using male privilege) were a few of the dynamics comprising the gender relations we were able to identify using this analytic approach (Greaves et al., 2007).

Although no participants directly reported experiencing any form of interpersonal violence in their relationships, this analysis of three couples using the Power and Control Wheel analytic framework allowed us to identify gender relations patterns in and around women's tobacco use that were consistent with dysfunctional elements of power and control. As such, this study stands as an example of a women-centered approach to gender relations analyses. In summary, the Power and Control Wheel draws attention to eight dimensions of gender relations that reflect power differences and is a useful analytical tool for developing understandings about how power is (and is not) negotiated in various contexts.

Using Critical Perspectives on Masculinities and Femininities

Howson's (2006) framework of gender relations also provides a useful theoretical lens for the analyses of qualitative data in that he identifies plural forms of femininities and masculinities within a critical feminist framework that situates all femininities as subordinate to hegemonic masculinity. In light of current social norms that stigmatize mothers who smoke but tolerate fathers who smoke, we believed that this framework provided an appropriate theoretical lens for facilitating our understanding of gender relations in this context (Bottorff et al., 2010).

We began our analyses with independent close readings of women's interviews, focusing on segments of the transcripts where women addressed men's smoking. We reviewed these segments in detail, comparing and contrasting data from all participants to identify patterns in women's constructions of men's smoking. In particular, the data were explored for representations of femininities and masculinities as described by Howson (2006).

The use of this analytic approach produced insights into how gender relations in the domestic context were characterized by women relying on discourses of *emphasized* femininities (accommodating hegemonic masculinity) or *ambivalent* femininities (strategically resisting or cooperating with hegemonic masculinity) as they contrasted their role in the family with that of their male partners. The three themes we delineated that comprised women's responses to men's continued smoking were characterized by gender relations that involved women defending men's smoking, regulating men's smoking, or accepting men's smoking as an artifact of their autonomy. The women's constructions of men's smoking reflected an underlying tension that included discourses related to the good father and to hegemonic masculine ideals, something that "good fathers" shouldn't do, but, inversely, something that men deserve. We interpreted the combinations of compliance, resistance, and cooperation with dominant hegemonic principles as representing a gender relations style that Howson (2006) had labeled *ambivalent* femininity (challenging the foundation of the gender order). Specifically, there was compliance in accepting and affirming men's breadwinner and protector status underpinning constructions of men's needs to smoke, but resistance and questioning about how men who smoked might best embody their roles as fathers. In addition, the deep concerns women expressed about the effect of smoking on their partner's health and the health of their children evoked evidence of ambivalent femininities that prescribed women's roles in taking care of the health of the men and children in their lives (Lee & Owens, 2002). In Howson's terms, this concern could also be interpreted as women responding with compliance and accommodation to men's lack of interest or expertise in self-health. In summary, using Howson's (2006) and Connell's (2005) gender relations theories as analytical frameworks provided useful analytical tools that helped reveal how women who align with idealized femininities can contribute to the reproduction of dominant masculinities in their everyday lives.

Future Directions

It is clear that continued efforts are needed to develop methods to examine the style and quality of the interactions that occur in the relationships between men and women, and among men and among women, as they perform socially constructed gendered health practices, and to explore the health implications of these interactions for men and women. The approaches to examining gender relations described in this chapter can be applied to other health and illness contexts and, we believe, provide important directions for furthering the development of gender relations methods.

In moving gender relations methods forward, we propose three key considerations. First, researchers focusing on gender relations in heterosexual couple-dyads to build understandings about health practices should ensure that the research methods used make audible the voices of men and women. This enables privileging gender relations as the mediator and/or outcome of health and illness practices, rather than subverting to competing victim discourses so often associated with this type of research. This approach will also help us avoid the binaries that pit women's and men's health research against one another (Broom, 2009). Furthermore, as gender relations researchers, by including both men and women we can focus on the interconnectedness of men's and women's health in increasingly sophisticated ways to advance the design of gender-appropriate programs and policies. Integral to this work is the interrogation of hegemony that positions women as the primary providers of family health amid men's estrangement from nurturing and self-health, and prevailing norms such as those that suggest married men live longer whereas being in a heterosexual relationship can be a significant health risk for women. In deconstructing such norms around gender relations we will be able to explain varying alignments and health practices within and across couples.

Second, gender relations health research should not be exclusively occupied by or preoccupied with heterosexual relations, but rather the methods should be robust enough to thoughtfully explore health within an array of intimate relationships (e.g., gay, lesbian, bisexual) as well as with those who are transitioning (i.e., transsexual). For example, grounded theory may hold potential for exploring shifts in gender relations, and the health implications during transitions among transgendered individuals, including their intimate relationships. And finally, gender relations research should also be conceptualized and applied to other peer and family relations. For example, although our FACET research was clearly linked to family health issues, future studies might explicitly integrate a wider array of characters (e.g., peers, siblings, relatives) to better account for the intersections of gender relations and health and illness practices. Examples might include intergenerational perspectives about health practices or the impact of peer gender relations at various historical and life course points. In widening the scope for multiple perspectives to be heard, the health and illness issues that gender relations can meaningfully engage are greatly increased.

In summary, a better understanding of gender relations has much to offer by extending health research beyond reporting one-sided accounts and/or distilling gender differences between women and men. Efforts to study the intersection between gender relations with individual and community health provide an important way to acknowledge the breadth of human experience, address temporal and changing cultural contexts, direct attention to an underrecognized component of health, and provide the insights needed to inform gender-sensitive programs and policies. The development of appropriate methods for conducting research on gender relations is essential to this endeavor.

References

Bottorff, J. L., Kalaw, C., Johnson, J. L., Chambers, N., Stewart, M., Greaves, L., et al. (2005). Unraveling smoking ties: How tobacco use is embedded in couple interactions. *Research in Nursing and Health, 28,* 316–328.

Bottorff, J. L., Kalaw, C., Johnson, J. L., Stewart, M., & Greaves, L. (2005). Tobacco use in intimate spaces: Issues in the study of couple dynamics. *Qualitative Health Research, 15,* 564–577.

Bottorff, J., Kalaw, C., Johnson, J. L., Stewart, M., Greaves, L., & Carey, J. (2006). Couple dynamics during women's tobacco reduction in pregnancy and post-partum. *Nicotine & Tobacco Research, 8,* 499–509.

Bottorff, J. L., Oliffe, J., Kelly, M. T., Greaves, L., Johnson, J. L., Ponic, P., et al. (2010). Men's business, women's work: Gender influences and fathers' smoking. *Sociology of Health and Illness, 32,* 583–596.

Broom, D. H. (2009). Men's health and women's health: Deadly enemies or strategic allies. *Critical Public Health, 19,* 269–277.

Connell, R. (2005). *Masculinities* (2nd ed.). Berkeley: University of California Press.

Domestic Abuse Intervention Programs. (2008). *The Duluth Model: Power and Control Wheel.* Retrieved May 25, 2010, from http://www.theduluthmodel .org/wheelgallery.php

Ferree, M. M., & Hall, E. J. (2000). Gender stratification and paradigm change. *American Sociological Review, 65,* 475–481.

Greaves, L., Cormier, R., Devries, K., Bottorff, J., Johnson, J., & Kirkland, S. A. D. (2003). *Expecting to quit: A best practices review of smoking cessation interventions for pregnant and postpartum girls and women.* Vancouver, BC, Canada: BC Centre of Excellence for Women's Health.

Greaves, L., Kalaw, C., & Bottorff, J. L. (2007). Case studies in power and control related to tobacco use during pregnancy. *Women's Health Issues, 17,* 325–332.

Howson, R. (2006). *Challenging hegemonic masculinity.* London: Routledge.

Johnson, J. L., Greaves, L., & Repta, R. (2009). Better science with sex and gender: Facilitating the use of a sex and gender-based analysis in health research. *International Journal for Equity in Health, 8,* 14. Retrieved December 5, 2010, from http://www.equityhealthj.com/content/8/1/14

Knafl, K., & Ayres, L. (1996). Managing large qualitative data sets in family research. *Journal of Family Nursing, 2,* 350–365.

Krieger, N. (2003). Genders, sexes, and health: What are the connections—and why does it matter? *International Journal of Epidemiology, 32,* 652–657.

Lee, C., & Owens, R. (2002). *The psychology of men's health series.* Philadelphia: Open University Press.

Lyons, A. (2009). Masculinities, femininities, behaviour and health. *Social and Personality Psychology Compass, 3,* 394–412.

Mumtaz, Z., & Salway, S. (2009). Understanding gendered influences on women's reproductive health in Pakistan: Moving beyond the autonomy paradigm. *Social Science & Medicine, 68,* 1349–1356.

Oliffe, J. L., & Phillips, M. (2008). Depression, men and masculinities: A review and recommendations. *Journal of Men's Health, 5,* 194–202.

Oliffe, J. L., Robertson, S., Kelly, M., Roy, P., & Ogrodniczuk, J. (2010). Connecting masculinity and depression among international male university students. *Qualitative Health Research, 20*(7) 987–998.

Ortiz, S. (2001). How interviewing became therapy for wives of professional athletes: Learning from a serendipitous experience. *Qualitative Inquiry, 7,* 192–220.

Racher, F., Kaufert, J., & Havens, B. (2000). Conjoint research interviews with frail, elderly couples: Methodological implications. *Journal of Family Nursing, 6,* 367–379.

Robertson, S. (2007). *Understanding men and health: Masculinities, identity and well-being.* Maidenhead, UK: Open University Press.

Saltonstall, R. (1993). Healthy bodies, social bodies: Men's and women's concepts and practices of health in everyday life. *Social Science & Medicine, 36,* 7–14.

Schippers, M. (2007). Recovering the feminine other: Masculinity, femininity, and gender hegemony. *Theory and Society, 36,* 85–102.

Schofield, T., Connell, R. W., Walker, L., Wood, J., & Butland, D. (2000). Understanding men's health and illness: A gender-relations approach to policy, research, and practice. *Journal of American College Health, 48,* 247–256.

Smiler, A. P., & Epstein, M. (2010). Measuring gender: Options and issues. In J. C. Chrisler & D. R. McCreary (Eds.), *Handbook of gender research in psychology* (Vol. 1, pp. 133–157). New York: Springer.

Smith, J. A., & Robertson, S. (2008). Men's health promotion: A new frontier in Australia and the UK? *Health Promotion International, 23,* 283–289.

Smith, J. W. (2000). Addiction medicine and domestic violence. *Journal of Substance Abuse Treatment, 19,* 329–338.

Tolhurst, R., Amekudzi, Y. P., Nyonator, F. K., Squire, S. B., & Theobald, S. (2008). "He will ask why the child gets sick so often": The gendered dynamics of intra-household bargaining over health care for children with fever in the Volta Region of Ghana. *Social Science & Medicine, 66,* 1106–1117.

Valentine, G. (1999). Doing household research: Interviewing couples together and apart. *Area, 31,* 67–74.

Warren, C. (2002). Qualitative interviewing. In J. Gubrium & J. Holstein (Eds.), *Handbook of interview research: Context and method* (pp. 83–101). Thousand Oaks, CA: SAGE.

Westmass, J., Wild, T. C., & Ferrence, R. (2002). Effects of gender in social control of smoking cessation. *Health Psychology, 21,* 368–376.

Developing a Gender Role Socialization Scale

11

Brenda Toner

Taryn Tang

Alisha Ali

Donna Akman

Noreen Stuckless

Mary Jane Esplen

Cheryl Rolin-Gilman

Lori Ross

We have developed a Gender Role Socialization Scale (GRSS) for women to address the internalization of prescribed gender role messages for women that may affect well-being. Female gender role socialization may be conceptualized as an enduring social construct in which women's lives can be contextualized (Lips, 1993; Worell & Remer, 1992). Currently, there are a number of mental health concerns that are more prevalent in women than in men, including depression, eating disorders, somatoform disorders, and most phobias (American Psychiatric Association, 1994). Therefore, it is imperative that research be undertaken to examine the various factors that may account for these differences between women and men. We acknowledge that this binary view of gender and health has theoretical and methodological limitations. We would argue, however, this traditional view and methodology is "alive and well" and continues to influence our well-being.

In our clinical experience, we have found that there is a lack of assessment and outcome measures that address gender and societal prescriptions for women. We suggest that this scale can be used as a tool for assessing or exploring the degree to which women have internalized prescribed gender role messages and how these messages may be affecting their health and well-being. The scale can also be used to examine the relationship between internalized gender role messages and the various types of mental health concerns that women experience, in order to facilitate the development of prevention and treatment protocols. As well, the GRSS can serve an important empirical function as a predictive or as an outcome measure in psychotherapy research with female clients. Moreover, this scale is applicable to female clients presenting with different symptoms because it does not focus on specific symptoms or diagnostic categories.

Gender Role Socialization Scale for Women

Please read the following statements and indicate how each one applies to you at this time in your life. *Please circle only one number for each item.* There are no right or wrong answers to these statements.

1) Strongly Disagree	2) Disagree	3) Slightly Disagree	4) Neutral	5) Slightly Agree	6) Agree	7) Strongly Agree
1. If I don't accomplish everything I should, then I must be a failure.						
1	2	3	4	5	6	7
2. I am to blame if I have low self-esteem.						
1	2	3	4	5	6	7
3. If I don't get what I need, it is because I ask for too much.						
1	2	3	4	5	6	7
4. What I look like is more important than how I feel.						
1	2	3	4	5	6	7
5. I feel embarrassed by my own sexual desires.						
1	2	3	4	5	6	7

1) Strongly Disagree	2) Disagree	3) Slightly Disagree	4) Neutral	5) Slightly Agree	6) Agree	7) Strongly Agree

6. I feel that I must always make room in my life to take care of others.

1	2	3	4	5	6	7

7. I will never be happy if I am not in a romantic relationship.

1	2	3	4	5	6	7

8. Compared to men, I am less able to handle stress.

1	2	3	4	5	6	7

9. If I am unhappy, it is because I am too hard to please.

1	2	3	4	5	6	7

10. If I take time for myself, I feel selfish.

1	2	3	4	5	6	7

11. If I do not like my body, I am to blame.

1	2	3	4	5	6	7

12. If other people let me down, it is because I expect too much.

1	2	3	4	5	6	7

13. I have only myself to blame for my problems.

1	2	3	4	5	6	7

14. I can't feel good about myself unless I feel physically attractive.

1	2	3	4	5	6	7

15. If I ever feel overwhelmed, it must mean that I am incompetent.

1	2	3	4	5	6	7

16. I feel that I must look good on the outside even if I don't feel good on the inside.

1	2	3	4	5	6	7

17. I feel that the needs of others are more important than my own needs.

1	2	3	4	5	6	7

18. No matter how I feel I must always try to look my best.

1	2	3	4	5	6	7

(Continued)

(Continued)

1) Strongly Disagree	2) Disagree	3) Slightly Disagree	4) Neutral	5) Slightly Agree	6) Agree	7) Strongly Agree
19. I don't feel that I can leave a relationship even when I know that it is not satisfying.						
1	2	3	4	5	6	7
20. I feel that I am not allowed to ask that my own needs be met.						
1	2	3	4	5	6	7
21. I don't like to say nice things about myself.						
1	2	3	4	5	6	7
22. Whenever I see media images of women, I feel dissatisfied with my body.						
1	2	3	4	5	6	7
23. I feel that I must always put my family's emotional needs before my own.						
1	2	3	4	5	6	7
24. I feel as though I should be less sexually forward than men.						
1	2	3	4	5	6	7
25. If a relationship fails, I usually feel that it is my fault.						
1	2	3	4	5	6	7
26. If I take time for myself, I feel guilty.						
1	2	3	4	5	6	7
27. Whenever I am eating, I am always thinking about how it will affect my body size.						
1	2	3	4	5	6	7
28. I often give up my own wishes in order to make other people happy.						
1	2	3	4	5	6	7
29. I feel as though I can't reveal the struggles in my life.						
1	2	3	4	5	6	7
30. In a relationship, I feel I must always put my partner's needs before my own.						
1	2	3	4	5	6	7

Item Generation

In the item generation phase, our goal was to be as inclusive as possible in developing a set of candidate items for consideration in the GRSS. Candidate items were derived from multiple sources including the following:

1. BEPKO & KRESTAN (1990)

An important source of candidate items for the scale was generated from the book *Too Good for Her Own Good*, by Claudia Bepko and Jo-Ann Krestan (1990), two family therapists and experts in the area of gender issues. Bepko and Krestan discussed society's "Code of Goodness" for women (i.e., the internalization of gender role messages for women). Based on their clinical experience, they suggested that there are five major rules for being a "good woman." These are included as the first five of the following themes, which reflect the internalization of gender role socialization for women, and in the sample candidate items that reflect the domains covered in the GRSS. The last three themes, innate differences, sexuality, and self-blame, and the corresponding sample candidate items, were generated from other sources, which we discuss in later sections.

- BE ATTRACTIVE

  #34 "I can't feel good about myself unless I feel physically attractive."

- BE A LADY

  #45 "I should never look like I am losing control even if everything is going wrong."

- BE UNSELFISH AND OF SERVICE

  #72 "I generally focus my energy on the needs of others at the cost of satisfying my own needs."

- MAKE RELATIONSHIPS WORK

  #11 "I will never be happy if I am not in a romantic relationship."

- BE COMPETENT WITHOUT COMPLAINT

  #61 "In order to feel confident, I must be able to handle many responsibilities without feeling overwhelmed."

- INNATE DIFFERENCES

  #8 "Because I was born female, I am more emotional than most men."

- SEXUALITY

  #67 "I feel as though I should be less sexually forward than men."

- SELF-BLAME

  #2 "I am to blame if I have low self-esteem."

The first author (B. Toner) identified messages from this book, and the research team translated the messages into potential candidate items for the scale. Where possible, these items were then categorized according to the five rules. Five team members in our research group independently categorized the candidate items into Bepko and Krestan's (1990) domains, achieving 93% agreement. In some cases, however, items overlapped into more than one domain. On items in which there were discrepancies, a consensus was reached by majority agreement.

2. GENERAL POPULATION

Candidate scale items were also generated from a large sample ($N = 330$) of women and men from the Ontario Science Centre, which is a science museum frequented by both residents of and visitors to Toronto. Participants were a representative sample of adult women and men from the population. The qualitative responses to two questions were content analyzed. These questions were (1) "Describe the characteristics and behaviours which you believe this society would like to see in women" and (2) "Describe the characteristics and behaviours which you feel would be ideal in women." These messages about women were identified and brought to the team for translation into possible candidate items.

3. CLINICAL AND RESEARCH EXPERIENCE

We used our expertise as researchers and clinicians in the field of women's mental health to generate candidate items. Since we wanted a scale that could reflect a continuum of expressions for women that cut across diagnostic entities, we looked at the theoretical and empirical literature on eating disorders, anxiety, functional bowel disorders (FBDs), depression, and relationship concerns. Issues and concerns relevant to clients, particularly gender role messages, were noted and discussed with the team and transformed into candidate scale items.

4. CLIENTS

We also wanted to generate candidate items that accurately represented concerns expressed by women seeking therapy. As part of a larger study investigating depression in therapy clients, data were collected using the Silencing the Self Scale (STSS; Jack & Dill, 1992). This scale includes an open-ended question that is completed by participants who agree with the statement "I never seem to measure up to the standards I set for myself." Participants responded to the open-ended question "Please list up to three of the standards you feel you don't measure up to." The participants were 40 consecutive clients attending the Women's Therapy Centre at the Centre for Addiction and Mental Health (CAMH) for individual psychotherapy presenting with a variety of mental health issues including depression, anxiety, and self-esteem issues. The statements written by clients were presented to the team, along with possible transformations of the statements into potential scale items. For example, the client statement "Have to be productive *all* the time or else I fail—I can't do it!" was presented along with the possible scale item "I have to be productive all the time." Together, the team went through the clients' statements and generated candidate items for the scale from this list.

The "self-blame" theme was generated based on the research team's expertise in psychosocial factors influencing women's emotional well-being. We postulated that self-blame is also an important component of women's gender role socialization. This theme was found in the qualitative statements written by participants from the Ontario Science Centre, and in the qualitative statements from clients attending the Women's Therapy Centre.

5. POPULAR LITERATURE

Our team consulted a random selection of current, popular women's magazines including *Homemakers, Vogue, Chatelaine, Redbook, Glamour, Ladies' Home Journal, Good Housekeeping, Cosmopolitan, InStyle,* and *Marie Claire* and various self-help books to examine societal messages for women. Each team member examined the written and photographic content of two magazines and generated a list of messages that women are given from the popular press. Some of the messages for women gleaned from these sources were that a woman should not be happy unless she is "Queen Bee"; dissatisfaction with one's body; playing down one's success; silencing one's voice; that a woman should be grateful for any relationship she is in; that if a woman "screws up" she need only blame herself; and that if a woman tries hard enough she should be able to do something herself. These messages were discussed among the team members and then converted into statements and candidate items for the scale through group consensus.

Item Generation and Refinement

1. EXPERTS IN WOMEN'S ISSUES

A team of 12 experts in gender issues who serve on the executive council (researchers, educators, clinicians) of Division 35 (Psychology of Women) in the American Psychological Association and therapists from the Women's Therapy Centre at the University of Toronto teaching hospitals reviewed a candidate set of 62 items. These experts rated each candidate item on a scale from 0 to 10, with 0 indicating that the item definitely should not be included in the scale and 10 indicating that the item definitely should be included in the scale. Experts were also asked to examine each item for clarity, ambiguous meaning, more than one meaning in a sentence, and double negative statements. They were asked to write any suggested changes in the space below the items as well as any additional themes or items that they believed should be included in the scale. An additional suggested theme was sexuality (e.g., "I feel embarrassed by my own sexual desires").

2. CROSS-CULTURAL APPLICABILITY

Our intent was to generate candidate items that have broad cultural applicability. Consequently, we consulted with experts from Switzerland, Hong Kong, and the Caribbean to produce a more culturally sensitive scale. These cultural experts consisted of female graduate students and faculty members from different academic disciplines who provided input regarding language and cultural relevancy and the types of issues raised by the items. Based on this feedback, we altered, added, and deleted candidate items from the prospective scale. In addition, candidate items from the GRSS were administered to Chinese female university students and working women in Hong Kong. Results from these two target groups provided further input for item refinement of the GRSS.

Our informants from Switzerland, Hong Kong, and the Caribbean provided insight into cultural issues we might have missed had we limited ourselves to a monocultural definition of gender role socialization. Moreover, we were forced to reevaluate candidate items for idioms that may have little cultural relevance outside of North America. For example, among other changes, the Swiss experts suggested several additional items reflecting women's inferiority to men (e.g., "I don't feel comfortable appearing smarter than men") and ideas regarding gender roles (e.g., "I feel I am not a 'good woman' if a career is more important to me than having children"). One change based on feedback from the Caribbean experts was altering the candidate item "I should never look like I am losing control even if everything is falling apart" to "I should never look like I am losing control even if everything is going wrong." These experts felt that some women may not be familiar with the phrase "falling apart." We also changed "I am naturally more emotional than most men" to "Because I was born female, I am more emotional than most men" because in the Caribbean the word *naturally* is equivalent to *of course* and not *biologically* as we had intended. Based on feedback from the Hong Kong experts and target groups, one item we changed was "I feel responsible for my family's well-being" to "I feel responsible for the day-to-day care of my family," and one item we deleted was "To be a good woman I always have to be sensitive to the needs of others." In the former, it was felt that in Chinese culture, both women and men are responsible for familial concerns but that it was mainly women who provided care on a day-to-day basis. In the latter change, the Hong Kong experts felt that this item would not differentiate between women and men in Chinese culture.

3. CLIENTS

Since we are interested in developing the GRSS as an assessment and outcome measure for use in therapy, it was important to receive feedback on candidate scale items from women receiving therapy. Six women receiving group intervention at the Women's Therapy Centre provided responses to the candidate items on the scale. Three of the women completed the GRSS both before and after the support group intervention focusing on strengthening self-esteem, thus enabling us to assess change. The other three women were administered the GRSS only at the end of group intervention and were asked to reflect on which items therapy had helped them to change and the degree to which they had changed. On approximately half of the candidate items, all the women indicated that there was at least some shift in their internalization of gender role messages. Of these candidate items, over 75% of the changes were in the moderate to marked range (conceptualized as 3 or more points on a 7-point scale). We did not make any changes to the candidate items because it was felt that they were all applicable as potential items for assessment.

CHALLENGES IN THE ITEM DEVELOPMENT STAGE

From the beginning we have been challenged with how to operationalize and measure the internalization of gender role messages for women. One issue was whether we were going to measure gender role conflict or gender role socialization. We decided to focus on the internalization of female gender role socialization for several reasons. First, we considered gender role socialization to be the larger construct and conflict to be a component of the gender role socialization of women. Certainly it is possible for gender role messages to be unhealthy for women but not necessarily conflicting. Second, we did not want to prescribe our notions of conflict on women who may not see a conflict in their lives. Third, it was difficult to create items to tap into the construct of conflict. Conflict that is inherent in a message could not be incorporated within one item because we would end up with a double-barreled statement.

An ongoing challenge we face involves the level of awareness of the issues among clients before and after therapy. Ideally, a feminist-oriented intervention can help women to explore and identify their internalization of gender role socialization messages, how these affect their lives, and possible avenues for change. However, given therapy's focus on developing insight and issues, it is quite possible that women's scores on the GRSS may increase before they decrease. That is, therapy might increase a client's awareness of gender role messages for women and how they apply to her life, resulting in high endorsement of the internalization of gender role socialization. However, it is hoped that by the end of therapy there will be greater variation in women's internalization of these messages.

ITEM SELECTION AND PRELIMINARY VALIDATION

We followed Jackson's (1970) multistage method of scale development, which stresses assessing validity at each stage. Research participants consisted of women and men from a community sample, undergraduate university students, and clients from several clinics throughout the University of Toronto teaching hospitals. All participants were administered the following measures:

1. *Gender Role Socialization Candidate Items*—82 items.

2. *Situational Scenarios*, descriptive scenarios designed to assess the degree to which participants' behavior correlates with their responses to the candidate items on the GRSS. The team wrote a number of scenarios that reflected gender role socialization themes and through group consensus selected four representative scenarios. Our cultural experts from Switzerland, Hong Kong, and the Caribbean also provided feedback regarding the scenarios, and changes were made accordingly. These scenarios were included to test for concurrent validity in selecting items for the GRSS and for providing a preliminary concurrent validation for the GRSS.

3. *Bem Sex Role Inventory–Short Version* (Bem, 1981), a 30-item scale designed to measure the degree to which individuals identify with traditional gender roles. This is included to test for convergent validity.

4. *Marlowe-Crowne Social Desirability Scale* (Crowne & Marlowe, 1960), designed to test the candidate items and the subsequent final scale for social desirability contamination.

Results

We have completed the scale selection and validation phases of this study. Data from 700 female participants, nearly evenly split between university, clinical, and community settings, were analyzed to produce a reliable scale of 30 items from the original pool of 82 candidate items. In addition to the candidate items, validating measures were also administered to participants, including (1) Situational Scenarios designed to assess the degree to which participants' behavior correlated with their responses on the candidate items, (2) Bem Sex Role Inventory to test for convergent validity, and (3) Marlowe-Crowne Social Desirability Scale to test for social desirability contamination.

As an initial step in our analyses, we examined the frequency distribution of the responses to each item, and those in which more than 60% of the responses were on a single point of the 7-point Likert scale were eliminated. Items were eliminated if there was a significant proportion (at least 7%) of "not applicable" responses endorsed by participants. Candidate items that correlated greater than .30 with the Marlowe-Crowne scale were eliminated. Further items were eliminated due to redundancy if they correlated greater than .60 with other candidate items. Items with the simplest phrasing were chosen through group consensus. We were very cognizant of ensuring that a priori themes were still represented in the remaining items.

We performed principal components factor analyses with the remaining candidate items, specifying different rotation methods and component selection criteria. The most parsimonious results suggested two main factors comprising 42 items. Through group consensus, additional items were eliminated that were ambiguous, redundant, double-barreled, or thought to prompt dichotomous rather than continuous responses. The remaining 30 items were subject to further principal components analysis, and once again, the most parsimonious results suggested two main factors accounting for 42% of the variance. The first factor reflects a mix of most of the a priori gender role socialization themes, and the second factor reflects mostly the theme "be unselfish and of service."

All missing values and "not applicable" responses were replaced with the item mean. Seven participants were eliminated from analyses because they had greater than 80% missing data. Thus, the total sample was 693 women (231 university; 278 community; 184 clinical). The mean age was 32.62 (standard deviation = 11.93, ranging from 18 to 76 years). Two hundred thirty-eight (34%) were married/common-law; 385 (56%) were single; 68 (10%) were separated or divorced or widowed. Annual household income was on a range, but there were over 200 missing responses because this variable was not asked on the original demographics form at the beginning of data collection. This was also the case with the occupation variable. The sample was educated: 13 (2%) had less than high school; 67 (10%)

completed high school; 18 (3%) had some college; 77 (11%) completed college; 191 (28%) had some university; 187 (27%) completed university; and 135 (19%) completed graduate studies. In terms of ethnicity, 125 (18%) indicated they were "Canadian," and 232 (34%) indicated they were European (*there are 12 other ethnic categories that have been reduced from a much larger number of categories based on participants' open-ended responses*).

Cronbach's alpha indicated that both the factors and the overall scale are highly reliable, with alphas of .90 for both factors and .93 for the overall scale. The 30-item scale correlates negatively (−.256) with the Marlowe-Crowne scale, indicating that higher social desirability is associated with lower endorsement of gender role socialization. Although this correlation is statistically significant, generally a correlation less than .30 with the Marlowe-Crowne scale is considered acceptable. The scale also correlated with the Situational Scenarios in the predicted directions. Finally, the scale was correlated negatively (−.361) with the masculinity subscale of the Bem Sex Role Inventory and was uncorrelated with the femininity subscale.

We acknowledge that constructions of gender are culture specific and illustrate societal values that do not necessarily reflect individual differences. In summary, we have developed a scale with excellent psychometric properties to measure the internalization of gender role messages for women. We hope that other researchers will continue to validate the 30-item GRSS with new samples of female participants and further examine the health impact of the new scale.

References

American Psychiatric Association. (1994). *Diagnostic and statistical manual of mental disorders* (4th ed.). Washington, DC: Author.

Bem, S. (1981). *Manual for the Bem Sex-Role Inventory.* Palo Alto, CA: Consulting Psychologists Press.

Bepko, C., & Krestan, J. (1990). *Too good for her own good.* New York: Harper and Row.

Crowne, D., & Marlowe, D. (1960). A new scale for social desirability independent of psychopathology. *Journal of Consulting Psychology, 24,* 349–354.

Jack, D. C., & Dill, D. (1992). The Silencing the Self Scale: Schemas of intimacy associated with depression in women. *Psychology of Women Quarterly, 16,* 97–106.

Jackson, D. (1970). A sequential system for personality scale development. In C. D. Spielberger (Ed.), *Current topics in clinical and community psychology 61* (p. 96). New York: Academic Press.

Lips, H. M. (1993). *Sex and gender: An introduction.* Mountain View, CA: Mayfield.

Worell, J., & Remer, P. (1992). *Feminist perspectives in therapy: An empowerment model for women.* Chichester, UK: John Wiley & Sons.

Part IV

Policy, Process, and Products

Despite thoughtfully applying methods amid aspirations for advancing the health of boys, girls, men, and women, we are often left contemplating and/or explicitly asking to address the "So what?" question. Caught between a rock (clinical practice) and a hard place (health policy), often meandering without a coherent map, researchers try to connect or stay connected to key stakeholders as a means of sharing their research findings in hopes of making a difference. In addressing the "So what?" question, the final three chapters offer key insights to global, macro policy issues, as well as some of the process and product challenges and considerations around knowledge exchange that can emerge.

While this important content resides at the end of this book, it is clear that the issues described in this section have featured early on in stand-alone studies, as well as in programs of research. In Chapter 12, Toni Schofield eloquently lays out how methods play a major role in bringing gender and health into being as a policy topic or problem. In guiding us through some fascinating historical and contemporary terrain, Schofield reveals how research and policymaking are dynamically interactive in mutually assigning understandings to health problems and their remedies. While detailing the challenges and shortcomings in this regard, she also suggests some important ways forward. Specifically, a project detailing alcohol consumption patterns is used to illustrate the usefulness of a dynamic approach to gender as a social process for distilling health inequalities between and among men and women in specific social settings or contexts. Moreover, Schofield also suggests how this frame might shed important light for better understanding and addressing the worldwide shortage of health care providers.

Drawing on an example from the British Columbia Centre of Excellence for Women's Health, Nancy Poole describes, in Chapter 13, the nuances and benefits of virtual communities of practice (vCoP). She makes a compelling case that by bringing researchers and end users together, vCoP make possible important continuing dialogue and recurring articulation of what constitutes knowledge and its application. The synthesis of information and the generation of new knowledge reveal how these learning communities add to the store of knowledge from their location of clinical, policy, and traditional cultural wisdom.

In Chapter 14, we map some connections between methods and knowledge exchange in differentiating how descriptive and intervention-based products are intricately connected to the study design and methods, before discussing some pathways for gender, sex, and health knowledge exchange. Specifically, peer-reviewed publications and virtual pathways are briefly described in highlighting key considerations for how research products can be marketed to maximize our knowledge exchange efforts.

Gender, Health, Research, and Public Policy **12**

Toni Schofield

This chapter discusses the relationship between prevailing representations and understandings of "gender and health" in national and international health policy contexts and the dominant research approaches and methods adopted in the formulation of such policy. Policymaking and research, the chapter proposes, may be understood as dynamic social processes that interact and bring meaning—including that of gender and health—into being. The chapter argues that the ways in which research and policy combine have significant implications for how gender and health are understood and addressed by policymakers both nationally and internationally. Based on a critical overview of current gender and health policies, the chapter suggests that prevailing representations are conceptually and empirically limited—an outcome derived in large part from particular research-based formulations that dominate the provision of evidence in policymaking. Advancing policy and strategies to address the problem of gender and health, then, demands different policy-based understandings and formulations of it that, in turn, require innovations in frameworks and methods used in researching the problem.

Research Evidence in Gender and Health Policy

How policymakers understand gender and health depends very considerably on how it has been examined, analyzed, and discussed by researchers.

Research "approaches and methods," in fact, play a major role in bringing gender and health into being as a policy topic or problem. They do not simply and passively reflect preexisting policy representations and understandings. The World Health Organization's (WHO's) website on gender and health (WHO, 2010a) is a good example. It provides information sheets that document and discuss the relationship between gender and a range of health-related issues (blindness, health and disasters, mental health, road traffic injuries, tuberculosis, HIV/AIDS, tobacco, aging, and malaria) to demonstrate that gender can be bad for your health whether you're a man or a woman. Drawing on *scientific evidence* derived mainly from epidemiological or large-scale quantitative studies that examine *sex differences in health outcomes,* the information sheets document and explain that these differences illustrate the ways in which "socially determined norms and roles for each sex can give rise to *inequities between men and women in health status and access to health care"* (emphasis added). So, for example, the consumption of tobacco in all its forms is 4 times greater among men than women globally because of prevailing sex-differentiated "social norms and roles" related to smoking. As a result, the lethal impact of tobacco use is markedly greater among men—who made up 3.4 million of the estimated 4.2 million tobacco-related premature deaths worldwide in 2000 (WHO Department of Gender and Women's Health, 2003b). Women, on the other hand, according to the WHO Department of Gender and Women's Health (2002), bear the lion's share of blindness throughout the world—64% of the total number of blind people are women. Much of this burden is preventable and shouldered by low-income countries, such as those in Asia and Africa, where barriers to accessing preventive services are greatest. Because of sex-differentiated norms and roles related to preventive health service access in these countries, according to the WHO information sheet, women experience tougher constraints on access than do men. On a global basis, women are also more likely to be living with HIV/AIDS, with the death rates associated with the condition showing an increasing predominance of women (WHO Department of Gender and Women's Health, 2003a). The reasons for this are complex, but as the WHO information sheet explains, it is the "gender norms and values" that accord men greater sexual freedom, including freedom from responsibility for pregnancy and sexually transmitted infection, and that underpin women's higher rates of the condition.

The WHO's (2010a) gender and health website concludes that these kinds of "gender differences" need to be eliminated because they produce "gender inequalities" in health outcomes that are "avoidable and unnecessary." To the extent that such inequalities are identifiable as "avoidable and unnecessary," the WHO (1990) proposes a distinction it developed between inequalities and inequities. The former refer to measurable health disparities in relation to individuals and populations while the latter refer to an ostensible subset of these—those that are "unnecessary, avoidable, unfair and unjust." Underpinning the distinction between inequality and inequity is the idea that health inequalities can be either natural or social. Where they are social, they are "unnecessary, avoidable, unfair and unjust," and a cause for social intervention. However, as the author of the original WHO (1990) report on health equity has recently commented, the distinction between inequality and inequity is no longer relevant in policy terms: inequality, she writes, "carries the same connotations of unfairness and injustice as the term 'inequities'" (Whitehead, 2007, p. 473). She proposes that there is now widespread consensus that social inequalities are the major determinants of health inequalities and that the way forward involves examination of a range of actions that might be adopted in "tackling social inequalities in health." Accordingly, the distinction between inequality and inequity no longer has any real analytical currency in research and policy terms in health (Schofield, 2007).

This new approach to health inequality and inequity in research and policy, however, has not yet percolated to the WHO's (2010a) website on gender and health. It still makes a distinction between gendered health inequalities and inequities. Yet at the heart of its conceptualization of both is *the measurable sex differential in health outcomes.* The WHO's gendered policy interventions proceed on the basis of women and girls, and men and boys, as two reproductively distinct groups whose biological sexual difference is basically compounded by social "norms and roles." It is these sex-differentiated "norms and roles," in effect, that are understood to be the fundamental cause of the problem, and the target of WHO policy interventions proposed for redressing it. For instance, in those low-income countries where women and girls are much less likely to access services to treat eye conditions that produce blindness, the WHO information sheet on the gendered nature of the condition suggests that the "norms and roles" responsible involve the failure of local male-dominated communities, governments, and other relevant agencies to take notice of, and act on, this inequity. The solution to the problem, at least at the level of research, is "to test methods to rectify the imbalance" (WHO Department of Gender and Women's Health, 2003, p. 2), but it is not evident what these methods might be and how they might be tested. In other words, the research frameworks and methods that presumably will be used to identify and analyze the specific social "norms and roles" that generate the problem and that, therefore, will be inextricably related to finding the solution are not made transparent.

The Two-Way Street Between Policy and Research in Gender and Health

Though the WHO has been increasingly challenged as the world's preeminent health policymaking agency (Walt, 1998; Walt & Gilson, 1994), it retains enormous scientific authority in relation to its analysis of, and policy recommendations about, global health problems and their solutions (Brown, Cueto, & Fee, 2006), including those related to gender and health. It is for this reason that this chapter began with a brief analysis of one of the WHO's main websites on gender and health. One of the fundamental features of the WHO's approach to gender and health that emerges from this analysis is *the mutually constitutive relationship between research and policy.* Such a relationship, this chapter proposes, is not confined to the WHO. In relation to gender and health, it prevails in a wide range of national policymaking contexts. What is particularly significant about the relationship is the way in which the problem of gender and health, and interventions for redressing it, is represented. The prevailing representation, as discussed above, is certainly an advance on previous health policy and research approaches that were oblivious to gender and its associated inequities. Yet it is also characterized by serious limitations that pose major obstacles to the development of policy and research that may be more effective in redressing gender and health inequities internationally. The following discusses these limitations but first responds to the question of what it means to propose that there is a mutually constitutive relationship between research and policy in relation to gender and health.

First, it is important to recognize and understand that public policymaking is a *dynamic social process* that involves identifying and responding to the problems of political constituencies. This is not achieved in a simple and straightforwardly linear or mechanical way whereby policymakers are neutral and objective respondents to, and rational choosers of, policy "objects" already established and proposed by constituencies. Rather, according to what some describe as a *social constructivist* perspective, policymakers, both elected and appointed, are but one—albeit a very significant one—of a number of players involved in complex interactions that bring policy problems and solutions into being, often in unpredictable ways (Burton, 2002). One of the main mechanisms by which they do so, as Carol Bacchi (1999) explained over 10 years ago, is through the ways in which they represent or "frame" the policy problem—the *discourses* or ideas about how the problems and solutions are understood (Lewis, 2005, p. 10).

In most policy arenas, understandings and representations of problems and solutions are shaped by a range of factors, but knowledge bases and research frameworks play an especially powerful role (Schofield, 2009). They are usually operationalized in policymaking through the use of specific knowledge or evidence to substantiate the reality of the policy problem and to suggest directions for interventions to address it.

As recent policy analysis suggests, it is the *technocratic* collection of frameworks and conceptual tools, informed largely by positivist science and supplied by a veritable army of *technical* experts, that prevails in framing policy problems and solutions (Schofield, 2009). Problem solving that draws on such an approach typically focuses on *linear cause-and-effect relationships and measurable patterns and outcomes.* Policymakers adopt such an approach because they believe that it not only ensures the calculability of results but also secures objectivity since the opportunity for interpretive, and therefore partisan, judgment is believed to be minimized (Christensen & Laegreid, 2007).

In health policy, particularly in relation to gender and health, it is epidemiology and large-scale quantitative studies of "health behaviors" that usually prevail in "rendering health inequalities real and actionable" (Schofield, 2007, p. 108). As we have already seen in relation to the WHO's (2010a) website on gender and health, epidemiology is the dominant scientific framework and method that brings "the problem" of gender and health into being by establishing measurable inequities in the rates of health conditions and impairments between the sexes. Such an approach has been widely adopted in a range of national policymaking contexts, especially in relation to men's health (Smith & Robertson, 2008). In Australia, the United States, and the Irish Republic, for example, men's health is constructed by a contrast with "women's health" (Schofield, 2010). What emerges as central to its representation is a robust binarism that relies mainly on statistical fabrication. From this perspective, women's health is basically constituted as a sex-based aggregate of measures related to women's reproductive illnesses and diseases, to their use of health services, and to their mortality, morbidity, disability, and "lifestyle" practices (such as alcohol and tobacco use, and diet and exercise regimes). Corresponding with this representation is a collection of the same sorts of indicators but applied to men as a sex-based category—men's health. It is the *margins of difference in the measurements between the two categories that are foundational for prevailing gender and health discourse.* If the magnitudes between the two are unequal, then so, too, are the health statuses of men and women. Differential magnitudes signal the presence of a "gender-specific" health issue. The absence of such difference, on the other hand, suggests gender neutrality and, in turn, no cause for gender-specific public interventions such as gender-specific policies, programs, and services.

This discourse, however, does not confine itself to biological sex differences. It has freely incorporated social understandings of men and women, forging a hybrid of biology and culture to create sex-based public health constituencies. Men, then, are constituted by the combination of male reproductive characteristics and engagement in the "male role" or masculine practices that are socially determined. The latter are distinguished by their contrast with the "female role" and feminine practices. Just as this approach imagines human embodiment as dimorphic, so too does it represent the social practices of human beings as taking "the shape of a dichotomy between all-women and all-men" (Connell, 2002, p. 36). It proposes a match or homology between embodiment and culture. This binary is what is understood as gender. Its incorporation of "the social" is selective and partial, representing men and women as wholly distinct and mutually exclusive categories of people, and gender as the relationship that connects them as such. It is this approach that informs the "gender norms and roles" analysis that characterizes the WHO's policy on gender and health.

Advancing an Alternative Approach to Gender and Health in Policy and Research

Recent sociological contributors to understanding gender, health, and inequality, however, propose that the "norms and roles" approach discloses some serious fissures in its conceptualization that render its soundness as a foundation for formulating solutions or interventions to address the problem of gendered health inequity seriously questionable. The "norms and roles" approach to gender, it is suggested, derives primarily from the theory of *gendered socialization* that developed in the 1970s and that understood gender primarily as a *category* of sex difference (Connell, 2009). As explained above, according to this categorical conceptualization, gender refers to the biological reproductive distinction between human beings that is matched by a sociocultural division between maleness or masculinity and femaleness and femininity. In other words, gender is represented as a kind of binary homology between reproductive biology and culture. From this perspective, "norms and roles" are the social mechanisms by which this division or difference is produced and reproduced.

Sociological critics of this view propose that gender is a much more complex phenomenon (Annandale & Clark, 1996; Connell, 2009; Schofield, 2010). Central to the critique is the idea that while it is empirically correct to say that there are significant differences between men and women, it is also empirically indisputable that men and women share many similarities. The binarist social explanation of "norms and roles" and categorical differences does not and cannot explain these similarities. Moreover, in adopting a category-based approach to the problem of gender and health inequality, it does not account for the *differences among men and among women.* The social norms and roles framework adopts differentiation from the "other" or "opposite sex" as its conceptual foundation. At the same time, however, when applied to health policy, it routinely not only acknowledges but emphasizes the idea of a *plurality* or multiple differences among both men and women. Certain groups of men and women are typically identified as bearing a particular health burden: indigenous people, those from minority ethnic backgrounds, African Americans (in the United States), people with disabilities, gay men and lesbians, people of low socioeconomic status, and those in rural locations.

These differences are real and significant, but positing them as central to gendered health inequalities creates conceptual tensions for the social norms and roles approach. On the one hand, to the extent that all men as a whole are represented as having comparable or worse health than women as a whole, and vice versa, the norms and roles framework establishes a *generalized* health interest among men and among women. Yet on the other hand, while it also proposes that there are differences among men or among women, only *specific groups* among each sex have comparable or worse health than their "opposite sex" (Schofield, Connell, Walker, & Wood, 2000). Such a representation is intrinsically contradictory because both are not simultaneously tenable in the absence of a rational account of how this is possible, as the U.S. feminist Iris Marion Young (1997) explained to us in relation to the development of identity politics in the U.S. women's movement in the 1980s. In brief, Young argued that "identity politics" raised conceptual and political problems because it drew on identity categories among women such as *lesbian, Aboriginal, African American, housewife, professional,* and *non-English-speaking* that either left out some individuals who call themselves women or distorted the experience of some of them (Young, 1997). In effect an "identity politics" approach to conceptualizing gender rendered impossible the idea of women as a unit with a common interest (Schofield, 2004, p. 9). The task for feminist theory and politics, according to Young, was to formulate a rigorous critical foundation for the idea of women as simultaneously pluralized and unified. In the absence of such a formulation there would be no coherent, theoretical basis for specifically feminist politics involving organized collective action including making claims on public resources (Schofield, 2004).

At the heart of Young's (1997) critique of identity politics is a major conceptual challenge to arbitrary, categorical constructions of collectivities such as men and women, and the differences between and among them. It articulates a new and critical perspective toward our understanding of gender that rejects simplistic binarist formulations evident in the social norms and roles approach. An example of the application of this critical perspective of the social norms and roles approach to gender and health is found in an Australian government-commissioned review and report of the scholarly research on gender and men's health (Connell et al., 1999). It found that the overwhelming body of peer-reviewed research focused on sex differences in biological health outcomes, such as mental health and disease conditions, bodily impairments and injuries, and "health behaviors" such as diet, physical activity, drug and alcohol consumption, and even the incidence of infection from chopstick use and dog bites! Most of these studies adopted large quantitative or epidemiological methods. As the report explained, however, sex difference studies seriously misrepresent the empirical reality of the relationship between gender and health:

> A finding of "sex difference" need not imply a difference between all men and all women. In fact it usually does not. Quite small differences, among a minority of the population, may produce statistically significant differences in overall rates or averages. . . . [Yet] large policy implications may be drawn which are not warranted by the

actual research. Policymakers must be concerned about the size of the effects, as well as the statistical significance level they reach. . . . [Further,] many studies searching for sex differences find none. "No difference" is, in fact, the usual finding in research on psychological characteristics of women and men. . . . [It] is also the finding in a good proportion of Australian research on health. (Connell et al., 1999, p. 26)

In the face of the report's critical review of the relevant literature, combined with wide-ranging community-based consultation, it concluded that

in some ways men as a group are worse off. . . . But in other respects, men as a group are not worse off. . . . [Indeed] the evidence is clear that there are significant health issues that have to do with the positions of men [and women] in gender relations. (Connell et al., 1999, p. 33)

In response to the conceptual and empirical limitations of the social norms and roles approach to gender and health inequality outlined above, critics have proposed that research and policy in the field of gender and health inequality would be more effectively advanced by adopting a new understanding of gender—as a *dynamic biosocial process* rather than the differential between sex-based categories (see, for example, Connell, 2009; Schofield, 2010). By contrast with its binarist counterpart, this approach views gender as a verb rather than a noun. Gender comprises particular patterns of activity or *structures of practice* that bring us into being as men and women, sometimes markedly differentiated from each other and other times not differentiated at all (Connell, 2009). At the heart of the process is the way in which *the biological reproductive distinction is socially mobilized in determining who gets to do what, where, and when; under what conditions; and with what consequences or outcomes, including access to participation in economic, social, and political life and the material and symbolic resources associated with it* (Schofield, 2004). In relation to health, as the Australian government-commissioned report recommended,

we need to . . . enable a move towards analysis of the mechanisms underlying health effects, and identification of the precise social location of the problems—both being requirements for effective policies. (Connell et al., 1999, p. 34)

What might such an approach look like in practice in relation to health research and policy? It is evident that no one model can be proposed here because of the sheer diversity of health and health care issues and the complexities of the gender dynamics involved in them. Nevertheless, several possibilities emerge. One pertains to the development of a dynamic gender-based model for developing effective policy to address so-called mainstream health problems. There is no shortage of such issues, but one that is presently being researched for the purposes of more effective policy intervention involves alcohol use and harm minimization among young adults. This is a large Australian Research Council–funded study undertaken with public health agencies in two of Australia's most populous states and a large private national human services organization for university students. It is well established that the health effects of alcohol use among young adults in many parts of the affluent world are deleterious, but they are documented as being much worse among young men. At the same time, exploratory sociological research suggests that some young women are increasingly exhibiting adverse drinking-related health impacts that are comparable to those of their male counterparts (Lindsay, 2010). Clearly, the sorts of policy interventions most likely to be effective in addressing and redressing the problem need to have an understanding of the gender dynamics of young people's drinking. Accordingly, in consultation with their research partners, the university researchers have devised a study that focuses on the drinking practices of young men and women in a variety of social settings: when, where, and with whom they drink; for what purposes; in what quantities; with what consequences; and so on. But the study also discriminates *among* young men and women primarily by socioeconomic status, ethnicity, and region (urban vs. rural). While a large survey is to be conducted, much of the research will be based on interviews and focus group discussions with young people themselves.

It is by operationalizing such an approach and method that the study expects to identify the patterns of similarities and differences between and among young men and women in order to identify how gender works in relation to the drinking practices of socially differentiated young people and, in turn, to understand how drinking works in bringing young people into being as young men and women who are socially differentiated. Central to this enterprise will be a focus on the *relations* that prevail between men and women, and among them, when they drink in specific social settings. From a health policy perspective, the study expects to locate the barriers to and opportunities for minimizing alcohol-related harm among young adults. From a sociological research perspective, it hopes to enrich current knowledge and understanding of the ways in which a particular arena of social practice—alcohol use—works in engaging with the biological reproductive distinction among young people in distinguishing them as gendered people. In doing so the study will also contribute to advancing what we mean by a dynamic biosocial approach to gender, the centrality of the relationality between and among men and women, how such an approach differs from the prevailing category-based perspective, and how it is more effective as a scientific foundation for health policy development and interventions.

A further example to illustrate the application of a dynamic gendered approach to "mainstream" health (and health care) policy is that of health workforce shortages. As the WHO has reported, health workforce shortages are expected to pose major challenges to health and health care on a global basis. Low-income countries, especially those in sub-Saharan Africa, are predicted to be the worst affected (WHO, 2010b). While policymakers are informed about the ominous numerical shortfall in the health workforce and where its most adverse effects are most likely to be felt, there is a dearth of research regarding the social dynamics responsible for generating the problem (Schofield, 2009). One of the most outstanding features of the health workforce worldwide is its gendered character. The participation of men and women in the health workforce is dramatically unequal, with women far outnumbering men overall but men dominating the apex of what is a profoundly hierarchical industry and institution. Curiously, this fact has escaped most research undertaken to inform and guide policymakers in trying to solve the problem.

A dynamic gendered framework, applied to a national context, would recognize that the health workforce actually comprises people engaged in a predominantly institutionalized and gendered social process of providing health care. The problem of health workforce shortages, then, requires examination of how this process is gendered, or how gender works in the organization of health care provision, specifically in relation to the similarities and differences between and among men and women regarding their participation in the health workforce. Systematic investigation of the process would mobilize an approach that operationalizes questions such as what are the similarities and differences between and among men and women in relation to who does what, where, when, under what conditions, with what consequences, and so on. In doing so, such a project would focus much of its data collection on what the members of the workforce have to say about their participation in the diverse and specific locations in which they work. Analysis of the findings would focus on the gendered patterns of similarities and differences yielded by the investigation to map the process and understand its central dynamics specifically in relation to the barriers and opportunities that health workforce members face in sustaining their participation and in cooperating with policymakers to work in areas of greatest demand.

Conclusion

Research and policymaking in health are dynamically interactive, mutually constituting their understanding of health problems and of their strategies to address and resolve them. Research and policy in relation to gender and health have been dominated by approaches and methods that have understood the problem of health inequity largely in terms of margins of difference in rates of health outcomes or indicators between the sexes, and the ways in which social norms and roles create these differentials. As this chapter has explained, such an approach is characterized by serious conceptual and empirical limitations that pose major challenges to the development of effective policy and strategy to address and redress gender-based health inequity. Developing effective policy and strategies to address the problem, then, demands innovations in theoretical frameworks and methods used to research and understand the problem. This chapter proposes that a dynamic approach to gender as a social process and how it operates in generating health inequalities between *and* among men and women in specific social settings or contexts will provide a more sound scientific foundation for understanding the barriers and opportunities that men and women face in advancing their health and health care on an equitable basis.

References

Annandale, E., & Clark, J. (1996). What is gender? Feminist theory and the sociology of human reproduction. *Sociology of Health and Illness, 18*(1), 17–44.

Bacchi, C. (1999). *Women, policy and politics: The construction of policy problems.* London: SAGE.

Brown, T. M., Cueto, M., & Fee, E. (2006). The transition from "international" to "global" public health and the world. *Historia, Cience, Saude Manguinhos, 13*(3), 623–647.

Burton, C. (2002). Introduction to complexity. In K. Sweeney & F. Griffiths (Eds.), *Complexity and healthcare: An introduction* (pp. 1–18). Abingdon, UK: Radcliffe Medical Press.

Christensen, T., & Laegreid, P. (2007). *Transcending new public management: The transformation of public sector reforms.* Aldershot, UK: Ashgate Press.

Connell, R. W. (2002). *Gender.* Cambridge, UK: Polity.

Connell, R. (2009). *Gender in world perspective* (2nd ed.). Cambridge, UK: Polity.

Connell, R. W., Schofield, T., Walker, L., Wood, J., Butland, D. L., & Fisher, J. (1999). *Men's health: A research agenda and background report.* Canberra, Australia: Commonwealth Department of Health and Aged Care.

Lewis, J. M. (2005). *Health policy and politics: Networks, ideas and power.* Melbourne, Australia: IP Communications.

Lindsay, J. (2010). Young Australians and the staging of intoxication and self-control. *Journal of Youth Studies, 12*(4), 373–386.

Schofield, T. (2004). *Boutique health? Gender and equity in health policy.* Australian Health Policy Institute Commissioned Paper Series 2004/08, University of Sydney.

Schofield, T. (2007). Health inequity and its social determinants: A sociological commentary. *Health Sociology Review, 16*(2), 105–114.

Schofield, T. (2009). Gendered organizational dynamics: The elephant in the room for Australian allied health workforce policy and planning? *Journal of Sociology, 4*(15), 383–400.

Schofield, T. (2010). Men's health. In E. Annandale & E. Kuhlmann (Eds.), *The handbook of gender and healthcare* (pp. 239–255). Basingstoke, UK: Palgrave Macmillan.

Schofield, T., Connell, R. W., Walker, L., & Wood, J. (2000). Understanding men's health and illness: A gender-relations approach to policy, research and practice. *Journal of American College Health, 48*(6), 247–256.

Smith, J. A., & Robertson, S. (2008). Men's health promotion: A new frontier in Australia and the UK? *Health Promotion International, 23*(3), 283–289.

Walt, G. (1998). Globalisation of international health. *The Lancet, 351*(9100), 434–437.

Walt, G., & Gilson, L. (1994). Reforming the health sector in developing countries: The central role of policy analysis. *Health Policy and Planning, 9*(4), 353–370.

Whitehead, M. (2007). A typology of actions to tackle social inequalities in health. *Journal of Epidemiology and Community Health, 61*(6), 473–478.

World Health Organization. (1990). *The concepts and principles of equity in health.* Copenhagen, Denmark: WHO Regional Office for Europe (EUR/ICP/RPD 414).

World Health Organization. (2010a). *Gender.* Retrieved December 27, 2010, from http://www.who.int/topics/gender/en

World Health Organization. (2010b). *The global shortage of health workers and its impact.* Fact Sheet No. 302. Retrieved December 27, 2010, from http://www.who.int/mediacentre/factsheets/fs302/en/index.html

World Health Organization Department of Gender and Women's Health. (2002). *Gender and blindness.* Retrieved December 27, 2010, from http://www.who.int/gender/other_health/en/genderblind.pdf

World Health Organization Department of Gender and Women's Health. (2003a). *Gender and HIV/AIDS.* Retrieved November 12, 2009, from http://www.who.int/gender/documents/en/HIV_AIDS.pdf

World Health Organization Department of Gender and Women's Health. (2003b). *Gender, health and tobacco.* Retrieved December 27, 2010, from http://www.who.int/gender/documents/Gender_Tobacco_2.pdf

Young, I. M. (1997). *Intersecting voices: Dilemmas of gender, political philosophy and policy.* Princeton, NJ: Princeton University Press.

Boundary Spanning 13

Knowledge Translation as Feminist Action Research in Virtual Communities of Practice

Nancy Poole

The advances in research on gender and health prompt us to consider, "Now what?" How do we share what we are learning and apply new knowledge to change policy and practice in health? In recent years, this question has been the focus of considerable attention in the broader health research world, in Canada and globally. The Canadian Institutes of Health Research employ the term *knowledge translation* to refer to "the methods for closing the gaps from knowledge to practice" (Straus, Tetroe, & Graham, 2009, p. 165). Many other terms are used to describe the processes related to raising awareness of research findings and promoting integration into health services practice and policy: *research utilization, dissemination* and *diffusion, knowledge transfer* and *uptake, knowledge exchange,* and *knowledge-to-action cycle.*

This chapter addresses the "Now what?" question through reflection on three foundational elements of knowledge translation: the nature of *knowledge* generated by gender and health research, the needs of the end users and the *context* in which they are located, and the emerging role of researchers in *facilitation* of research-to-action practices. The work of researchers at the British Columbia Centre of Excellence for Women's Health (BCCEWH) in engaging researchers and end users of research in virtual communities affords empirical examples. Virtual communities of practice (vCoP) are highlighted as useful mechanisms for translation of knowledge on gender and health research, given their foundation in participatory action research methods. Further, vCoP as inclusive forums for co-construction and translation of knowledge invite reexamination of the researcher's role as boundary spanner in facilitating knowledge translation on gender and health research.

The Nature of the Research to Be Translated

The field of substance use research is illustrative of the complexity of knowledge generated through active investigation of sex and gender influences on health and their interaction with other forms of difference and inequality. Uncovering knowledge through holistic gender analysis applied to health research, and determining the routes to translating this knowledge to action, is a complex process.

A recent review by BCCEWH researchers of the literature on the use of alcohol by girls and young women, and the health and social consequences of heavy and binge drinking by this population, offers insights to the complex interplay of factors influencing substance use and the challenges inherent in translating gender and health research to practice and policy. An international study examining gender-specific trends, using cross-cultural comparisons from 1998 to 2006 in 24 countries and regions, affirmed that drinking and drunkenness remained higher among boys than girls, but found that the gender gap was closing; girls appear to be catching up with boys in some countries (Simons-Morton et al., 2009). Binge drinking is more common among girls than boys aged 13 and 15 in Canada, as well as among 15-year-old girls (compared with boys of the same age) in Iceland, Norway, Spain, and the United Kingdom.

The literature also documents the higher vulnerability of girls and women to the negative health impacts of alcohol use—for example, elevated risks of developing liver disease, cardiac disease, gastrointestinal problems, breast cancer, osteoporosis, reproductive health problems, and addiction (National Institute on Alcohol Abuse and Alcoholism, 2003; Spear, 2002). To make sense of the health implications and pathways to alcohol use requires analysis of complex intersections among the health problems associated with drinking, as well as identification of broad, society-based gendered influences. Studies have highlighted the complex links between sexual assault and heavy drinking and other substance use, and noted adolescence as a time of particular risk of sexual assault for girls (Covington, 2008). Further, a recent study on the longitudinal associations among depression, obesity, and alcohol use disorders in young adults (McCarty et al., 2009) identified several gendered linkages, namely that women with an alcohol disorder at age 24 were more than three times as likely to be obese when they were 27. Women who were obese at 27 were more than twice as likely to be depressed when they were 30. And women who were depressed at 27 were at an increased risk for alcohol disorders at 30. Similarly, complex gendered pathways to substance use were found by researchers at the National Center on Addiction and Substance Abuse (2003) at Columbia University in a large multimethods study. They documented how key school and developmental transitions pose special risks for uptake of problematic substance use by girls, such as the early onset of puberty; the transition from elementary to high school, or from high school to college or university; and frequent moves from one home or neighborhood to another.

Research has also shown alcohol advertising to be a powerful form of gendered cultural conditioning. Alcohol marketing tailors sweet-tasting drinks to girls, apparently with some success: The 2008 Adolescent Health Survey in British Columbia found that girls were more likely than boys to have drunk "coolers" on the Saturday prior to the survey whereas boys were more likely to have drunk beer (Smith, et al., 2009). More insidious, researchers have documented how alcohol advertising in the guise of selling "health and freedom" actually connects alcohol and tobacco use with violence, sexual assault, sexual harassment, pornography, teenage pregnancy, addiction, and eating disorders (Kilbourne, 1999).

These examples of the interplay among trends in prevalence, sex-specific health consequences, and gendered pathways to, and influences on, alcohol use by girls and young women underline the need for fluid, collaborative, and reflexive mechanisms for transforming research into practice and policy. And indeed, emerging knowledge translation methodologies (Best et al., 2003; Graham & Tetroe, 2007; Greenhalgh, Robert, Macfarlane, Bate, & Kyriakidou, 2004; Kitson et al., 2008) are more complex, multisectoral, and multidirectional than the traditional, top-down "science push" to disseminate evidence to potential users, often through the presentation of systematic reviews, or "demand pull" that is driven by health professionals, consumers, and civil servants who seek specific information on which to base action (Lavis, Lomas, Hamid, & Sewankambod, 2006). However, growing awareness of the complexities of knowledge translation has not bridged the chasm separating most researchers and end users. Technical models, many with a focus on problem solving and knowledge management as ways to break down and disseminate knowledge, dominate approaches to knowledge translation (Sudsawad, 2007).

As a result, the literature continues to "reflect traditional post-positivist assumptions espousing discrete linear processes and reductionist conclusions" whereas "the human nature of social interaction KT [knowledge translation]" suggests that "implementation science will therefore perhaps forever be as much art as science" (McWilliam et al., 2009). For researchers at the BCCEWH, art and science can be seen to intersect in the dynamic, open-ended processes of feminist action research. Specifically, our commitment to effecting change in policies and practices in women's health builds on shared responsibilities for integrating contextualized evidence.

The End User of Gender and Health Research

It is fundamental to knowledge translation that researchers and end users come together in continuing dialogue and recurring articulation of what constitutes knowledge and its application. Contemporary knowledge translation frameworks in health research build on participatory models of knowledge construction and dissemination for the stated purpose of producing beneficial outcomes throughout the health care and health public policy systems. A second core step to "Now what?" reflections on gender and health research is to thoughtfully consider end users and their contextual challenges.

Often dualistic interactions between researchers and end users are conceptualized, studied, and promoted in knowledge translation efforts: researcher to policymaker, researcher to health care practitioner, researcher to health literacy expert. In contrast, the BCCEWH approach has always been firmly grounded in multisectoral collaborations, inclusive of partners from community, health services, and policy domains. This vision of multisectoral research collaboration was articulated by a group of 80 women's health researchers from across Canada in 1999, in the Fusion model (Greaves & Ballem, 2001). The model defines multidirectional knowledge exchange, along with deliberately reflexive explorations of the determinants of health, including sex and gender, inviting transdisciplinary action. In so doing, the Fusion model reaches back to the feminist consciousness-raising (CR) of the 1970s and moves forward on participatory action research (PAR) and feminist action research (FAR) processes to integrate multiple voices and forms of knowledge in health research. From the outset, the BCCEWH has undertaken and sponsored initiatives that are designed to overcome academic and bureaucratic obstacles and strengthen linkages between researchers and end users.

Barriers often cited regarding translation of research to inform this range of praxis include key challenges for end users, such as constraints of time, resources, capacity to appraise and translate research evidence, and resistance to changing what has always been done (Bowen, Martens, & The Need to Know Team, 2005; Estabrooks, Thompson, Lovely, & Hofmeyer, 2006; Jacobson, Butterill, & Goering, 2003). The relevance of these barriers to the end users of women's health research has been tested in a number of collective processes that led us to introduce a model for voluntary, short-term virtual communities as locations for communal ways to synthesize information and generate new knowledge while addressing the experience of information overload.

The use of technology has allowed for expanded involvement in the sharing of knowledge grounded in personal practice. Access to vCoP via desktop videoconferencing addresses travel, resource, and geographical constraints that inhibit involvement. The vCoP created since 2005 have examined evidence on a range of topics related to addictions support and policy integration, such as integrated approaches to working on violence, mental health, and substance use concerns; supportive system policies and practices for mothers with substance use problems facing child welfare interventions; and sex/gender and diversity-based analysis in animating the National Framework for Action to Reduce the Harms Associated with Alcohol and Other Drugs and Substances in Canada (see BCCEWH, 2007). Some 25 to 35 participants in each virtual community have worked within a framework of open dialogic deliberation for about 6 months, using web meetings and a shared online workspace (where documents are posted and online discussion boards are made available).

A current example of vCoP is one bringing together First Nations and Inuit service providers, health system planners, researchers, and health/political organizational representatives from seven jurisdictions across northern Canada for the purpose of generating and synthesizing knowledge on substance use treatment and support for First Nations and Inuit women at risk of having a child affected by fetal alcohol spectrum disorder. This learning community compiles written evidence in a virtual work space or collaboratory, and meets online monthly for 90 minutes to discuss academic and experiential contributions and add to the store of knowledge from clinical, policy, and traditional cultural wisdoms, as well as to strategize on individual and collective action and recommendations for government action.

The engaged multisectoral approach realized by vCoP extends the practice of feminist CR as it emerged in the 1970s (Shreve, 1989). The CR model typically involved a three-stage process in which individual experiences were shared with group members; discussion identified the common elements in group members' experiences and how that commonality related to the overall status of women; and, finally, an iterative process was used to strategize action, take action, and assess the impact of this action. Keating (2005) describes the contributions of this CR model as (1) making explicit the political implications of women's so-called personal lives, (2) introducing nonhierarchical and transformative spaces for thinking about and acting on one's own and each other's different situations, and (3) providing a model for creating knowledge and theory in a participatory and collective manner.

Keating (2005) proposes "coalitional consciousness building" as a contemporary CR model that pays close attention to the contexts in which experiences are articulated and played, engenders awareness of resistance to multiple oppressions, and explores barriers to and possibilities for coalitional action. This approach has relevance to the design of the vCoP sponsored by the BCCEWH. As is characteristic of feminist action research processes (Frisby, Magui, & Reid, 2009; Reid, Tom, & Frisby, 2006), vCoP specifically support inclusion, reflexivity, collective deliberation, challenge to dominant paradigms, and focus on action/integration into practice and policy. Participants are not left in binary engagements, or in the unidisciplinary, bounded, institutionalized territory associated with the nonspread of innovation (Ferlie, Fitzgerald, Wood, & Hawkins, 2005).

The outcomes achieved from the vCoP as mechanisms for knowledge translation align with the goals of feminist action research. To date, the tangible knowledge products from vCoP include information sheets; journal articles; webcasts with up to 100 subscribed participants; presentations at regional, provincial, and national conferences; policy recommendation summaries; and collaborative research proposals. Participants remark on how the technologically mediated spaces allow for inclusivity beyond their own workplace or immediate circle of influence, providing much-needed reinforcement of their insights into the influence of gender and direction for changes to practice and policy in their own contexts. Evaluations indicate that involvement in vCoP has been the catalyst for further reading, proactive initiatives on program changes, and empowerment that arises from feeling "respected, heard, and validated."

In addition to being supportive of co-construction of knowledge and reflexivity, central tenets of participatory action research, the vCoP play a key role in helping participants consider how resistance to attending to gender and health research plays out in global and local policy and treatment contexts. For example, participants who are service providers often describe resistance to applying sex-, gender-, and diversity-based analysis (SGBA); to mainstreaming gender-based responses; and to offering gender-specific programming in their settings. Overall, the substance use field in which they are located has functioned as if sex and gender differences were peripheral to understanding substance use and addiction. Consequently women have consistently been referred to as a "special population," marginal to a generic approach to substance use treatment, harm reduction, and prevention. The vCoP function as locations for clarifying broad and workplace-specific resistances, for interrogating key concepts such as "empowerment" in treatment, and for moving beyond a problem orientation to identify what is working, and what might work.

Within a virtual forum, distance and power relationships are bridged differently than in face-to-face knowledge exchange. The vCoP contribute to self-reflection and multidirectional discussion of how to creatively bring about change. This combination of diverse participants having multiple sources of knowledge, along with the "we-ness" created in democratic dialogue and reflection, can foster discourse about the making and taking of creative action in ways that are transformative as opposed to discouraging (Anzaldua, 2008). The vCoP become concerned with "contemporary conditions and possibilities for developing a kind of communicative freedom that open up fresh possibilities for working in the contested terrains that combat oppressive and limiting systems of thought" (Ghaye et al., 2008, p. 374). They are catalytic in moving beyond narrow examination of gender and health research that is detached from an integrative context and toward engagement of multisectoral end users in discourse that fully takes into account and affirms end user contexts.

The Researcher as Boundary Spanner in Knowledge Translation

The role of the researcher as facilitator of knowledge diffusion and translation in such praxis-focused processes needs consideration. The isolation and control the researcher experiences in contributing to an academic knowledge exchange forum, such as a peer-reviewed journal, are worlds apart from the interactivity of guiding a participatory deliberative dialogue, with multisectoral end users, working in challenging contexts, often dismissive of or hostile to applying gender lenses.

For over a decade, knowledge translation experts have been grappling with the nature and function of facilitation of knowledge translation processes (Kitson, Harvey, & McCormack, 1998; Nutley, Walter, & Davies, 2007; Rycroft-Malone et al., 2004; Scott & Snelgrove-Clarke, 2008). Yet engagement with how the uptake of research is impeded by broad systemic resistance to understanding and acting on gender differences has not been described as being in the purview of facilitation. Returning to the example of the substance use field, there are neither mechanisms for considering the influence of sex and gender on the experience of substance use and addiction, nor the "ubiquity and grip" (Bradley, 2007, p. 25) of gendered power relations in decision making in the field. The need for conscious facilitation of positive change to address the influence of gender on substance use, treatment, and drug policy has yet to be strongly endorsed. This has been described as the need "to choose deliberately" how to shift entrenched attitudes and paradigms in the substance use field, and for "revision, which means letting go of how we have seen in order to construct new perceptions" (Ettorre, 2004, p. 328).

The change agent aspect of facilitation in the knowledge translation process was identified as early as 1998 by Kitson et al. and further explored by this team of researchers over the past decade (see, for example, Harvey et al., 2002; Kitson et al., 2008). They conclude that the purpose of facilitation, in its most holistic conceptualization, involves "enabling individuals and teams to analyse, reflect and change their own attitudes, behaviour and ways of working" (Harvey et al., 2002, p. 580). They identify a diverse range of skills and personal attributes that may be required to perform the role of facilitator—networker, visionary, catalyst, credible source, innovator, understander of the system, pragmatist, outreach educator, risk taker, and lateral thinker, to name but a few. Little evidence exists, as yet, to indicate the relative importance of such attributes and skills in influencing knowledge uptake and change.

To some extent, the increasing pressure by funding agencies for researchers to be accountable for knowledge translation has given impetus to new explorations of the researcher's role. The Fusion model developed at the BCCEWH in 1999 contains core elements of what other researchers refer to as "engaged scholarship" (Van De Ven, 2007) as a means to close the research-to-practice and research-to-policy gap. This concept recognizes that the gap between "science push" and "user pull" methods of translating and applying evidence to solve problems can be addressed by relational processes. These processes may take different forms of negotiation and collaboration between researchers and practitioners in learning communities, but they must enable the involvement of researchers and end users at all stages in the study of complex problems—from the formulation of questions and research design to analysis of findings, to integration into practice and policy. As such, engaged scholarship parallels the concern of feminist action research with dialogue and information exchange that leverage and respect the different kinds of knowledge that participants bring to the research process.

Feminist scholar Mary O'Brien took on the challenge of describing engaged scholarship in a 1987 keynote conference presentation titled "Feminism as Passionate Scholarship" (O'Brien, 1989). She began that presentation as follows:

> A slippery notion is embedded in the word passion. Passion is by definition resistant to the notion of objectivity, embedded in conventional notions of scholarship. Perhaps what passion and scholarship have in common is context: passion never occurs in a vacuum—passion is passion for something—and neither does scholarship occur in a vacuum, all protestants of objectivity notwithstanding. (p. 245)

She went on to argue for engaged and ethically contextualized scholarship, realized not in individual but in collective pursuits. She describes the feminist practice of consciousness-raising as an innovative pedagogy and an effective collective praxis, a location where the passionate scholar and teacher can be engaged in the "political, practical, and pedagogical task directed to reforming and reproducing the world" (O'Brien, 1989, pp. 255–256). She speaks of "teaching and learning as both an intimate and a social dialectical process which must be passionately maintained in a collective endeavour" (p. 256) not for intellectual purposes, but for developing strategies for social change.

The collectivity of learning as a community endeavor is at the heart of engaged scholarship and feminist action research. It is this experience of researcher as both learner *and* catalyst for learning in a multisectoral process that characterizes the vCoP presented here. In the BCCEWH model for virtual learning communities, the researcher initiates and coordinates joint learning among representatives of different disciplines and sectors, fostering an "inquiry culture" (Mattsson & Kemmis, 2007), and simultaneously takes part in group efforts working toward integration of knowledge. The role involves a transgression of boundaries between research and society for the explicit purpose of linking up research, clinical wisdom, policy wisdom, and lived experience to identify ways to improve health. The vCoP are an embodiment of what have been described as transdisciplinary research processes (Godemann, 2008), involving aspects of boundary crossing, orientation to real-life problems, a participative understanding of research, and integration of different types of knowledge that contribute to the solution of socially relevant questions and open the way to further research (Godemann, 2008).

Now What?

Graham (2007) has proposed that knowledge translation is a dynamic and iterative process that includes synthesis, dissemination, exchange, and ethically sound application, and "this process takes place within a complex system of interactions between researchers and knowledge users which may vary in intensity, complexity and level of engagement depending on the nature of the research and the findings as well as the needs of the particular knowledge use." It has been argued here that high levels of engagement are warranted in the translation of knowledge on gender and health research. Specifically, the knowledge-to-action process must address and integrate three foundational elements: evidence of the complex interactions of sex, gender, and other health determinants; the contributions of multisectoral participants who come together to exchange and synthesize knowledge derived from their different contexts; and facilitation with collaborative and transformative intentions.

In educational and other contexts, it is the boundary spanner who "provides the participatory connection between separate and different communities of practice" (Scanlon, 2001). The vCoP described here have been designed to span locations, sectors, and the resource and attitudinal barriers that inhibit gender-based analysis. The researcher who invites participants into a forum for participatory action research on gender and health takes on the facilitation role of a boundary spanner, in that she or he works with multisectoral contributors to knowledge translation through processes intended to build trust and respect; contextualize experiential, clinical, and cultural knowledge; disseminate what is learned; challenge resistance to change; and promote integrative frameworks for action. This boundary spanning role evokes historical consciousness-raising practices, also concerned with multiple perspectives translated into social change, and provokes gender and health researchers to act as engaged and passionate scholars.

References

Anzaldua, G. (2008). La conciencia de la mestiza: Towards a new consciousness. In G. Anzaldua (Ed.), *Making face, making soul/haciendo caras: Creative and critical perspectives by feminists of color* (pp. 377–389). San Francisco: Aunt Lute Books.

Best, A., Stokols, D., Green, L., Leischow, S., Holmes, B., & Buchholz, K. (2003). An integrative framework for community partnering to translate theory into effective health promotion strategy. *American Journal of Health Promotion, 18*(2), 168–176.

Bowen, S., Martens, P., & The *Need to Know* Team. (2005). Demystifying knowledge translation: Learning from the community. *Journal of Health Services Research & Policy, 10*(4), 203–211.

Bradley, H. (2007). *Gender.* Cambridge, UK: Polity.

British Columbia Centre of Excellence for Women's Health. (2007). *Coalescing on women and substance use: Linking research, practice and policy.* Retrieved December 27, 2010, from http://www.coalescing-vc.org/

Covington, S. S. (2008). Women and addiction: A trauma-informed approach. *Journal of Psychoactive Drugs, SARC Supplement 5,* 377–385.

Estabrooks, C., Thompson, D., Lovely, J., & Hofmeyer, A. (2006). A guide to knowledge translation theory. *The Journal of Continuing Education in the Health Professions, 26*(1), 25–36.

Ettorre, E. (2004). Revisioning women and drug use: Gender sensitivity, embodiment and reducing harm. *International Journal of Drug Policy, 15*(5/6), 327–335.

Ferlie, E., Fitzgerald, L., Wood, M., & Hawkins, C. (2005). The nonspread of innovations: The mediating role of professionals. *Academy of Management Journal, 48*(1), 117–134.

Frisby, W., Magui, P., & Reid, C. (2009). The "f" word has everything to do with it. *Action Research, 7*(1), 13–29.

Ghaye, T., Melander-Wikman, A., Kisare, M., Chambers, P., Bergmark, U., Kostenius, C., et al. (2008). Participatory and appreciative action and reflection (PAAR)—Democratizing reflective practices. *Reflective Practice, 9*(4), 361–397.

Godemann, J. (2008). Knowledge integration: A key challenge for transdisciplinary cooperation. *Environmental Education Research, 14*(6), 625–641.

Graham, I. D. (2007). *Knowledge translation at CIHR.* Retrieved December 27, 2010, from http://www.cihr-irsc.gc.ca/e/33747.html

Graham, I. D., & Tetroe, J. (2007). Whither knowledge translation: An international research agenda. *Nursing Research, 56*(4), S86–S88.

Greaves, L., & Ballem, P. (2001). *Fusion: A model for integrated health research.* Vancouver, BC, Canada: British Columbia Centre of Excellence for Women's Health.

Greenhalgh, T., Robert, G., Macfarlane, F., Bate, P., & Kyriakidou, O. (2004). Diffusion of innovations in service organizations: Systematic review and recommendations. *Milbank Quarterly, 82*, 581–629.

Harvey, G., Loftus-Hills, A., Rycroft-Malone, J., Titchen, A., Kitson, A., McCormack, B., et al. (2002). Getting evidence into practice: The role and function of facilitation. *Journal of Advanced Nursing, 37*(6), 577–588.

Jacobson, N., Butterill, D., & Goering, P. (2003). Development of a framework for knowledge translation: Understanding user context. *Journal of Health Services Research & Policy, 8*(2), 94–99.

Keating, C. (2005). Building coalitional consciousness. *National Women's Studies Association, 17*(2), 86–103.

Kilbourne, J. (1999). *Deadly persuasion: Why women and girls must fight the addictive power of advertising.* New York: Simon and Schuster.

Kitson, A., Harvey, J., & McCormack, B. (1998). Enabling the implementation of evidence-based practice: A conceptual framework. *Quality in Health Care, 7*, 149–158.

Kitson, A., Rycroft-Malone, J., Harvey, G., McCormack, B., Seers, K., & Titchen, A. (2008). Evaluating the successful implementation of evidence into practice using the PARiHS framework: Theoretical and practical challenges. *Implementation Science, 3*(1), 1.

Lavis, J. N., Lomas, J., Hamid, M., & Sewankambod, N. K. (2006). Assessing country-level efforts to link research to action. *Bulletin of the World Health Organization, 84*(8), 620–628.

Mattsson, M., & Kemmis, S. (2007). Praxis-related research: Serving two masters? *Pedagogy, Culture & Society, 15*(2), 185–214.

McCarty, C. A., Kosterman, R., Mason, A., McCauley, E., Hawkins, D., Herrenkohl, T. I., et al. (2009). Longitudinal associations among depression, obesity and alcohol use disorders in young adulthood. *General Hospital Psychiatry, 31*(5), 442–450.

McWilliam, C., Kothari, A., Ward-Griffin, C., Forbes, D., Leipert, B., & South West Community Care Access Centre Home Care. (2009). Evolving the theory and praxis of knowledge translation through social interaction: A social phenomenological study. *Implementation Science, 4*(1), 26.

National Center on Addiction and Substance Abuse. (2003). *The formative years: Pathways to substance abuse among girls and young women ages 8–22.* New York: Author.

National Institute on Alcohol Abuse and Alcoholism. (2003). *Alcohol: A women's health issue.* Rockville, MD: U.S. Department of Health and Human Services.

Nutley, S. M., Walter, I., & Davies, H. T. (2007). *Using evidence: How research can inform public services.* Bristol, UK: Policy Press.

O'Brien, M. (1989). Feminism as passionate scholarship. In M. O'Brien (Ed.), *Reproducing the world* (pp. 245–257). San Francisco: Westview Press.

Reid, C., Tom, A., & Frisby, W. (2006). Finding the "action" in feminist participatory action research. *Action Research, 4*(3), 315–332.

Rycroft-Malone, J., Harvey, G., Seers, K., Kitson, A., McCormack, B., & Titchen, A. (2004). An exploration of the factors that influence the implementation of evidence into practice. *Journal of Clinical Nursing, 13*(8), 913–924.

Scanlon, L. (2001). *The Boundary Spanner: Exploring the new frontiers of a school-university partnership as a community of practice.* Retrieved December 27, 2010, from http://www.aare.edu.au/01pap/sca01718.htm

Scott, S. D., & Snelgrove-Clarke, E. (2008). Facilitation: The final frontier? *Nursing for Women's Health, 12*(1), 26–29.

Shreve, A. (1989). *Women together, women alone: The legacy of the consciousness-raising movement.* New York: Viking Press.

Simons-Morton, B., Farhat, T., ter Bogt, T. F. M., Hublet, A., Kuntsche, E., Gabhainn, S. N., et al. (2009). Gender specific trends in alcohol use: Cross-cultural comparisons from 1998 to 2006 in 24 countries and regions. *International Journal of Public Health, 54*(2), 199–208.

Smith, A., Stewart, D., Peled, M., Poon, C., Saewyc, E., & McCreary Centre Society. (2009). *A Picture of Health: Highlights from the 2008 BC Adolescent Health Survey.* Vancouver, BC, Canada: McCreary Centre Society.

Spear, L. P. (2002). Alcohol's effects on adolescents. *The Journal of the National Institute on Alcohol Abuse and Alcoholism, 26*(4), 287–291.

Straus, S. E., Tetroe, J., & Graham, I. D. (2009). Defining knowledge translation. *Canadian Medical Association Journal, 181*(3/4), 165–168.

Sudsawad, P. (2007). *Knowledge translation: Introduction to models, strategies and measures.* Madison, WI: National Center for the Dissemination of Disability Research.

Van De Ven, A. H. (2007). *Engaged scholarship: A guide for organizational and social research.* New York: Oxford University Press.

Design, Methods, and Knowledge Exchange

Connections and Pathways

John L. Oliffe

14

I n writing this chapter, I have two objectives. First, using an example drawn from the Investigating Tobacco and Gender research team (University of British Columbia, 2010b), I illustrate how early conceptual considerations for addressing research problems not only drive the study design and methods, but also determine the type of deliverable that can be reasonably promised for knowledge exchange. Second, I map some pathways for distributing descriptive and intervention research products through peer-reviewed publications, and briefly describe some recent experiences with developing my own website (www.menshealthresearch.ubc.ca) as a means to guide the virtual knowledge exchange efforts of others. In concluding the chapter, I suggest some principles of marketing to make gender, sex, and health research products more visible.

Connecting Design, Methods, and Knowledge Exchange Products

Typically, the impetus to writing a gender- and/or sex-based research proposal emerges from the belief that a problem or disparity exists, about which there is limited analysis or understanding. Predictably absent here are effective programmatic or systematic solutions to address the problem or emergent issue. It is early on in deconstructing a particular issue that gender- and sex-based research questions are posed. For example, smoking in pregnancy and the postpartum period has long been positioned as a women's health issue because anatomically and physiologically the female carries the fetus, and at birth the mother is the primary source of food and caregiving for the newborn. Health promotion messages often portray sex as both nature *and* nurture in locating women as the mediator of smoking during pregnancy and in the postpartum period. In addition, socially constructed ideals of femininity and gender typically support and extend these sex claims. Consider Image 14.1, from a 2009 United Kingdom–based National Health Service (NHS) campaign that was "designed to make the consequences of smoking during pregnancy feel immediate, in order to foster a strong and immediate motivation for pregnant women to quit, and stay quit" (Smokefree Resource Centre, 2009).

In this silhouette, the mother's smoke emerges not from the cigarette but from the fetus, which lies in wait, defenseless, fragile, and clearly in harm's way. The mother's right hand cradles *her* "baby bump" from which *their* smoke extrudes, while the left hand levers the cigarette to and from her pursed lips. The woman's hands seem contradictory in their actions, and amid the protection and harm imbued by the two opposing gestures, it is ever clear that the mother's smoking is the central issue and target of this campaign.

The epidemiological data can also affirm this as a women's issue, citing statistics that indicate as few as 15.8% of pregnant women who smoke

Image 14.1   NHS Smoking and Pregnancy Campaign

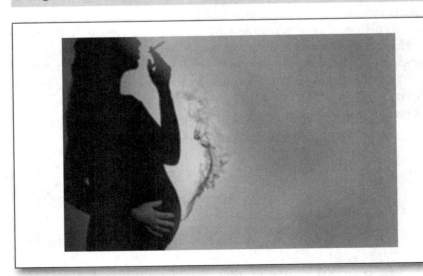

Source: UK-based National Health Service (NHS). http://smokefree.nhs.uk/resources/campaigns/smoking-and-pregnancy/

make a quit attempt, and only half of these are smoke-free when their child is born (Connor & McIntyre, 1999). Moreover, the estimated relapse rates for women who quit smoking during pregnancy are 25% within 1 month postpartum, 50% within 4 months postpartum, and 70% to 90% by 1 year postpartum (Fingerhut, Kleinman, & Kendrick, 1990; Mullen, Quinn, & Ershoff, 1990; Secker-Walker et al., 1995). Although this compelling evidence supports the notion of a women's health issue, men are also strongly implicated, given that 29% of fathers continue to smoke during their child-rearing years (Callard & Lavigne, 2005), and having a partner who smokes is a strong predictor of mothers returning to tobacco during pregnancy and the postpartum period (Fingerhut et al., 1990; Johnson, Ratner, Bottorff, Hall, & Dahinten, 2000; Klesges, Johnson, Ward, & Barnard, 2001; Mullen, Richardson, & Quinn, 1997; Ratner, Johnson, Bottorff, Dahinten, & Hall, 2000).

Foregrounding the interest about *who* smokes in pregnancy and the postpartum period are data confirming 15% of Canadian households have at least one person who smokes inside the home every day, and almost 10% of children under the age of 12 (about 379,000 children) are regularly exposed to secondhand smoke (SHS) at home. Associated with fetal and infant exposure to SHS are early pregnancy loss (Venners et al., 2004), low birth weight and associated risks, middle-ear infections, respiratory infections such as bronchitis and pneumonia, and sudden infant death syndrome (British Medical Association, 2004; Martinez, Wright, Taussig, & Group Health Medical Associates, 1994). Aside from the direct health risks for mothers and fathers who smoke, the well-being of a third party (or parties) is also clearly at risk when one or both parents smoke.

In distilling how gender and sex influence smoking in pregnancy and the postpartum period, the Families Controlling and Eliminating Tobacco group (University of British Columbia, 2010a), a subgroup of the iTAG team, investigated the interactions between mothers and fathers to learn how gender relations and family dynamics can impact tobacco use. What followed was a two-phase research program design. In Phase 1 we interviewed moms and dads separately about the household dynamics surrounding tobacco, focusing on the women's experiences during pregnancy and the postpartum period. We also examined the connections between masculinities and the smoking patterns of dads in pregnancy and the postpartum period (Bottorff, Oliffe, Kalaw, Carey, & Mróz, 2006; Oliffe, Bottorff, Johnson, Kelly, & LeBeau, 2010) and explored how gender ideals around the parenting of children up to 7 years of age influenced smoking practices (Bottorff et al., 2010). The team used qualitative methods including participant observations, individual interviews, and photo-elicitation, all of which have been detailed in Part III of this book. A key benefit of these methods for our research was the collection of rich data from which thick descriptions were developed to explain how masculinities and femininities and gender relations impacted smoking in pregnancy and the postpartum period.

While Phase 1 drew national funding support, it is important to acknowledge that, based on our qualitative design, we could only reasonably expect to describe the gender issues underpinning smoking in pregnancy and the postpartum period. Therefore, from the outset the end product of Phase 1 was intended to be *descriptive,* and our promissory note clearly delineated discovery as our aim. We also wanted to inform interventions but not build them—at least not yet! In Phase 2 we focused on designing, disseminating, and evaluating targeted print-based tobacco reduction *interventions.* The women's booklet, *Couples and Smoking* (downloadable at www.facet.ubc.ca), took into consideration household dynamics in targeting pregnant women and mothers to thoughtfully consider their couple-based interactions around tobacco. The men's booklet, *The Right Time, the Right Reasons* (also downloadable at www.facet.ubc.ca), highlighted men's testimonials about the challenges of tobacco reduction and cessation while detailing their motivations for wanting to be smoke-free fathers. In both interventions, we purposely avoided writing for "shock value" or espousing a "how to quit" booklet, in part because those messages saturate the market, but more so because we wanted to prompt contemplation for change among smokers by highlighting what we had learned from study participants in Phase 1.

The methods used in Phase 2 included focus group interviews conducted with moms, dads, and health care providers to design and refine the interventions, and survey questionnaires and quantitative analyses were used in the pilot testing to capture end users' evaluations. The interventions were decision aids, designed to be used as stand-alone products or adjuncts to practitioner counseling, assisting moms and dads to weigh up the benefits, risks, and scientific uncertainty of tobacco use (Brouwers, Stacey, & O'Connor, 2009). Within the context of pregnancy, our intent was to mobilize, support, and increase the effectiveness of moms' and dads' tobacco reduction and cessation efforts.

In briefly describing our research program, two key connections between study design and methods and knowledge exchange products are apparent. First, the research problem(s) or issues had to be fully understood and described before the intervention(s) could be designed and tested. For example, we were careful to avoid stigmatizing or blaming pregnant women and mothers or temporally compartmentalizing *women's* smoking as a pregnancy issue. Instead, we focused on couple interactions around smoking and pregnancy and the postpartum period. We also anchored smoking in pregnancy and the postpartum period as a fathers' issue, highlighting men's desire to be good role models, providers, and protectors, while pointing to how smoking diluted and disconnected many men from those masculine ideals.

It might be argued that description is the core business or, more pro-vocatively, the preoccupation and major limitation of much gender, sex, and health research. After all, Phase 1 of our study took 6 years. So, why did we not accept gender and sex as central and design a randomized con-trol trial to evaluate our intervention? Partly, it was because a suite of gender-savvy interventions from which to choose did not exist to guide the design, but more important perhaps, using generic principles to develop interventions without fully understanding the intertwined gendered issues, we risked reifying smoking in pregnancy and the postpartum period as a women's health issue. While the intent of the campaign that accompanied Image 14.1 was to promote the health of the woman and the fetus, we were convinced of the need to message both women and men about smoking in pregnancy and the postpartum period in nonmedical and nonjudgmental ways. This design decision also related, in large part, to the data collected in Phase 1, whereby participants were adamant that they already endured significant stigma, but wanted peer or professional guidance and support to reduce or quit smoking.

Second, we drew on diverse methodologies and methods to develop descriptive and intervention-based products, and sequentially transition from one to the other. Oftentimes, researchers and, in some cases, particu-lar study topics seem to stall, falling short of interventions. This can be a conscious decision whereby the research program vision does not include "in-house" development and testing of interventions. For example, point-ing to how diverse masculinities and femininities emerge in relation to particular illnesses or health practices can be the sole aim of some gender and health research. Indeed, not all research should be dedicated to serving today's decision makers because the feedstock of methods, theory, and empirical innovation most often emerges from descriptive research (Lomas, 2009). Researchers can also take the middle ground between descriptive and intervention products by targeting clinicians and/or policymakers with their findings as a means to informing (as distinct from designing) inter-ventions. However, as Lomas eloquently cautions, researchers have a ten-dency to overestimate the value of *their* facts in clinical decision making. Meta-analyses and systematic or scoping reviews, along with examples for applying theory, can also be an effective conduit between description and intervention by synthesizing the current evidence or illustrating analytic frames to prompt and preempt the need for specific interventions. For example, Courtenay's (2000) article, "Constructions of Masculinity and Their Influence on Men's Well-Being: A Theory of Gender and Health," has been cited more than 700 times, and a literature review by Galdas, Cheater, and Marshall (2005) addressing men's health help-seeking behavior has also been widely cited by researchers, clinicians, and policymakers. Articles such as these can be highly influential in guiding the work of others.

While appreciating that research programs do not always envision or cannot extend their operations to include interventions, the limits of description and diversity have emerged amid the need to apply gender, sex, and health research. In large part, this is dictated by funding agencies and their obligations to donors as well as those who provide and consume health care. Population health trends are increasingly linked to service provision, and the political, public, and professional expectations about accessing effective health care demand more than theorizing or thick description about how gender and sex connect to various health issues. Said another way, inevitably the question is asked: What can we do with descriptive knowledge to improve the health of boys and girls and men and women? So while an array of research products is key to advancing gender, sex, and health research, the need to deliver gender- and sex-savvy interventions that thoughtfully address the problems "we" describe is ever present. Regardless of whether that vision is distilled early on or emergent in design, the ability to creatively draw from a suite of research methods is central to having the capacity to develop thick description, and to design and evaluate intervention-based products.

Old and New Pathways for Knowledge Exchange

The distribution channels for knowledge exchange are constantly changing, and key considerations include how, where, and to whom the study findings should be disseminated (Lavis et al., 2003). While acknowledging that many pathways exist for knowledge exchange, in what follows I have focused on two commonly used mediums in an effort to guide other gender, sex, and health researchers. First, I address some key considerations for publishing in peer-reviewed journals. Second, briefly described are recent experiences with developing a men's health research website (www.menshealthresearch.ubc.ca) along with broader considerations about virtual means to extending the capacity for knowledge exchange.

PEER-REVIEWED PUBLICATIONS: NOTHING IS WRITTEN UNTIL IT IS READ

Publishing in peer-reviewed journals continues to be a benchmark indicator for chronicling the outcomes and gauging the usefulness of specific studies, as well as the researchers' ability to deliver end products from their work. Empirical methods, theory, and review articles can be developed from most studies, and, ideally, in publishing this assortment of writings, the awareness and interest of students, researchers, clinicians, and policymakers are garnered. However, the increasing number of peer-reviewed health journals amid debates about the virtues of open access has added to the complexities for deciding where best to publish.

Our review of specialty journals focused on gender, sex, and health research (see Table 14.1) is organized chronologically by year of inception and includes specificities about impact factors, focus, and access. Men's health journals emerged more recently than women's, and this accounts, in part, for the diverse impact factors, a measure that reflects the average number of citations of the total articles within a publication. While scholars continue to debate the significance of bibliometric measures, the impact factor is often used to signal the relative importance of a journal within its field, and journals with higher impact factors are deemed more important than those with lower ratings. The overall lower impact factors of the specialty journals listed in Table 14.1 might also reflect the relative newness of gender, sex, and health research. However, these specialty journals are important information repositories, fundamental to building capacity by showcasing what, as well as how, gender, sex, and health research is done.

Table 14.2 lists some journals that regularly publish but do not specialize in gender, sex, and health research. These journals focus on body systems or diseases (e.g., endocrine system, heart disease), specific disciplines (e.g., nursing, medicine, psychology), and/or target audiences (e.g., clinicians, researchers, policymakers). One benefit of publishing in these locales is that

Table 14.1   Specialty Journals

Journal	Impact Factor	5-Year Factor	Focus	Open Access
Women & Health since 1975	.941	1.436	Medical focus on women's health, does not theorize gender. Publishes original papers and critical reviews containing highly useful information for researchers, policy planners, and all providers of health care for women.	Yes (fee based)
Journal of Women's Health since 1992	1.943	1.935	Medical focus on women's health. Publishes articles on diseases or conditions that hold greater risk for or are more prevalent among women.	Yes (fee based)

(Continued)

Table 14.1 (Continued)

Journal	Impact Factor	5-Year Factor	Focus	Open Access
BMC Women's Health since 2001	No JCR index		Publishes original peer-reviewed research articles in all aspects of the health and health care of adolescent girls and women, with a particular focus on the prevention, diagnosis, and management of fertility disorders and diseases of gynecological and breast origin.	Yes (fee based)
International Journal of Men's Health since 2002	No JCR index		Publishes multidisciplinary, multicultural, empirical, theoretical, applied, and historical contributions focusing on men's health issues, as well as critical reviews.	No
Journal of Men's Health since 2004	No JCR index		A comprehensive, accessible resource of knowledge addressing policy and patient care issues and offering sex and gender information about men's health, disease, and illness issues.	No
Gender Medicine: The Journal for the Study of Sex and Gender Differences since 2004	No JCR index		Focuses on the impact of sex differences in normal human physiology, and the pathophysiology and clinical features of disease.	No (Publication costs including peer review, copyediting, layout, printing, postage, and online hosting/ archiving are recovered in part through author fees.)

Journal	Impact Factor	5-Year Factor	Focus	Open Access
American Journal of Men's Health since 2007	.471		Resource for frontline men's health care providers and patient educators, policy development specialists, researchers, and scholars. Manuscripts address male-specific diseases and health conditions; masculinity and the social constructions of masculinity.	No

Note: JCR = *Journal Citation Reports.*

articles can reach diverse audiences and influence "others" who might not explicitly engage gender and sex in their work. Manuscripts focused on gender and/or sex and health can also be strategically reworked to engage "new" readers. For example, theorizing around social constructions of masculinity and cardiac rehabilitation might engage sociology and health audiences, whereas the practice implications drawn from the same study can be packaged for a journal that targets clinicians. While I am not suggesting that the same findings be published more than once, writing to engage varying perspectives within a gender and/or sex frame to broaden "our" reach is not only good use of data; it can garner important dialogue within and between researcher groups that might ordinarily be estranged.

Central to debates about the virtues of peer-reviewed publications is the issue of open access. Advocates of open-access journals argue that scholarly journals be made available online to the reader without financial, legal, or technical barriers other than those related to gaining access to the Internet itself (Suber, 2010). Key benefits of open access include the availability of articles for taxpayers, patients, and the general public, a strategy that ideally results in articles being downloaded and cited by more readers, and better integrated into the knowledge base. Opponents of the open-access model argue that the pay-for-access model is necessary to adequately compensate the publisher for its work in maintaining a scholarly reputation, arranging for peer review, and editing and indexing articles. The best of both worlds is also available for purchase at varying rates with some journals, whereby the author or authors pay a fee to make their article freely available to others online (see Tables 14.1 and 14.2). While the specificities of open access continue to shift (e.g., hybrid vs. delayed open access), authors need to be cognizant of funding guidelines and policies in reassessing decisions about where to publish. While not the primary

Table 14.2 Journals That Publish but Do Not Specialize in Gender or Sex and Health Articles

Journal	Impact Factor	5-Year Factor	Focus	Open Access
Social Science & Medicine since 1979	2.710	3.615	An international and interdisciplinary forum for the dissemination of social science research on health. Publishes material relevant to any aspect of health from a wide range of social science disciplines (anthropology, economics, epidemiology, geography, policy, psychology, and sociology).	No
Sociology of Health & Illness since 1979	1.845	2.89	An international medical sociology journal that publishes sociological articles on all aspects of health, illness, medicine, and health care. Welcomes empirical and theoretical contributions in the form of original research reports or review articles.	Yes (fee based)
Health: An Interdisciplinary Journal for the Social Study of Health, Illness and Medicine since 1997	1.32	1.63	A broad-ranging interdisciplinary journal related to health and the social sciences. Focuses on the changing place of health matters in modern society.	No
Journal of Health and Social Behavior since 2004	2.35	4.536	A medical sociology journal that publishes empirical and theoretical articles that apply sociological concepts and methods to the understanding of health and illness and the organization of medicine and health care.	No

Journal	Impact Factor	5-Year Factor	Focus	Open Access
Addiction since 1884	4.244	5.185	Scope spans human clinical, epidemiological, experimental, policy, and historical research relating to any activity that has addictive potential. Publishes some sex-based differences research.	Yes (fee based)
American Heart Journal since 1925	4.28	4.1	Investigation, scholarly review, and opinion concerning the practice of cardiovascular medicine. Encourages submission of negative clinical studies, reports on study designs, and studies involving the organization of medical care.	No
American Journal of Health Behavior since 1977	1.357	1.629	Focused on the relationships among personal behavior, social structure, and health highlighting behavioral science principles and strategies to assist in designing and implementing programs to prevent disease and promote health.	No
American Journal of Health Studies since 1984	No JCR index		Publishes comprehensive literature reviews, meta-analyses, theory-driven intervention studies, comprehensive case studies, and thoughtful commentaries on health education and health promotion.	No

Note: JCR = *Journal Citation Reports.*

evaluative criteria to guide those decisions, it can be useful to search databases (e.g., Web of Science, Google Scholar) to see how often, as well as by whom, your published articles are cited. The Directory of Open Access Journals, which lists some options (http://www.doaj.org/), can also assist authors in deciding where to publish.

Open-access issues prevail as key considerations for new, as well as more experienced, researchers. Given that much of the descriptive work in gender and health is dedicated to emancipation through privileging people's illness experiences and/or making visible underserved populations, publishing in open-access journals might be considered integral to that enterprise. Of course, no journal can guarantee an audience for your work, and alternatives to peer-reviewed publications include executive summaries and community reports that can be written and distributed directly to target specific audiences. I used this strategy in a study examining the role of prostate cancer support groups (PCSGs) in health promotion. Specifically, a report summarizing our published study findings was disseminated via hard copy and PDF (downloadable from www.menshealthresearch.ubc.ca) as a strategy for ensuring the public, including men who experience prostate cancer and their families, could access information about the services PCSGs provide. Likewise, brief reports can engage other target audiences, including health care professionals. Thoughtfully considering where, how, and what to publish early on in each project, while considering the overarching goals of the research program, is integral to communicating study findings both within and around peer-reviewed journals.

VIRTUALLY WHERE?

One emergent medium for knowledge exchange is the Internet, and increasingly researchers invest time and money to develop a virtual presence for recruiting study participants, inviting input/dialogue from visitors, showcasing their research, and making available descriptive and intervention products derived from their work. For example, the goal for developing the men's health research site (www.menshealthresearch.ubc.ca) was to raise awareness about our research program and redirect visitors to published articles as well as provide them with downloadable content drawn from our work. While content development and navigation for the site were primary considerations, it was only by regularly analyzing the data collected by Google Analytics, a free service that monitors and reports website traffic, that we were able to evaluate our progress and refine the design accordingly. Figure 14.1, the Google Analytics dashboard, displays some of the many data available about the first month's traffic to the site, including the number of visitors by date, country of origin, entry pathway, and time spent per visit. Most interesting was the sudden increase in the number of visitors around the middle of April, a by-product of a mass e-mail sent to colleagues announcing the launch of our site along with the hyperlink. While the traffic to the site was encouraging, the bounce rate indicates that 35% of the 240 visitors entered and exited the home page without reviewing any other content. After analyzing all the data in the

Figure 14.1   Google Analytics™ Dashboard

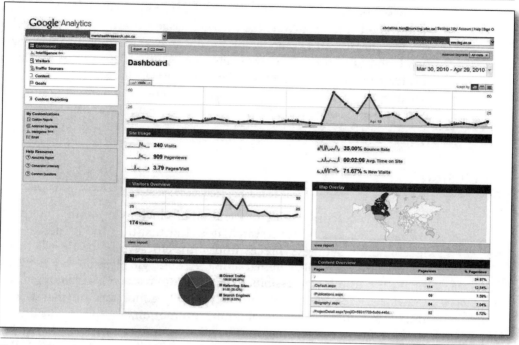

Source: Google.

report, we focused on strategies for increasing the traffic to the site, and adjusted the design by (1) linking our PubMed abstracts and (2) making available downloaded content directly from the site.

In terms of increasing the traffic to the site, search engine optimization (SEO), a process for maximizing search engine referrals, included exchanging links with other compatible men's health sites and assigning key words, metatags, and descriptors for each of the website sections and pages. A site map of our website was also submitted to various search engines, signaling the most important pages. In an effort to attract return visitors, a "web feed" feature, a system that allows subscribers to sign up to see new content as it is published to the site, can also be added.

While adjustments to the website are ongoing, we have also begun to consider evidence around the gendered use of the Internet, in assessing if and how men-centered interventions can be effectively distributed through this medium. For example, men use the Internet more intensively for news and entertainment while education- and health-related information is accessed more often by women (Office for National Statistics, 2009). In addition, Web 2.0—which refers to interactive information sharing and includes web-based communities, social networking sites, podcasts, wikis, and blogs—is touted as facilitating online individual agency in the uptake of health promotion messages especially among younger visitors (Robinson & Robertson, 2010). That said, Facebook, one of the biggest and best-known Web 2.0 platforms, attracts more women (56%) than men in the United States. These Internet usage patterns indicate that the web in general, and Facebook specifically, may reach more women than men with health promotion interventions (Smith, 2010). While touching on a few fundamental issues about "virtual" knowledge exchange, it is clear that there is great complexity, yet also great potential, for extending our individual and collective reach to engage diverse online audiences.

Conclusion

In affirming descriptive and intervention products as key to the enterprise of gender, sex, and health research, it is clear that the product design and dissemination pathways directly impact the efficacy of our efforts. Only a few academics specialize in marketing, yet strategic plans are key to maximizing the visibility, accessibility, and uptake of research. Said another way, knowledge exchange efforts are increasingly contingent on marketing's four Ps: product, place (distribution), promotion, and price. Ideally, the products are developed in concert with community members, key stakeholders, and potential distributors, as Nancy Poole (in Chapter 13 of this volume) suggests. However, the plan and vision, and much of the energy required to achieve even the most modest knowledge exchange goals, typically reside with the principal researcher and/or research team. Therefore, effective leaders are strategic in courting collaborators and stakeholders across research programs while drawing on the investigative team's expertise to make good on the promissory notes pertaining to knowledge exchange. In this respect, distributors and product promotion experts will feature and ideally take the lead in their specialty area. While these linkages are often made based on the researcher's track record, ideally the capacity to effectively engage partners to address the four Ps will grow with time, trust, and the strategic avoidance of "drive-by" collaborations.

References

Bottorff, J. L., Kelly, M. T., Oliffe, J. L., Johnson, J. L., Greaves, L., & Chan, A. (2010). Tobacco use patterns in traditional and shared parenting families: A gender perspective. *BMC Public Health Journal, 10,* 239.

Bottorff, J. L., Oliffe, J. L., Kalaw, C., Carey, J., & Mróz, L. (2006). Men's constructions of smoking in the context of women's tobacco reduction during pregnancy. *Social Science and Medicine, 62*(12), 3096–3108.

British Medical Association. (2004). *Smoking and reproductive life: The impact of smoking on sexual, reproductive and child health.* London, Edinburgh: British Medical Association, Board of Science and Education and Tobacco Control Resource Centre.

Brouwers, M. C., Stacey, D., & O'Connor, A. M. (2009). Knowledge translation tools. In S. E. Straus, J. Tetroe, & I. D. Graham (Eds.), *Knowledge translation in health care: Moving from evidence to practice* (pp. 35–45). West Sussex, UK: Blackwell.

Callard, C., & Lavigne, C. (2005). *A world No Tobacco Day message from Canada's health professionals.* Physicians for a Smoke-Free Canada: The Canadian Dental Association. Retrieved December 5, 2010, from http://www.cda-adc .ca/en/cda/news_events/media/news_releases/2005/pdfs/wntd2005.pdf

Connor, S. K., & McIntyre, L. (1999). The socio-demographic predictors of smoking cessation among pregnant women in Canada. *Canadian Journal of Public Health, 90,* 352–355.

Courtenay, W. H. (2000). Constructions of masculinity and their influence on men's well-being: A theory of gender and health. *Social Science and Medicine, 50,* 1385–1401.

Fingerhut, L. A., Kleinman, J. C., & Kendrick, J. S. (1990). Smoking before, during, and after pregnancy. *American Journal of Public Health, 80*(5), 541–544.

Galdas, P. M., Cheater, F., & Marshall, P. (2005). Men and health help-seeking behaviour: Literature review. *Journal of Advanced Nursing, 49,* 616–623.

Johnson, J. L., Ratner, P. A., Bottorff, J. L., Hall, W., & Dahinten, S. (2000). Preventing smoking relapse in postpartum women. *Nursing Research, 49,* 44–52.

Klesges, R. C., Johnson, K. C., Ward, K. D., & Barnard, M. (2001). Smoking cessation in pregnant women. *Obstetrics and Gynecological Clinics of North America, 28,* 269–282.

Lavis, J. N., Robertson, D., Woodside, J. M., McLeod, C. B., Abelson, J., & the Knowledge Transfer Study Group. (2003). How can research organizations more effectively transfer research knowledge to decision makers? *Milbank Quarterly, 81*(2), 221–248.

Lomas, J. (2009). Foreword—Improving research dissemination and uptake in the health sector: Beyond the sound of one hand clapping. In S. E. Straus, J. Tetroe, & I. D. Graham (Eds.), *Knowledge translation in health care: Moving from evidence to practice* (pp. xii–xvi). West Sussex, UK: Blackwell.

Martinez, F. D., Wright, A., Taussig, L., & Group Health Medical Associates. (1994). The effect of paternal smoking on the birthweight of newborns whose mothers did not smoke. *American Journal of Public Health, 84,* 1489–1491.

Mullen, P. D., Quinn, V. P., & Ershoff, D. H. (1990). Maintenance of nonsmoking postpartum by women who stopped smoking during pregnancy. *American Journal of Public Health, 80*(8), 992–994.

Mullen, P. D., Richardson, M. A., & Quinn, V. P. (1997). Postpartum return to smoking: Who is at risk and when? *American Journal of Health Promotion, 11,* 323–330.

Office for National Statistics. (2009). *National Statistics Omnibus Survey.* Retrieved from http://www.statistics.gov.uk/default.asp

Oliffe, J. L., Bottorff, J. L., Johnson, J. L., Kelly, M. T., & LeBeau, K. (2010). Fathers: Locating smoking and masculinity in the postpartum. *Qualitative Health Research, 20,* 330–339.

Ratner, P. A., Johnson, J. L., Bottorff, J. L., Dahinten, S., & Hall, W. (2000). Twelve-month follow-up of a smoking relapse prevention intervention for postpartum women. *Addictive Behaviors, 25,* 81–92.

Robinson, M., and Robertson, S. (2010). Young men's health promotion and new information communication technologies: Illuminating the issues and research agendas. *Health Promotion International, 25,* 363–370.

Secker-Walker, R. H., Solomon, L. J., Flynn, B. S., Skelly, J. M., Lepage, S. S., Goodwin, G. D., et al. (1995). Smoking relapse prevention counseling during prenatal and early postnatal care. *American Journal of Preventive Medicine, 11*(2), 86–93.

Smith, J. (2010, January 4). *December data on Facebook's US growth by age and gender: Beyond 100 million.* Retrieved December 5, 2010, from http://www.insidefacebook .com/2010/01/04/december-data-on-facebook%e2%80%99s-us-growth-by-age-and-gender-beyond-100-million/

Smokefree Resource Centre. (2009). *Campaigns: Pregnancy.* Retrieved December 5, 2010, from http://smokefree.nhs.uk/resources/campaigns/smoking-and-pregnancy/

Suber, P. (2010). *Open access overview.* Retrieved December 10, 2010, from http://www.earlham.edu/~peters/fos/overview.htm

University of British Columbia. (2010a, June 19). *FACET: Families Controlling and Eliminating Tobacco.* Retrieved December 5, 2010, from http://www.facet.ubc.ca

University of British Columbia. (2010b, December 3). *iTAG: Investigating Tobacco & Gender.* Retrieved December 5, 2010, from http://www.itag.ubc.ca

Venners, S. A., Wang, X., Chen, C., Wang, L., Chen, D., Guang, W., et al. (2004). Paternal smoking and pregnancy loss: A prospective study using a biomarker of pregnancy. *American Journal of Epidemiology, 159,* 993–1001.

Afterword

John L. Oliffe and Lorraine Greaves

The impetus for this book came from our recognition that gender, sex, and health research has thoughtfully addressed important and diverse issues, and indeed is essential to achieve good, ethical science necessary to improving health. Yet it is still all too often found occupying the periphery of health research. How do we change this going forward?

Parts I and II of this volume highlighted the history, contexts, and relevance, along with an array of design considerations and options whereby sex and/or gender can deliberately, strategically, and rightfully be considered central to health research. In this context the "So what?" question does not yield nearly as much as the proactive rephrasing "So what can sex and gender reveal about health and particular disease and illness issues?"

The six-part offering in Part III provided a palette of methods for delivering on that potential. Contextualized within diverse health and illness issues, the gender and sex methods described revealed an eclectic assortment of tools from which to choose. By no means are all possibilities captured or fully represented here; instead, prospects and pathways for getting started are raised. Indeed, rather than attempting to prescribe a chronology or combination, the offerings in Part III afford many ways and means for addressing sex, gender, and health issues.

Part IV mapped some policy, process, and product terrain that is less often explicitly connected to methods. Yet, again, threaded through these chapters are important considerations about how gender and sex research connects to wider political considerations, community partnerships, and product development.

There are two additional considerations that we want to leave you with. First, the advancement of gender, sex, and health research is contingent on sustaining an ongoing dialogue about concepts, theories, design, and methods. While we might engage in this enterprise by explicitly self-labeling as experts in men's health, women's health, or gender and health, and/or as feminists, masculinists, or social or bench scientists, there is a great deal to be gained from stepping out (even if only for a moment!) of those compartments and categories. Through meaningfully connecting with others within the enterprise of gender, sex, and health research and consciously developing and embracing transdisciplinary approaches, the influence and impact of our collective work may be realized sooner rather than later.

Second, capacity building may be best achieved by a commitment to a clear goal of mainstreaming gender in addition to continuing to develop specialized knowledge and experience in sex, gender, and health, so that gender and sex permeate the design and doing of all health research and ultimately clinical practice and policymaking. To that end, sharing this volume widely with both researchers and research users might be a strategic step toward achieving that goal.

Author Index

Aaron, S. D., 60
Abbas, N., 48
Abel, P., 164–165
Abelson, J., 232
Addis, M. E., 18
Adkins, L., 132
Adler, P., 107
Adler, P. A., 107
Agate, R. J., 89
Alain, L., 153
Alexander, V. D., 130
Al-Khatib, S. M., 153
Allen, L., 129
Aloisi, A. M., 93
Alonso, P., 93
Amaratunga, C., 10
Amekudzi, Y. P., 179
Amos, A., 130
Anderson, G., 43
Andersson, N., 23
Andrew, M. K., 146
Angus, J., 132
Annandale, E., 39, 41, 44, 208
Anzaldua, G., 220
Aragons, N., 31–32
Arber, S., 146
Archer, L., 117
Aries, E., 161
Armstrong, E. A., 46
Arnold, A. P., 87, 90, 91
Arora, K., 116, 140
Artazcoz, L., 112
Auger, A. P., 56–57
Auger, C. J., 89
Ayres, L., 183

Bacchi, C., 206
Balaban, E., 86
Bale, T. L., 56–57
Ballem, P., 10, 218

Banks, I., 165
Barbeau, E. M., 44
Barnard, M., 229
Barrett, A. E., 27
Barrett-Connor, E., 51, 52
Baruchel, S., 129
Bass, B., 153
Bassett, M. T., 43
Bate, P., 217
Batien, B. D., 65, 78
Bayer, N., 65, 68–70
Beach, F. A., 86, 88
Becker, H. S., 129–130
Becker, J. B., 86–87, 91, 93
Beere, C. A., 24
Belcher, S. M., 93
Bem, S. L., 24, 32, 65, 80, 198
Bennett, W., 115
Benoit, C., 41, 45, 55
Bepko, C., 193
Bergmark, U., 221
Berkley, K. J., 91
Berman, H., 129
Bernard, H. R., 106–107, 115, 118–119
Bernier, J., 7, 20, 27, 55
Berwick, M., 32
Best, A., 217
Beyer, C., 89
Bibb, G. S., 146
Bierman, A. S., 152
Bird, C. A., 153
Bird, C. E., 22, 31, 39, 51, 70
Birgenheir, D. G., 65, 78
Black, D., 26
Blalock, H. M., 66, 73
Blaustein, J. D., 91
Blimkie, C. J., 49
Boland, M. A., 145

Bollman, R. D., 145, 153
Bond, T. G., 75
Booth, T., 129
Booth, W., 129
Borkhoff, C. M., 22, 94
Bottorff, J. L., 28, 121, 129, 131, 176, 180–181, 183–184, 229
Boucekkine, C., 48
Bourdieu, P., 131–132, 140
Bowen, S., 218
Boyd, J., 88
Boydell, K. M., 156
Boyle, M. H., 156
Bracke, P., 77
Bradley, C. J., 43
Bradley, H., 221
Brady, D., 118
Brady, M. S., 32
Brain, K., 164
Brammer, M., 49
Braveman, P. A., 44
Bredin, K., 90
Bridgman, P. W., 66
Broom, D. H., 186
Brouwers, M. C., 230
Brown, T. M., 206
Brunelle, P. L., 92
Brutsaert, D., 92
Bryant, L., 114
Buchholz, K., 217
Budge, C., 169–170
Bulliard, J., 31
Buonomano, D. V., 94
Burgess, J., 118
Burns, N., 156
Burris, M., 128–129
Burton, C., 206
Bus, L., 93
Bush, T., 52
Bushnell, C. D., 92

Butera, K. J., 107
Butland, D. L., 175, 178, 209–210
Butler, J., 24, 28, 30
Butterill, D., 218
Bweklwy, K. J., 86–87, 91, 93
Bye, L. M., 117
Byrne, B. M., 68
Byrnes, J. P., 45

Cadman, D. T., 156
Callard, C., 229
Carere, R. G., 92
Carey, J., 28, 183, 229
Carkoglu, A., 130
Carovano, K., 129
Carpenter, M., 45
Carryer, J., 169–170
Carter, C. I., 116, 140
Casey, M. A., 118
Cash, J., 128
Cervoni, N., 95
Chaabouni, S., 48
Chabot, C., 113, 118, 121
Chambers, N., 180–181, 183
Chambers, P., 221
Champagne, B., 89
Champagne, F. A., 95
Chan, A., 229
Charchar, F. J., 89
Charlton, J., 156
Cheater, F., 231
Chen, C., 229
Chen, D., 229
Chen, J. T., 56
Chen, L., 145
Chideya, S., 44
Cho, R., 153
Choi, N., 24
Chouinard, V., 152
Chow, D., 10
Christakou, A., 49
Christensen, T., 207
Christiaens, W., 77
Christoffersen, A., 54
Christos, P. J., 32
Clark, J., 208
Clark, M. D., 24
Clark, N., 55
Clark-Ibanez, M., 129
Clarkson, R. S., 93
Cleary, A., 45
Clinch, J., 60

Cloutier-Fisher, D., 153
Clow, B., 7, 20, 27, 55
Coates, J., 117, 161
Cockcroft, A., 23
Cohan, M., 117–118
Cohane, G. H., 18
Cohen, D., 121
Cohen, R. M., 88
Coit, D. G., 32
Colley, A., 65, 80
Collins, F. S., 42–43
Connell, R. W., 26–27, 131, 175, 176–177, 178, 179, 207, 208, 209–210
Connor, S. K., 229
Cooper, H., 146
Corbett, M., 45
Corbin, J. M., 55
Cormier, R., 54, 55, 180
Correa-de-Araujo, R., 45
Cote, R., 65, 68–70
Courtenay, W. H., 42, 167, 231
Covington, S. S., 216
Cowell, C. T., 49
Cox, B., 31
Coyne, K. S., 96
Craft, R. M., 93
Craig, B. A., 70
Crenshaw, K. W., 54
Cresswell, J. W., 107
Cronin, A., 130
Cronk, C. E., 146
Crooks, V. A., 152
Crowne, D., 198
Cubbin, C., 44
Cueto, M., 206
Cummins, S., 44
Cunningham-Burley, S., 130
Curtis, L. H., 153

Dahinten, S., 229
Dales, R. E., 60
D'Alessio, A. C., 95
D'Anella, A., 115
Datta, A., 117
David, L., 24
Davidson, K. W., 77
Davies, H. T., 221
Davis, I., 49
Davis, P. G., 88
Day, K., 164
De Ayala, R. J., 66
de Beauvoir, S., 24

De Koninck, M., 10
de la Chapelle, A., 19
de Vries, G. J., 56–57, 87, 89, 97
Death, A., 92
DeHart, D. D., 46
del Mar Garca Calvente, M., 112
Delamont, S., 106
Delgado, A., 112
Dence, C., 92
Denys, D., 93
Devries, K., 180
Dewhirst, T., 130
Dhamoon, R., 54–55
Diamond, M., 91
Dickinson, M., 130
Diemer, M. A., 23–24
Dill, D., 194
Dillabough, J., 132
Dominiczak, A. F., 89
Donahoe, P. K., 48
Donner, L., 146
Drapeau, A., 153
Drennan, J., 118
Drexler, H., 92
Dudley, M., 156
Duffy, L. R., 129
Dulac, C., 95, 96
Dunn, G. A., 56–57
Dvorsky, G., 12, 29–31, 33
Dworkin, R. H., 96
Dworkin, S. L., 55
Dyck, I., 132, 152

Eckel, L. A., 91
Edwards, D., 162, 165
Edwards, M. S., 43
Egerter, S., 44
Eglin, P., 162
Einstein, G., 86, 88, 93, 95
Eisler, R. M., 24
El-Khayat, H. A., 93
Ellaway, A., 44
El-Wakad, A. S., 93
Emerson, R. M., 119
Emslie, C., 117
Epstein, I., 129
Epstein, M., 176
Epstein, S., 57
Erens, B., 112
Ershoff, D. H., 229
Estabrooks, C., 218
Ettorre, E., 221
Eusterschulte, B., 89

Fairclough, N. L., 162
Farhat, T., 216
Fausto-Sterling, A., 20, 33–34, 88
Fee, E., 206
Fenton, K. A., 112
Ferlie, E., 220
Ferree, M. M., 178
Ferrence, R., 176
Fetterman, D. M., 106
Field, P. M., 86
Fielding, J., 130
Fields, J., 117
Finch, J., 117
Fingerhut, L. A., 229
Fiocco, A., 93
Fischer Aggarwal, B. A., 52
Fish, E. N., 92, 94
Fish, J., 46
Fisher, J., 209–210
Fishman, J. R., 4, 6
Fitzgerald, J., 128, 130, 140
Fitzgerald, L., 220
Fitzpatrick, P., 145
Flaherty, B., 130
Fletcher, R. H., 70
Fletcher, S. W., 70
Florio, T., 156
Flynn, B. S., 229
Fonarow, G. C., 153
Fontana, A., 115
Forbes, D., 217
Forger, N. G., 56–57
Foucault, M., 162
Fowler, R. A., 152
Fox, C. M., 75
Frank, G. R., 88
Fremont, A., 153
Fretz, R. I., 119
Frey, J. H., 115
Friedman, A., 31
Friestad, C., 44
Frisby, W., 220
Frith, H., 129
Frohlich, K., 130–131
Frohman, L., 129
Fujiwara, T., 50
Fuqua, D. R., 24
Furberg, C., 52

Gabhainn, S. N., 216
Gable, R., 24
Galasinski, D., 165
Galdas, P. M., 231

Galvin, M., 45
Gannon, K., 164–165
Gao, M., 92
Garfinkel, H., 162
Garrett, R., 132
Garvin, T., 153
Gaudet, D., 92
Geary, N., 86–87, 91, 93
Geiger, H. J., 70
Gerall, A. A., 87
Gesler, W. M., 44
Ghaye, T., 221
Gibson, B. E., 132
Gilbert, F. S., 95
Gilmore, J. H., 49
Gilson, L., 205
Gitt, A. K., 65, 71
Given, B. A., 65, 75–76
Given, C. W., 43, 65,
    75–76
Gjertsen, F., 156
Glass, K., 112, 121
Glazier, R. H., 22, 94
Glover, L., 164–165
Godemann, J., 223
Goering, P., 218
Goffman, E., 162, 166
Goldenberg, S., 107, 115
Goodwin, G. D., 229
Gorman, J. M., 93
Gottfried, M., 23–24
Gough, B., 162, 164, 165,
    166–167
Goy, R. W., 86, 87, 91
Grady, D., 52
Graham, H., 130
Graham, I. D., 215, 217, 223
Grant, K. R., 41
Greaves, L., 5, 10, 11, 18, 20–21,
    23, 27, 28, 40, 47, 56, 86,
    107, 111–112, 116, 121, 130,
    156, 175, 176, 180–181,
    183–184, 218, 229
Grech, E. D., 71
Green, L., 217
Greenhalgh, T., 217
Greenland, S., 71
Greenspan, J. D., 93
Griffin, C., 162
Grisham, W., 89
Gropler, R. J., 92
Grosz, E., 85
Guang, W., 229

Gubitz, G., 65, 68–70
Gurau, A., 92
Gustavsson, P., 31–32

Haglund, M., 130
Haines, R. J., 116, 130–131, 131,
    138, 140
Halari, R., 49
Halberstam, J., 26
Hall, E. J., 178
Hall, W., 229
Halpin, M., 131
Hambleton, R. K., 75
Hamid, M., 217
Hamilton, L., 46
Hammill, B. J., 153
Hampson, E., 86–87, 91, 93
Hancock, A., 54–55
Handelsman, D. J., 92
Hankivsky, O., 10, 54–55, 55, 156
Haqq, C. M., 48
Haraway, D. J., 29
Harcourt, D., 129
Harding, G., 96
Hargreaves, J., 33
Harjola, V. P., 92
Harkin, T., 92
Harper, D., 129
Harris, G., 86
Harrison, B., 130
Harrison, C. M., 118
Harvey, G., 221
Harvey, J., 217, 221
Hatton, G. I., 95
Haugen, A., 63
Havens, B., 181
Hawker, G. A., 22, 94
Hawkins, C., 220
Hawkins, J. R., 48
Haworth-Brockmann, M., 7, 20,
    27, 55, 146
Hay, M., 91
Hayden, E. C., 92
Hayduk, L. A., 78
Heckathorn, D. D., 109
Heer, T., 65, 71
Heikes, E. J., 117
Heisley, D. D., 129
Helms, B., 24
Heng, D., 145
Herman, J. P., 86–87, 91, 93
Hernandez, A. F., 153
Herrero, P., 92

Herrington, D., 52
Hershler, R., 145
Hertzman, C., 145
Herzog, A. G., 93
Hester, S., 162
Hewer, A., 63
Hill, J. H., 117
Hill Collins, P., 54
Hillstrom, H., 49
Hladunewich, M. A., 152
Hochadel, M., 92
Hofmeyer, A., 218
Hogler, W., 49
Holcomb, S. M., 61
Holmes, B., 217
Hopper, J., 49
House, J. S., 44
Howard, J., 156
Howlett, E., 118
Howson, A., 33
Howson, R., 177, 179,
    184–185
Hublet, A., 216
Hughes, J., 12, 29–31, 33
Hughes-Benzie, R., 90
Hulley, S. B., 52
Hume, D., 67
Humphries, K. H., 92
Hunt, K., 39, 41, 44, 117
Hussey, W., 129
Hutchby, I., 162
Hutchinson, S., 117–118
Hyde, A., 118
Hydén, L.-C., 117
Hytten, K., 156

Ifkovits, E., 49
Ikezuki, Y., 50
Inglis, D., 49
Isfeld, H., 146
Iuliano-Burns, S., 49
Iyer, A., 45, 112

Jack, D. C., 194
Jackson, D., 198
Jacobson, N., 218
Janes, D., 145, 147
Jategaonkar, N., 130
Jefferson, G., 166
Jenkins, R., 156
Jimenez, S., 93
Johnson, A. M., 112
Johnson, J. A. 145

Johnson, J. L., 11, 18, 20–21, 23,
    27, 28, 40, 44, 47, 56, 85–86,
    109, 111–112, 113, 115, 116,
    121, 138, 140, 156, 175, 176,
    180–181, 183, 229
Johnson, K. C., 229
Jost, A., 48
Judge, T. A., 65, 72–75
Juenger, C., 65, 71
Jurkowski, J. M., 129
Juurlink, D. N., 152

Kaibuchi, K., 90
Kalaian, H. A., 65, 75–76
Kalaw, C., 28, 180–181,
    183–184, 229
Kamei, Y., 50
Kandrack, M., 41
Kannel, W. B., 51
Kantor, E., 43
Katz, J., 32
Kaufert, J., 181
Kazanjian, A., 153
Kearns, R. A., 44
Keating, C., 219
Kelk, N., 156
Kelly, M. T., 122, 131, 176, 229
Kelly, S., 156
Kelly, U. A., 55
Kemmis, S., 223
Kemp, A. F., 49
Kendrick, J. S., 229
Kilbourne, J., 217
Killion, C. M., 128–129
Kim, J., 118
Kimchi, T., 95, 96
Kimmel, M., 45
Kirkland, S., 77
Kirkland, S. A. D., 180
Kisare, M., 221
Kissinger, P., 121
Kitson, A., 217, 221
Kitwood, T., 90
Kleinman, J. C., 229
Klepp, K., 44
Klesges, R. C., 229
Klitzing, S. W., 128
Knaak, K., 18
Knafl, K., 183
Knickmeyer, R. C., 49
Knight, R., 115
Knox, S. S., 52–53
Kobayashi, K., 153

Koehoorn, M., 107
Koenig, B. A., 4, 6
Komajda, M., 92
Konigsberg, L. W., 61
Kontos, P., 132
Kosiak, B., 45
Kostenius, C., 221
Kosterman, R., 216
Kothari, A., 217
Kreder, H. J., 22, 94
Krestan, J., 193
Krieger, N., 43, 44,
    56, 62, 175
Krueger, R. A., 118
Krystal, A. D., 93
Kuntsche, E., 216
Kvale, S., 116
Kyriakidou, O., 217

Labad, J., 93
LaBresh, K. A., 153
Laegreid, P., 207
Lagacé, C., 145
Lanes, S. F., 67
Lannin, D. R., 43
Lantz, P. M., 44
Lavigne, C., 229
Lavis, J. N., 217, 232
Lawler, S., 131
Lawrence, K., 57
Leadbeater, B., 112, 121
LeBeau, K., 229
Lee, C., 42, 185
Leech, T. G. J., 24
Leipert, B., 217
Leischow, S., 217
Lemieux, S., 156
Lepage, S. S., 229
Lepkowski, J. M., 44
Leppert, J., 57
Lerner, D. J., 51
Levecque, K., 77
Levine, M., 118
Levy, S. J., 129
Lewis, J. M., 206
Li, J., 49
Li, P., 152
Liang, L., 153
Liao, M., 52
Lichtenstein, B., 117
Lin, A. E., 90
Lin, W., 49
Lin, Y., 43

Lindsay, J., 211
Lindström, L., 57
Links, P. S., 156
Lips, H. M., 189
Little, J., 155
Liu, P., 92
Livingston, B. A., 65, 72–75
Lloyd-Richardson, E. E., 130
Locke, B. D., 23–24
Loftus-Hills, A., 221
Logan, G. D., 78
Lomas, J., 217, 231
Looney, C. B., 49
Lope, V., 31–32
López-Abente, G., 31–32
Lorber, J., 17, 30, 39
Louise, A., 145
Lovely, J., 218
Ludlow, L. H., 23–24
Lupien, S. J., 93
Lynch, J. W., 44
Lyons, A. C., 26, 28, 175–178

Macfarlane, F., 217
Macintyre, S., 44
Maggi, S., 145
Magill, C., 129
Magui, P., 220
Mahalik, J. R., 23–24
Maheu, F., 93
Mahomed, N. N., 22, 94
Maiteny, P., 118
Majumdar, S., 145
Maltby, J., 65, 80
Mann, S., 89
Marcella, S., 115
Marchi, K. S., 44
Marlowe, D., 198
Marsaglio, W., 117–118
Marshall, P., 231
Martens, P., 218
Martin, E., 33
Martinez, F. D., 229
Mason, A., 216
Mason, J., 106
Mason, K., 121
Massey, D. B., 44
Mathews, H. F., 43
Mattsson, M., 223
Mauss, M., 132
Maynard, L. M., 49
McCabe, G. P., 70

McCall, L., 55
McCarthy, M. M., 56–57
McCarty, C. A., 216
McCorkle, R., 65, 75–76
McCormack, B., 217, 221
McDonagh, K., 129
McEwen, B. S., 86, 88, 91, 93
McFadden, M., 164
McInnis, M. G., 93
McIntyre, A., 129
McIntyre, L., 229
McKeever, P., 129, 132
McLeod, C. B., 232
McLeod, J., 132
McManus, S., 112
McNeil, S., 146
McNiven, C., 145, 147
McPhaul, M. J., 19
McWilliam, C., 217
Measham, F., 164
Mehdizadeh, A., 60
Mehlum, L., 156
Melander-Wikman, A., 221
Menchon, J. M., 93
Merlo, E., 92
Mero, R. P., 44
Merry, H., 146
Merzenich, M. M., 94, 95
Mesmeules, M., 145
Messerschmidt, J. W., 131, 26–27
Metzler, M., 44
Mikulski, B. A., 92
Miller, D. C., 45
Miller, K., 132
Miller, V. M., 91
Milner, T. A., 93
Minuk, J., 65, 68–70
Miqueo, C., 112
Mitchell, J., 43
Mittleman, M. A., 52–53
Mitura, V., 145, 153
Moatakef-Imani, M. B., 93
Modney, B. K., 95
Mogil, J. S., 93
Mollerup, S., 63
Moore, D. S., 70
Moore, H. L., 72
Moran-Ellis, J., 130
Morettin, D., 153
Morgenstern, H., 71
Mosca, L., 52
Motsei, M., 118
Moynihan, C., 26

Mróz, L., 28, 107, 109, 115, 118, 229
Mulhern, G., 65, 80
Mullen, K., 26
Mullen, P. D., 229
Mullings, L., 46, 54
Mumtaz, Z., 179
Murphy-Eberenz, K., 93
Musick, M. A., 44
Mykhalovskiy, E., 19, 130–131

Namaste, V., 25
Neri, G., 90
Nguyen, T. V., 49
Nichter, M., 130
Nieminen, M. S., 92
Nilsson, K. W., 57
Noble, J. B., 26
Nordquist, N., 57
Nottebohm, F., 86–87
Nutley, S. M., 221
Nyonator, F. K., 179

Oakley, A., 115
O'Brien, M., 222
O'Connor, A. M., 230
Offord, D. R., 156
Ogrodniczuk, J., 176
Öhrvik, J., 57
Ojemann, L., 43
Oliffe, J. L., 25, 28, 107, 109, 111–112, 115, 116, 118, 129, 131, 176, 229
Oliveria, S. A., 32
Oliver, S. A., 32
Omran, M. A., 93
O'Neil, J., 24
Orland-Barak, L., 55
Orth-Gomer, K., 52–53
Ortiz, S., 181
Östlin, P., 45, 112
Ostry, A., 107, 145
Osuga, Y., 50
Ouahid, S., 48
Owens, R., 185

Papanek, H., 4
Pardue, M. L., 3, 39, 49, 86, 91–93
Parr, H., 152, 156
Parsons, B., 88
Patrick, D., 44, 107, 111–112, 116
Pattyn, E., 77

Paul-Ward, A., 129
Pavis, S., 130
Payne, J. L., 93
Pederson, A., 7, 20, 27, 55
Peirce-Sandner, S., 96
Peled, M., 217
Pérez-Gómez, B., 31–32
Peterson, L. R., 92
Petraitis, C., 115
Petrovic, M., 93
Pfaff, D. W., 88
Phillips, D. H., 63
Phillips, M., 176
Phillips, S., 65, 68–70
Phillips, S. P., 8
Philo, C., 156
Phoenix, C. H., 87
Pilgrim, C., 89
Pilote, L., 92
Pini, B., 114, 117
Pink, S., 140
Pinto, R., 152
Pohar, S., 145
Poland, B., 130–131, 132
Poland, B. D., 131, 138
Pollán, M., 31–32
Pomerantz, A., 166
Pong, R., 145, 156
Ponic, P., 121, 176
Poon, C., 217
Popper, K. R., 67
Potter, J., 162, 165, 168
Powers, L. S., 128
Prastawa, M. W., 49
Prkachin, K., 44, 113, 121
Pross, D. C., 153
Pu, A., 92
Puderer, H., 145, 147

Quinn, V. P., 229
Quiton, R. L., 93

Racher, F., 181
Radloff, L. S., 75
Rae-Grant, N. I., 156
Raisman, G., 86
Rammsayer, T. H., 73
Ramsdale, D. R., 71
Ramzan, B., 114
Rapkin, A. J., 93
Rasgon, N., 93
Rasquin, P., 86, 88

Ratner, P. A., 229
Rauch, F., 49
Rector, T., 153
Reddy, G., 21
Redwood-Jones, Y. A., 130
Rehkopf, D. H., 56
Reid, C., 55, 220
Reijneveld, S. A., 146
Reinharz, S., 114
Reisert, I., 89
Remer, P., 189
Repta, R., 11, 18, 20–21, 23, 27, 40, 47, 56, 86, 156, 175
Revicki, D. A., 96
Rhodes, T., 128, 130, 140
Rich, A. C., 30
Richard, B., 153
Richardson, M. A., 229
Ridge, D., 117
Rieder, A., 57
Rieker, P. P., 22, 31, 39, 51, 70
Riggs, B., 52
Rinn, J. L., 48
Risman, B. J., 116
Rissman, E. F., 89
Robert, G., 217
Roberts, C., 43
Roberts, S. S., 92
Robertson, D., 232
Robertson, S., 169, 176, 178, 207, 240
Robinson, M., 169, 240
Roche, A. F., 49
Rock, M., 130–131
Rockwood, K., 146
Rogers, H. J., 75
Romeo, R. D., 93
Rose, G., 140
Rosenberg, M., 107, 111–112, 116, 153
Rosenberg, M. W., 147
Ross, N., 153
Roy, P., 176
Roy, P. S., 93
Rubia, K., 49
Rubinow, D. R., 93
Ruiz-Cantero, M. T., 112
Ryberg, D., 63
Rycroft-Malone, J., 221

Sabur, N., 152
Saewyc, E., 217
Salganik, M. J., 109

Saltonstall, R., 176
Salway, S., 179
Sanchez, S., 130
Sangl, J., 45
Sapolsky, R. M., 97
Saposnik, G., 65, 68–70
Sarvela, P. D., 146
Scallan, E., 145
Scanlon, L., 223
Schachar, R. J., 78
Schafer, W. D., 45
Schanen, C., 89
Schechtman, K. B., 92
Schiebinger, L. L., 19
Schiele, R., 65, 71
Schippers, M., 26–27, 177–179
Schmidt, P. J., 93
Schofield, T., 175, 178, 205, 206, 207, 208–209, 209–210, 212
Schramek, T. E., 93
Schulman, K. A., 153
Schulz, A. J., 46, 54
Schulz, R., 65, 75–76
Scordalakes, E. M., 89
Scott, R. P. J., 23–24
Scott, S. D., 221
Scribner, R., 121
Secker-Walker, R. H., 229
Seckl, J. R., 95
Seda, O., 92
Seem, S. R., 24
Seeman, E., 49
Seers, K., 221
Segalas, C., 93
Segall, A., 41
Seidler, V., 166
Semenciw, R., 31
Semrouni, M., 48
Sen, G., 45, 112
Sewankambod, N. K., 217
Seymour-Smith, S., 167
Shah, T., 153
Sharma, S., 95
Shatla, R. H., 93
Shaw, L. L., 119
Shea, A. M., 153
Shea, B., 23
Shilling, C., 33
Short, R. V., 86
Shoveller, J. A., 44, 107, 111–112, 113, 115, 116, 118, 121
Shreve, A., 219
Shumka, L., 41, 45

Sigmundson, H. K., 91
Simerly, R. B., 89
Simon, V., 50–51
Simons-Morton, B., 216
Singh, S. N., 92
Sjöberg, R. L., 57
Skar, M., 130
Skeggs, B., 132
Skelly, J. M., 229
Skidmore, J. R., 24
Sleney, J., 130
Smaje, C., 146
Smiler, A. P., 176
Smith, A., 217
Smith, A. B., 49
Smith, E. P., 88
Smith, J., 240
Smith, J. A., 178, 183, 207
Snelgrove-Clarke, E., 221
Snowe, O. J., 92
Snyder, M., 48
Sobo, E. J., 105–106, 116–119, 121
Soliman, N. A., 93
Solomon, L. J., 229
Song, J., 49
Soobader, M., 44
Soon, J. A., 118
Soto, P. F., 92
Spade, D., 33–34
Sparks, R., 130–131
Spear, L. P., 216
Spear, S., 121
Specker, B., 88
Spencer, J. L., 93
Spitzer, D., 10
Squire, S. B., 179
Stacey, D., 230
Staines, P., 145
Stephens, C., 169–170
Stern, J. M., 95
Stevens, B., 129
Stevens, S. S., 66
Stewart, D., 88, 93, 217
Stewart, M., 28, 77, 180–181, 183
Stine, W. W., 66
Stokols, D., 217
Stoltenberg, S. F., 65, 78
Stommel, M., 65, 75–76
Strack, R. W., 129
Strahorn, P., 89
Straus, S. E., 215
Strauss, A. L., 55
Suarez, L., 51

Suber, P., 235
Subramanian, S. V., 56
Sudsawad, P., 217
Suppes, P., 66
Swaminathan, H., 75
Swanson, F. H., 43
Swanson, M. S., 43
Swartz, K. L., 93
Sweetman, P., 127, 129
Swift, J., 26
Szatmari, P., 156

Takahashi, H., 88
Takeuchi, T., 50
Tannen, D., 161
Tannock, R., 78
Tao, Z. W., 129
Taussig, L., 229
Taveggia, T. C., 70
Taya, S., 90
Taylor, D., 156
Taylor, N., 130
Taylor, S., 162
Teghtsoonian, K., 77
ter Bogt, T. F. M., 216
Tetroe, J., 215, 217
Theobald, S., 179
Thomas, J., 105, 107
Thompson, D., 218
Tilleczek, K., 156
Tinkler, P., 129–130
Titchen, A., 221
Tolhurst, R., 179
Tom, A., 220
Tomaszewski, M., 89
Tomoum, H. Y., 93
Toublanc, J. E., 48
Towae, F., 65, 71
Towne, B., 49
Townsend, C. O., 65, 69
Tremblay, J., 92
Troche, S. J., 73
Trudeau, K. J., 77
Tsutsumi, O., 50
Tu, M., 93
Turk, D. C., 96

Upshur, R. E. G., 132
Uvnäs-Moberg, K., 52

Valentine, G., 182
Vallejo, J., 93
Van De Ven, A. H., 222

van Praag, L., 77
van Roosmalen, E., 77
Vandemheen, K. L., 60
Varcoe, C., 55
Venners, S. A., 229
Vertinsky, P. A., 33
Vetsa, Y. S., 49
Viswanathan, M., 66
Vives-Cases, C., 112
Volpe, T., 156
Vulink, N. C., 93

Wacquant, L. J. D., 131
Wade, J., 89
Walker, L., 175, 178, 209–210
Wall, J., 45
Walt, G., 205
Walter, I., 221
Wang, C. C., 128–129, 129, 130
Wang, H., 52–53
Wang, L., 229
Wang, X., 229
Ward, C. H., 24
Ward, K. D., 229
Ward-Griffin, C., 217
Warren, C., 182
Waterman, P. D., 56
Waters, B., 156
Waters, E. M., 93
Watkins, R., 90
Watson, J., 26
Waxman, H. A., 92
Weaver, I. C., 95
Weber, R. P., 163
Weir, L., 19
Weismann, M. M., 93
Weksberg, R., 90
Wells, J. C., 49
West, C., 23, 28–29
Westenberg, H. G., 93
Westmass, J., 176
Wetherell, M., 162, 164
White, H. R., 27
White, P., 130
Whitehead, M., 205
Whittle, S., 25
Wick, J. G., 4, 6
Wickstrom, M., 153
Wienbergen, H., 65, 71
Wiggins, S., 165
Wild, T. C., 176
Wildgen, J., 121

Wilensky, A., 43
Wilkinson, S., 165
Williams, A., 153
Williams, C. L., 117
Williams, D. R., 42–43
Williams, S. J., 132
Willott, S., 162
Wilson, E., 156
Wilson, K., 147
Wilson, M., 73
Wingard, D. L., 51
Wingfield, J., 89
Wisemandle, W., 49
Wizemann, T. M., 3, 39,
    49, 86, 91–93
Wolcott, H. F., 105–107, 111

Wolf, D. L., 105, 116
Wood, A. M., 65, 80
Wood, G. E., 93
Wood, J., 175, 178, 209–210
Wood, M., 220
Woodside, J. M., 232
Wooffitt, R., 162
Woolsey, R. L., 92
Worell, J., 189
Wright, A., 229
Wright, J. G., 22, 94
Wrightsman, L., 24

Xerri, C., 95
Xiang, Y., 128
Xu, J., 90, 96

Yang, L. Y., 89
Yates, S. J., 162
Yi, W. K., 129
Yin, R. K., 106
Young, E. A.,
    86–87, 91, 93
Young, I. M., 209
Young, L. E., 153
Young, N. L., 132
Young, W. C., 87

Ziebland, S., 117
Zifchock, R. A., 49
Zimmerman, D. H.,
    23, 28–29
Zinnes, J. L., 66

Subject Index

Accountability of gender, 28–29
Acute heart failure, 92
Adolescent alcohol use, 216–217
Age, 45
AIDS, 5, 204
Alcohol studies, 210–211, 216–217
Alcoholism, 78–79
Ambivalent femininity,
    177, 184–185
Androgen deprivation
    therapy, 25
Androgen receptors, 88
Anti-Mullerian hormone, 47–48
Artificial wombs, 29
Australia, 11, 210–211
Autodriving, 129
Autoimmune diseases, 92–93

Beach, Frank, 88
Bem Sex Role Inventory,
    32, 65, 80–81
*Better Science With Sex and
    Gender: A Primer for Health
    Research*, 11
Bias
    description of, 70
    differential item
        functioning, 75
    gender, 22
Biological differences, 5, 91
    See also Sex differences
Biological sex. *See also* Sex
    animal studies of, 86–87
    binary notion of, 87
    definition of, 85–86, 91
    environmental factors, 95–96
    experiences that affect,
        94–95, 97
    gender effects on, 94
    genetic influences, 89–91

hormone receptor
    distribution, 88–89
measurement of, 85–97
reproductive functions of, 86
research paradigms for, 87–91
social influences on, 97
Birth control pill, 29
Bodily hexis
    age-based elements of, 138
    description of, 132
    gendered, 134–140
    habitus effects on, 132
    smoking, 133–134, 136
Brain
    experiential effects on, 94–95
    sex differences in, 93–94
    synaptic remodeling of, 94
British Columbia Centre of
    Excellence for Women's
    Health (BCCEWH),
    202, 215, 224
"Broken window index," 121

Canada
    secondary analysis of
        mortality gap between
        urban and rural
        Canadians, 145–156
    sex and gender analysis
        in, 10–11
Canadian Institutes of Health
    Research, 109, 120, 121, 215
Capacity building, 244
Cardiovascular disease, 52–53
Causal assumptions, 66–67
Center for Epidemiological
    Studies–Depression
    scale, 75–77
Chance, 70
Chromosomes, 19, 48, 85, 89–90

Chronological age, 45
Class, 44–46
Clinical trials, 5
Cloning, 29
Coalitional consciousness
    building, 219
Comparative approach to
    research, 92–93
Compulsive heterosexuality, 30
Concept measurements
    description of, 66
    gender differences in, 75–77
Confounding, 70–72
Congenital adrenal
    hyperplasia, 90, 94
Consciousness-raising, 218–219
Constrained choice,
    gender as, 22–23
Content analysis, 161–164
Continental philosophy, 162
Conversation analysis, 162
"Conversational" interviews, 115
Coronary heart disease, 51
Cultural capital, 132

Depression, 32, 57, 75–76, 93
Differential item functioning, 75
Direct observation, 106–107
Directory of Open Access
    Journals, 237
Discourse analysis
    description of, 162
    gender applications of, 165
    health-related applications
        of, 164–165
    history of, 162
    hormone replacement therapy
        case study, 169–170
    social interactions studied
        using, 167–169

253

transcriptional entries
    used in, 167–169
value of, 171
Discursive practices, 165–166
Discursive psychology, 162
Discursive resources,
    164–166, 171
Diseases, sex differences in,
    19–20, 51, 92–93
Diversity, 8–9
"Doing gender," 29
Dyad summary, 182–183
Dynamic gendered
    framework, 212

Embodied gender, 28–29
Emphasized femininity,
    27, 177, 184
Environment
    biological sex affected
        by, 95–96
    health affected by, 43–44, 57
Epidemiology, 207
Epigenetic research, 56–57
Estrogen receptors, 88
Ethnicity, 42–43
Ethnography, 106, 121
Ethnomethodology, 162
Evidence-based medicine, 96

Families Controlling and
    Eliminating Tobacco
    (FACET), 180–186, 229–230
Female masculinity, 26
Female role, 207
Femaleness, 26
Femininity
    ambivalent, 177, 184–185
    Bem Sex Role
        Inventory, 80–81
    critical perspective
        on, 184–185
    definition of, 26–27
    emphasized, 27, 177, 184
    health behaviors affected
        by, 27, 176
    hegemonic, 177
    heterosexual influences on, 30
    protest, 177
    relational theory of, 178
    socially constructed
        ideals of, 228
    societal perceptions of, 24

Feminist action research,
    218, 220, 222
Fetishization, 129
Fieldwork
    advantages of, 105, 121
    considerations when
        conducting, 120–121
    definition of, 105
    example of, 179
    feasibility of, 120
    focus groups, 118–121
    history of, 106
    insider–outsider
        relations in, 105
    interview strategies and
        techniques used
        in, 114–120
    observational
        strategies, 106–114
    power relations arising
        during, 121
    recruitment for, 112
    sexually transmitted infection
        study, 107, 109–114, 116
    strength of, 122
Focus groups, 118–121, 230

Gay men's health, 5
Gender
    accountability of, 28–29
    antecedents of, 72–75
    as binary variable,
        69, 72, 79, 208
    Bird and Rieker's model of, 22
    category-based
        approach to, 208
    as constrained choice, 22–23
    contextual nature of, 18, 39–41
    critical appraisals of, 7
    definition of, 20–21, 208, 210
    dynamic biosocial process
        view of, 210
    effects of, 68–72
    embodied, 28–29
    "fault line" of, 4–6
    health behaviors and, 69
    impulsivity and, 78–79
    institutionalized, 21–22
    Internet use and, 239
    medical system's recognition
        of variance in, 33
    norms and roles
        approach, 208–209

as performance, 28–29
quantification of, 7
"race" and, 43
relational nature of, 27–28
sex and, 31–33, 40, 51–53, 94
sex differences and, 21
sex-based studies
    addition of, 51–53
smoking and, 130–140, 229
social aspects and context of,
    18, 31, 176
in workplace, 21
Gender analysis, 7, 10
Gender attitudes, 80
Gender bias, 22
Gender differences
    concept measurements
        affected by, 75–77
    gene-environment research
        framework for
        studying, 56–57
    in health, 22, 31–32, 65, 68–69
    impulsivity effects, 79
    plurality of, 208
    researcher–participant, 117
    studies of, 68–69
Gender hegemony, 27, 179
Gender identity, 24–25, 30, 80
Gender measurement
    causal assumptions, 66–67
    gender role orientation, 72–75
    overview of, 65–68
    theoretical assumptions
        associated with, 73
Gender relations
    analytical tools used in, 182–185
    conceptualizations of, 176–178
    description of, 27–28, 175
    dyad summary, 182–183
    FACET project, 180–186,
        229–230
    family applications of, 186
    future directions for, 185–186
    grounded theory
        applications, 186
    health and, 176
    in health research, 178–185
    men's health and, 179
    methods for, 180–185
    Power and Control
        Wheel, 183–184
    power in, 178
    women's health and, 179

Gender role(s)
definition of, 23, 80
dualistic understanding of, 23
dyadic, 23
hierarchy of, 28
internalizing of, 23
measurement of, 23–24
physician-patient interactions
affected by, 22
postgenderism beliefs
regarding, 29
Gender role orientation, 72–75
Gender role socialization scale
cross-cultural applicability,
196–197
description of, 189–190
feedback regarding, 197
illustration of, 190–192
items, 193–198
refinement, 195–198
results, 199–200
validation of, 198
Gender stereotypes, 80
Gendered bodily hexis, 134–140
Gendered cultural
conditioning, 217
Gendered effects, 77–79
Gendered socialization, 208
Gendered workforce, 212
Gene-environment
research, 56–57
General Accounting Office, 11
Grounded theory, 162, 186

Habitus
bodily hexis affected by, 132
Bourdieu's theory
of, 131–132, 140
cultural capital and, 132
social fields and, 131
social reproduction of, 132
Health
factors that affect, 9
gender differences in,
22, 31–32, 55
gender effects on, 41, 50
gender relations and, 176
gendered effects and, 77–78
geographical influences
on, 42–43
masculinity effects on, 26
sex effects on, 19–20, 50
sexual identity effects on, 46

social determinants of. See Social
determinants of health
Health behaviors
femininity effects on, 27, 176
gender and, 69, 176
health policy and, 207
masculinity effects
on, 26, 45, 176
Health Canada, 10, 11, 116
Health inequalities, 204–205
Health outcomes, 204, 209
Health policy
case study investigations, 210–211
description of, 203
gender and, 205–207
research and, 203–206
Health promotion, 228, 238
Health research
end user of, 218–221
fieldwork. See Fieldwork
frameworks for. See Research
frameworks
gender inequality in, 205
gender relations in, 178–185
gene-environment, 56–57
generic approach to, 4
heterosexuality in, 30
institutionalized gender
effects on, 21
intersectional, 53–55
multilevel modeling, 56
photography use in, 129
secondary analysis of
mortality gap between
urban and rural
Canadians, 145–156
sex as variable in, 49–50
social determinants of health
incorporated into, 41–42
systems modeling, 56
visual methods used in. See
Visual methods
Hegemonic femininity, 177
Hegemonic masculinity,
26, 32, 177
Heterosexual privilege, 46
Heterosexuality, 30
Hijra, 21
HIV, 204
Homophobia, 46
Hormone receptors, 88–89
Hormone replacement
therapy, 169–170

Identity politics, 209
Impulsivity, 78–79
Inclusion and difference
paradigm, 58
In-depth interviews, 112
Institutionalized gender, 21–22
Internet, 238–240
Intersectionality, 53–55
Intersex bodies, 20, 33
Interviews
description of, 114–115
focus group, 118–121, 230
note-taking during, 119–120
qualitative, 119
semistructured, 116–118
unstructured, 115–116

Journals, 233–237

Knowledge exchange
design, methods, and products
for, 227–232
Internet for, 238–240
pathways for, 232–240
peer-reviewed publications,
232–238
Knowledge translation
components of, 223
definition of, 215
end users of gender and health
research, 217
methodologies, 217
research for, 216–218
researcher as boundary
spanner in, 221–223
Knowledge-to-action
process, 223

Lordosis, 86

Male role, 207
Maleness, 26
Marginalized masculinity, 177
Masculinity
Bem Sex
Inventory, 80–81
complicit, 177
critical perspective on,
184–185
definition of, 25–26
discursive resources
use of, 165–166
female, 26

health affected by, 26, 45, 176
hegemonic, 26, 32, 177
heterosexual influences
    on, 30
marginalized, 177
men's health affected by, 166
mental health and, 27
relational theory of, 178
smoking and, 138
social context of, 18
societal perceptions of, 24
subordinate, 177
Measure, 66
Measurement error, 79–80
Melanoma, 31
Membership categorization
    analysis, 162
Men
    coronary heart disease
        in, 51
    gendered bodily hexis during
        smoking by, 135–136
    societal views on, 21
    tobacco use by, 130
Men's health
    focus on, 5, 207
    gender relations effect
        on, 179
    masculine practices
        that affect, 167
Men's talk, 161
Menstrual cycle, 93
Mental health
    depression, 32, 57, 75–76, 93
    gendered effects and, 78
    masculinity and, 27
Mental health disorders, 189
Michael Smith Foundation for
    Health Research, xvii
Mullerian-inhibiting
    hormone, 48
Multilevel modeling, 56
Myocardial infarction, 20, 92

National Institutes of Health
    (NIH), 10, 11
Naturalistic observation,
    106, 111, 128
Neurotransmitters, 95
NEXUS, vii
Nonreactive observation, 107
Norms and roles approach,
    208–209

Observational
    strategies, 106–114
Open-access journals,
    235, 237–238
Opportunities for health, 8
Ovarian cycle, 93
Ovarian hormone therapy, 52

Parthenogenesis, 29
Participant observation, 111, 121
Participant-driven
    photography
    description of, 128–129
    smoking study, 130–140
Participatory action research,
    128–129, 218, 220
Patriarchy, 4
Peer-reviewed publications,
    232–238
Performance, gender as, 28–29
Personalized medicine, 96
Pheromones, 95
Photo-elicitation
    interviewing, 129
Photography, 128–129
Photovoice, 128–129
Physician-patient
    interactions, 22
Place, 43–44
Policymaking, 11
Postgenderism, 29–30
Power and Control
    Wheel, 183–184
Prostate cancer support
    groups, 238
Protest femininity, 177
Public policy
    alternative approaches,
        208–212
    description of, 203
    framing of, 206–207
    gender and, 205–207
    linear cause-and-effect
        relationships, 206–207
    research and, 203–206
    social constructivist
        perspective, 206

Qualitative content
    analysis, 162–163
Qualitative interviews, 119
Quantitative content
    analysis, 162–163

Race, 42–43
Random error, 70
Rapport building, 107
Reactive observation, 106–107
Reflexivity, 55
Relationships
    gender relations
        influence on, 27
    technological influences on, 29
Reproductive hormones
    description of, 86–87
    developmental organization
        by, 87–88
    receptors for, 88–89
Research design
    description of, 12, 18
    ethical implications of, 57–58
    gendered nature of, 19
Research frameworks. See also
    Health research
    gene-environment, 56–57
    intersectionality, 53–55
    multilevel modeling, 56
    social determinants of health
        included in, 46–47
    systems modeling, 56
Research proposals, 227

Same-sex reproduction, 29
Search engine optimization, 239
Secondary analysis of mortality
    gap between urban and
    rural Canadians, 145–156
Self-descriptions, 9
Semistructured interviews,
    116–118
Sex. See also Biological sex
    anatomical differences
        based on, 20
    as binary biological
        category, 18–19
    biological form and
        function of, 49–50
    conceptualization
        of, 19–20
    covariates that affect, 49
    cultural differences in, 20
    definition of, 19, 47
    gender and, 31–33,
        40, 51–53, 94
    health affected by, 19–20
    health promotion
        messages, 228

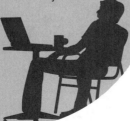
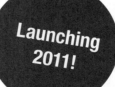